For Angela

Contents

Preface

Patient safety is the foundation of good patient care. The unnerving fact that healthcare can harm us as well as heal us is the reason for suggesting that patient safety is the heart of healthcare quality. Effectiveness, access to care, timeliness and the other dimensions of quality are all important. But when a member of your family goes into hospital or receives other healthcare then above all you want them to be safe. There is something horrifying about being harmed, or indeed causing harm, in an environment of care and trust. Both for patients and staff, safety is the emotional heart of healthcare quality. I also believe in terms of understanding, improvement and day-to-day running of healthcare that safety is a touchstone and guide to the care that is given to the patients; the clinician or the organization that keeps safety to the fore in the midst of the many other often competing priorities achieves something remarkable and provides the care that we would all want to receive.

Why though, even if you accept this perspective, should you read a book on patient safety? The first reason is very simple: the importance of the topic. As you will see if you read on, there is compelling evidence that, while healthcare brings enormous benefits to us all, errors are common and patients are frequently harmed. The nature and scale of this harm is hard to comprehend. It is made up, worldwide, of hundreds of thousands of individual tragedies every year, in which patients are traumatized, suffer unnecessary pain, are left disabled or die. Many more people have their care interrupted or delayed by minor errors and problems; these incidents are not as serious for patients but are a massive and relentless drain on scarce healthcare resources.

A second reason is that for all the books, reports, articles and Websites devoted to patient safety, there is still no straightforward overview of the field. The books that are available are mostly multi-author edited texts which, while they bring a rich diversity of perspective, are not primarily aimed at explaining the basic principles, characteristics and direction of the field. My aim has been to show the landscape of patient safety: how it evolved, the research that underpins the area, the key conceptual issues that have to be addressed, and the practical action needed to reduce error and harm and, when harm does occur, to help those involved.

Third, patient safety is a meeting point for a multitude of other topics. The relevant literature is difficult to grasp, being scattered, diverse and multidisciplinary in nature. Much of it is published in areas, such as cognitive psychology and ergonomics, which are unfamiliar to medicine. Worse still, many of the topics fundamental to progress in patient safety are themselves the subjects of huge literatures and much debate. For instance, a substantial amount of work has been carried out, from a number of different perspectives, on the factors that produce safe, high performing teams. The same could be said of expertise, decision making, human error, human factors, information technology, leadership, organizational culture ... the list goes on and on.

A fourth reason is to show that patient safety is, very simply, a tough problem in cultural, technical, clinical and psychological terms, not to mention its massive scale and heterogeneity. Healthcare is the largest industry in the world and extraordinarily diverse in terms of the activities involved and the manner of its delivery. We are faced with hugely intractable, multifaceted problems, which are deeply embedded within our healthcare systems. Understanding this is both an intellectual and a practical challenge. One of the greatest obstacles to progress on patient safety is, paradoxically, the attraction of neat solutions, whether political, organizational or clinical.

The nature of the book

I hope that this book can be read by anyone either interested or involved in healthcare, as an introduction to patient safety or to deepen their knowledge of specific topics. I have tried to write a clear and comprehensive overview of the major themes while not shying away from the difficulties, controversies and challenges. To my mind the attempt, in many papers and conferences, to present all quality and safety issues in the simplest possible terms has been a disaster and a major obstacle both to progress generally and specifically to the engagement of clinicians. I have also tried to make the book a gateway into the field. Some truly wonderful books and papers have been written about patient safety, or topics relevant to it, and I have tried to show my own sources of inspiration and learning and direct people to them.

A book of this kind is inevitably highly selective and some decisions have to be made about what to cover and in how much detail. I have tried, as far as possible, to address generic issues that cross specialties and disciplinary boundaries, rather than examine a series of specific clinical topics. I believe this approach brings a greater understanding and enables the reader to take the basic principles and apply them in whatever setting they work in. I have, however, included illustrations and specific clinical examples wherever possible, aiming to balance and illuminate the more general points. Patient safety is still largely confined to hospital medicine and to the developed world, and the book reflects this. Safety in primary care, mental health, care given in the home and patient safety in developing countries are vital issues, but work on them has hardly begun.

The second edition of this book is very different from the first, reflecting developments in both the field and my own understanding. In 2005 I was able to write that most safety improvement programmes were, to my mind, rather haphazard and without defined direction or purpose. That was true then, but no longer. The entire second half of this book discusses how healthcare can be made safer and contains a host of examples and illustrations of improvements to the safety and quality of care.

The book is designed to be read straight through, though readers who wish to address particular themes and topics can select specific sections. The first half of the book discusses the nature of safety and the essential understanding that is needed before improvements can be made The first section of three chapters addresses the history and evolution of patient safety and the vexed question of how safety relates to quality. Patient safety emerged from a particular historical context; understanding how it emerged is the best way, to my mind, to understand its character, strengths and limitations. The next three chapters address the nature and scale of harm, examining the research evidence, the role of reporting systems and the neglected topic of measurement of safety. Chapters 7 and 8 form another section devoted to understanding why errors and accidents happen, reviewing the concept of human error, the nature of accidents, perspectives on safety and methods of analysing incidents. The following two chapters consider the impact of errors and harm on the people involved, patients and their families in Chapter 9 and clinical staff in Chapter 10.

The chapters in the second half of the book, all in one way or another concern the reduction of error and the ultimate aim of safe, reliable healthcare. The fifth section opens with a discussion of ways in which clinical processes can be improved, rooted in well established methods of quality improvement in both healthcare and manufacturing industries. The next chapter considers the new, but potentially very fruitful, role of design in patient safety followed by a discussion of the critical role of information technology. Section 6, consisting of five chapters, complements these technological solutions by addressing the different ways that people, both patients and staff, can either erode or create safety, both as individuals and as teams. Two final chapters consider how all these component parts can be integrated to bring us safer organizations and safer healthcare systems.

The fact that a quarter of this book is devoted to the many ways in which people individually or within teams actively create safety reflects my own belief that anyone in any discipline and at any level in healthcare can improve the safety of care. Systems and processes are important but in the end people make the difference. I hope this book may be of some help to you.

Inspiration, acknowledgements and thanks

Many people, whether they know it or not, have helped in the writing of this book. In the first edition I listed a number of people who through their actions, their writings or their conversation had expanded my view or changed the way I think about patient safety. Even then it was a long list but now it is impossibly long and so I will simply say that the list of references and sources is testament to the richness of the patient safety literature and that I am indebted to everyone named there. As before, however, I will single out two people, Lucian Leape and James Reason, who require special mention both because of their influence on the field and the help they have given to me personally. Both have been an inspiration and unfailingly generous in their support and encouragement.

I also wish to thank the following people for their contribution to the book. Rachel Davis provided exemplary help, encouragement and tactful criticism during the writing; Katrina Brown, Susannah Long, Krishna Moorthy and Susanna Walker nobly read and commented on the entire manuscript, resulting in many more apposite examples, much greater clarity and the removal of a variety of errors and infelicities. Raj Aggarwal, Jonathan Benn, Susan Burnett, Nick Sevdalis and Jonny West provided specialist input to specific chapters. Most academic authors suffer from what a friend of mine called the benign neglect of academic editors; in complete contrast, Mary Banks has encouraged me throughout to write the book I wanted to write.

The book could also never have been written without the support and assistance of a number of people. Ara Darzi saw the potential of a unit dedicated to patient safety set within a department of surgery and has supported my work throughout my time in his department. My colleagues in the department and in the Imperial Centre for Patient Safety and Service Quality have been patient and tolerant of my immersion in this project. As every researcher knows, the time-consuming treadmill of searching for funding is a constant distraction from actually doing useful research. I am particularly grateful therefore to Sally Davies at the National Institute of Health Research and to Vin McCloughlin at the Health Foundation for their support over the years and for providing the stable funding environment in which our research has flourished and which has enabled this book to be written.

The incomparable P.G. Wodehouse dedicated one of his books to his daughter Leonora (queen of her species), without whose never-failing sympathy and encouragement, as he said, it would have been finished in half the time. I must thank my wife Angela for her sympathy and patience and for her encouraging remarks after bravely reading Chapter 1. Everything else I might thank her for is expressed in the dedication.

SECTION ONE
The Evolution of Patient Safety

CHAPTER 1
Medical harm: a brief history

Over the last ten years there has been a deluge of statistics on medical error and harm to patients, a series of truly tragic cases of healthcare failure and a growing number of major government and professional reports on the need to make healthcare safer. There is now widespread acceptance and awareness of the problem of medical harm and a determination, in some quarters at least, to tackle it. It seems that we are only now waking up to the full scale of medical error and harm to patients. Yet, awareness of medical harm and efforts to reduce it are as old as medicine itself, dating back to Hippocrates classic dictum to 'abstain from harming or wronging any man'.

The cure can be worse than the disease

Medicine has always been an inherently risky enterprise, the hopes of benefit and cure always linked to the possibility of harm. The word 'pharmakos' means both remedy and poison; the words 'kill' and 'cure' were apparently closely linked in ancient Greece (Porter, 1999). Throughout medical history there are instances of cures that proved worse than the disease, of terrible suffering inflicted on hapless patients in the name of medicine, and of well intentioned though deeply misguided interventions that did more harm than good. Think, for example, of the application of mercury and arsenic as medicines, the heroic bleeding cures of Benjamin Rush, the widespread use of lobotomy in the 1940s and the thalidomide disasters of the 1960s (Sharpe and Faden, 1998). A history of medicine as harm, rather than benefit, could easily be written; a one-sided, incomplete history to be sure, but a feasible proposition nonetheless.

Looking back with all the smugness and wisdom of hindsight, many of these so-called cures now seem to be absurd, even cruel. In all probability though, the doctors who inflicted these cures on their patients were intelligent, altruistic, committed physicians whose intention was to relieve suffering. The possibility of harm is inherent to the practice of medicine, especially at the frontiers of knowledge and experience. We might think that the advances of modern medicine mean that medical harm is now of only historical interest. However, for all its genuine and wonderful achievements, modern medicine too has the

Patient Safety, 2nd edition. By Charles Vincent. Published 2010 by Blackwell Publishing Ltd.

potential for considerable harm, perhaps even greater harm than in the past. As Chantler (1999) has observed, medicine used to be simple, ineffective and relatively safe; now it is complex, effective and potentially dangerous. New innovations bring new risks, greater power brings greater probability of harm and new technology offers new possibilities for unforeseen outcomes and lethal hazards. The hazards associated with the delivery of simple, well understood healthcare, of course remain. Consider, for example, the routine use of non-sterile injections in many developing countries. Before turning to the hazards of modern medicine however, we will briefly review some important antecedents of our current concern with the safety of healthcare.

Heroic medicine and natural healing

The phrase 'First do no harm', a later twist on the original Hippocratic wording, can be traced to an 1849 treatise 'Physician and patient' by Worthington Hooker, who in turn attributed it to an earlier source (Sharpe and Faden, 1998). The background to this injunction, and its use at that point in the development of Western medicine, lay in a reaction to the 'heroic medicine' of the early 19th century.

Heroic medicine was, in essence, the willingness to intervene at all costs and put the saving of life above the immediate suffering of the patient. As Sharpe and Faden (1998) have pointed out, when reviewing the history of iatrogenic harm in American medicine, it is this period that stands out for the violence of its remedies. Heroism was certainly required of the patient in the mid-19th century. For instance, in the treatment of cases of 'morbid excitement' such as yellow fever, Benjamin Rush, a leading exponent of heroic medicine, might drain over half the total blood volume from his patient. Yet Rush was heroic in his turn, staying in fever ridden Philadelphia to care for his sick patients. Rush explicitly condemned the Hippocratic belief in the healing power of nature, stating that the first duty of a doctor was 'heroic action, to fight disease'.

Physicians more trusting of natural healing on the other hand saw heroic medicine as dangerous, even murderous. Sharpe and Faden quote the assessment of J. Marion Sims, a famous gynaecological surgeon, writing in 1835 at the time of his graduation from medical school:

I knew nothing about medicine, but I had sense enough to see that doctors were killing their patients, that medicine was not an exact science, that it was wholly empirical and that it would be better to trust entirely to Nature than to the hazardous skill of the doctors.
(SHARPE AND FADEN, 1998: P. 8)

These extreme positions, of heroic intervention and natural healing, eventually gave way to a more conservative position, espoused by such leading physicians as Oliver Wendell Holmes, who attempted to objectively assess the balance of risk and benefit of any particular intervention. This recognizably modern approach puts patient outcome as the determining factor and explicitly broadens the physician's responsibility to the avoidance of pain and suffering, however induced – whether from the disease or the treatment.

Judgements about what constitutes harm are not straightforward and are irretrievably bound up with the personal philosophies of both physician and patient. To the sincere, if misguided, heroic practitioners, loss of life was the one overriding harm to be avoided and any action was justified in that pursuit. This was moderated by the more conservative position in striking a balance between intervening to achieve benefit and avoiding unnecessary suffering. Such dilemmas are of course common today when, for instance, a surgeon must consider whether an operation to remove a cancer in a terminally ill patient, which might prolong life, is worth the additional pain, suffering and risk associated with the operation. The final decision nowadays may rest with the patient and family, but they will be strongly influenced by medical advice. The patient too must decide whether to 'first do no harm' or whether to risk harm in the pursuit of other benefits. From this we can already see that there is no absolute state of safety that we can aspire to, but that safety must always be seen in the context of other objectives. Safety can, however, be prioritized and become an explicit goal instead; in contrast, for much of medical history, safety was an objective but one not backed by analysis and systematic action.

Hospitalism and hospital acquired infection

Dangerous treatments were one form of harm. However, hospitals could also be secondary sources of harm, in which patients acquired new diseases simply from being in hospital. By the mid-19th century, anaesthesia had made surgery less traumatic and allowed surgeons time to operate in a careful and deliberate manner. However, infection was rife. Sepsis was so common, and gangrene so epidemic, that those entering hospital for surgery were 'exposed to more chance of death than the English soldier on the field of Waterloo' (Porter, 1999: p. 369). The term 'hospitalism' was coined to describe the disease promoting qualities of hospitals, and some doctors believed they needed to be periodically burnt down. As late as 1863, Florence Nightingale introduced her *Notes on Hospitals*, as follows:

It may seem a strange principle to enunciate as the very first requirement in a Hospital that it should do the sick no harm. It is quite necessary, nevertheless, to lay down such a principle, because the actual mortality in hospitals, especially in those of large crowded cities, is very much higher than any calculation founded on the mortality of the same class of diseases amongst patients treated out of hospital would lead us to expect.
(SHARPE AND FADEN, 1998: P. 157)

Puerperal fever, striking mothers after childbirth, was particularly lethal and widely known to be more common in hospitals than in home deliveries. A small number of doctors in both England and America suspected that this was caused by transfer of 'germs' and argued that doctors should wash between an autopsy and a birth. These claims of the contagious nature of puerperal fever, and the apparently absurd possibility of it being transferred by doctors, were strongly rebutted by many, including the obstetrician Charles Meigs, who concluded his defence of his position with the marvellous assertion that 'a gentleman's hands are clean' (Sharpe and Faden, 1998: p. 154). Bacteria were apparently confined to the lower classes.

Dramatic evidence of the role of hygiene was provided by Ignaz Semmelweiss in Vienna in his study of two obstetric wards. In Ward One, mortality from infection hit a peak of 29% with 600–800 women dying every year, whereas in Ward Two mortality was 3%. Semmelweiss noted that the only difference between wards was that patients on Ward One were attended by medical students and those on Ward Two by midwifery students. When they changed places, mortality rates reversed. Following the rapid death of a colleague who cut his finger during an autopsy, Semmelweiss concluded that his colleague had died of the same disease as the women and that puerperal fever was caused by conveying putrid particles to the pregnant woman during examinations. He instituted a policy of hand disinfection with chlorinated lime, and mortality plummeted. Semmelweiss finally published his findings in 1857, after similar findings in other hospitals, but found it difficult to persuade his fellow clinicians and his beliefs were still largely ignored when he died in 1865 (Jarvis, 1994).

Lister faced similar battles to gain acceptance of the use of antiseptic techniques in surgery, partly from scepticism about the existence of microorganisms capable of transmitting infection. However, by the end of the 19th century, with experimental support from the work or Pasteur and Koch, the principles of infection control and the new techniques of sterilization of instruments were fairly well established. Surgical gowns and masks, sterilization and rubber gloves were all in use and, most importantly, surgeons believed that safe surgery was both a possibility and a duty. However, one hundred years later, with transmission of infection well understood and taught in every nursing and medical school, we face an epidemic of hospital acquired infection. The causes of these infections are complex, with antibiotic resistant organisms, hospital overcrowding, shortage of time and lack of easily available washing facilities all playing a part. However, as in Semmelweiss's time, a major factor is difficulty of ensuring that staff, in the midst of all their other duties, do not forget to wash their hands between patients.

Surgical errors and surgical outcome

Ernest Codman, a Boston surgeon of the early 20th century, was a pioneer in the scientific assessment of surgical outcome and in making patient outcome the guiding principle and justification of surgical intervention. Codman was so disgusted with the lack of evaluation at Massachusetts General Hospital that he resigned to set up his own 'End-Result' hospital. This was based on the, for Codman, commonsense notion that 'every hospital should follow every patient it treats, long enough to determine whether or not the treatment has been successful, and then to enquire "if not, why not" with a view to preventing similar failures in the future' (Sharpe and Faden, 1998: p. 29). Crucially Codman was prepared to consider, and more remarkably make public, the occurrence of errors in treatment and to analyse their causes (Box 1.1).

BOX 1.1 Codman's categories for the assessment of unsuccessful treatment

Errors due to lack of technical knowledge or skill;
Errors due to lack of surgical judgement;
Errors due to lack of care or equipment;
Errors due to lack of diagnostic skill;
The patient's unconquerable disease;
The patient's refusal of treatment;
The calamities of surgery or those accidents and complications over which we have no known control.

(FROM SHARPE AND FADEN, 1998)

From 1911 to 1916, there were 337 patient discharged from Codman's hospital, with 123 errors recorded. In addition to errors, he recorded 'calamities of surgery' over which he had no control, but which he believed should be acknowledged and made known to the public. He was unsparing of himself, noting, after ligating a patient's hepatic duct which led to their death, that he 'had made an error of skill of the most gross character and even during the operation had failed to recognize it' (Neuhauser, 2002).

Codman challenged his colleagues to demonstrate the efficacy of their procedures, and not rely solely on the prestige of their profession to justify their actions. Unless the methods of science were applied to the evaluation of outcomes, Codman contended, there was nothing to distinguish a surgeon from a genial charlatan. His denunciations of humbuggery, by which he meant putting income ahead of outcome, culminated in his presentation of a large cartoon at a meeting of the local Surgical Society. In the picture, an ostrich is shown with its head beneath a pile of golden surgical eggs depicting the lucrative practices threatened by objective evaluation and publication of findings. This episode caused uproar but, anticipating this, Codman had already resigned his post at Massachusetts General Hospital.

Although Codman was ostracized and ridiculed by many, his proposals were nevertheless adopted by the American Surgical Society, but the eventual 'minimum standards for hospitals' instituted after the First World War omitted two of the most crucial components: the analysis of outcomes and the classification of error. The Minimum Standard ran until 1952, until it was overtaken by the formation of the organization that eventually became the Joint Commission on Accreditation of Healthcare Organizations (JCAHO), the largest accrediting body in the United States (Sharpe and Faden, 1998).

Iatrogenic disease

In the early decades of the 20th century, the scientific understanding of disease was well advanced, the excesses of heroic treatments had been curbed, but few effective treatments were available. Entering medical school in 1933, Lewis Thomas reflected that the purpose of the curriculum was:

. . . to teach the recognition of disease entities, their classification, signs, symptoms, and laboratory manifestations and how to make an accurate diagnosis. The treatment of disease was the most minor part of the curriculum, almost left out altogether . . . nor do I remember much talk about treating disease at any time in the four years of medical school except by the surgeons, and most of their discussions dealt with the management of injuries, the drainage or removal of infected organs and tissues and, to a very limited extent, the excision of cancers.
(THOMAS, 1984: PP. 27–28)

When medicine could achieve relatively little, it was hardly surprising that medical harm was far from people's minds, though Thomas does describe some fairly hair-raising treatments for delirium tremens involving massive doses of paraldehyde.

In the 1920s, however, the potential harmful effects of medicine were explicitly recognized with the introduction of the term 'iatrogenic disease'. The term 'iatrogenic' comes from the Greek word for physician 'iatros' and 'genesis', meaning origin; iatrogenic disease is therefore an illness induced, in some way, by a physician. The first usage is credited to Bleuler's 1924 textbook of psychiatry and implied at that time a nervous problem induced as a result of a physician's diagnosis of a disease (Sharpe and Faden, 1998). Thus a diagnosis of heart disease, for instance, could make the patient extremely anxious and induce an iatrogenic neurosis. Clinicians were therefore extremely careful when discussing diagnoses to avoid distressing or depressing the patient unduly. This well intentioned paternalism is a far cry from today's insistence on disclosing risks of all kinds which of course, as Bleuler and others recognized, carries its own hazards.

With the advances of medical science in the mid-20th century, the term iatrogenic disease broadened in scope to include harm due to the medical intervention itself. The particular stimulus for this was the increasing use of penicillin and other antibiotics. In the post war years there was a massive expansion in the medicines available, the usage of drugs and the availability of hospital beds and hospital treatments. By the mid-1950s some doctors, notably David Barr and Robert Moser, were beginning to realize that there were potential hazards associated with the enormous increase in drug use and availability. Barr's paper 'The hazards of modern diagnosis and therapy' (Barr, 1956) set out some of the major risks, but largely in the spirit of pointing out that there was an inevitable price to pay for therapeutic advance. However, Moser (1959) went further in also considering the overuse of medical therapy, coining the phrase 'antibiotic abandon' to describe the use of penicillin for anything and everything. Moser's view of iatrogenic disease, at least by the time of his 1959 book, 'Diseases of medical progress', was subtly different from Barr's in that he viewed these diseases of progress as those that would not have occurred if sound therapeutic practices had been employed. There is a suggestion at least, in this view, that harm is not entirely an unavoidable by-product of medical success, but may also be due to unsound practice, in which treatments are given without clear indications and without due regard for the balance of risk and benefit. At that time however, as Sharpe and Faden point out, questions of the balance of risk and benefit lay largely with the clinician, with little if any consideration of the patient's perspective.

Systematic studies of the hazards of hospitalization

While iatrogenic harm had been noted, it was seldom systematically studied. One of the first explicit, systematic prospective studies of iatrogenic complications was carried out by Elihu Schimmel in 1960/61 at Yale University Medical School. In retrospect, although it had limited impact at the time, it can be seen as a landmark study of the quality and safety of medical care.

Schimmel, with the support of his departmental chairman, succeeded in mobilizing the junior doctors of three hospital wards to report and describe adverse episodes resulting from acceptable diagnostic or therapeutic measures deliberately instituted in the hospital. The use of an explicit definition of harmful episodes was remarkably progressive in outlook, but the study took care not to implicate the actions of clinical staff in any harm that might result from treatment; reactions due to error, and reactions from previous treatment, and situations that were only potentially harmful were excluded. Even when errors were omitted, the results were striking with 20% of patients experiencing one or more untoward episodes including 16 fatalities (Box 1.2 and

---

BOX 1.2 The hazards of hospitalization

The occurrence of hospital-induced complications in a university medical service was documented in the prospective investigation of over 1000 patients. The reported episodes were the untoward consequences of acceptable medical care in diagnosis and therapy. During the 8-month study, 240 episodes occurred in 198 patients. In 105 patients, hospitalization was either prolonged by an adverse episode or the manifestations were not resolved at the time of discharge. Thus, 20% of the patients admitted to the medical wards experienced one or more untoward episodes and 10% had a prolonged or unresolved episode. The severity of the 240 episodes was minor in 110, moderate in 82 and major in 48, of which 16 ended fatally.

Patients encountering noxious episodes had a mean total hospitalization of 28.7 days compared with 11.4 days in other patients. The risk of having such episodes seemed directly related to the time spent in the hospital. The number and variety of these reactions emphasizes the magnitude and scope of hazards to which the hospitalized patient is exposed. A judicious selection of diagnostic and therapeutic measures can be made only with knowledge of these potential hazards as well as the proposed benefits.
(ADAPTED FROM SCHIMMEL, 1964: P. 100)

Table 1.1). Schimmel's summary bears a remarkable resemblance in both content and tone to the findings of the major record reviews of adverse events of the 1980s and 1990s. Schimmel remarked that the economic loss and emotional disturbance suffered by many patients were beyond the scope of the study, yet could not be considered insignificant complications of their medical care. Today we still have yet to assess the full economic consequences of harm to patients and have barely addressed the emotional trauma.

In his conclusion, Schimmel both defends the practice of medicine and yet argues for much greater attention to risks. The difficulty of balancing potential benefit and potential harm, and the need for constant review and monitoring of that balance, both during a patient's treatment and as medicine evolves, is expressed with great clarity:

The classical charge to the physician has always been primum non nocere. *Modern medicine, however, has introduced procedures that cannot always be used harmlessly. To seek absolute safety is to advocate therapeutic nihilism at a time when the scope of medical care has grown beyond previous imagination and power. The dangers of new measures*

Table 1.1 Examples of fatal episodes

Agent or procedure	Manifestation of the episode	Age (years)	Underlying disease
Cystoscopy	Cardiac arrest	69	Chronic pyelonephritis
Thoracentesis	Ventricular fibrillation	76	Congestive heart failure
Esophagoscopy	Perforation	50	Cirrhosis
Barium enema	Cardiac arrest	89	Tuberculous peritonitis
Heparin (iv)	Retroperitoneal haemorrhage	66	Hypernephroma
Blakemore tube	Asphyxia	59	Cirrhosis
Digoxin	Ventricular fibrillation	40	Rheumatic heart disease
Sedatives	Staphylococcal pneumonia	73	Parkinsonism

Reproduced from *Quality & Safety in Health Care*, E M Schimmel. "The hazards of hospitalization". **12**, no. 1, 58–63, 2003, with permission from BMJ Publishing Group Ltd.

must be accepted as generally warranted by their benefits and should not preclude their useful employment. Until safer procedures evolve however, physicians will best serve their patients by weighing each measure according to its goals and risks, by choosing only those that have been justified, and by remaining prepared to alter the procedures when imminent or actual harm threatens to obliterate their good.
(SCHIMMEL, 1964: P. 100)

In 1981, Steel, Gertman, Cresenzi and Anderson set out to reassess Schimmel's findings in a medical service of a tertiary care hospital (Steel *et al.*, 1981). They noted that in the preceding 15 years the number and complexity of diagnostic procedures had increased markedly, the number of drugs in use had increased and the patient population had aged. Of 815 patients in their study, an incredible 36% suffered an iatrogenic illness, with 9% being major in that they threatened life or produced a major disability. Exposure to drugs was the main factor leading to adverse effects, with nitrates, digoxin, lidocaine, aminophylline and heparin being the most dangerous. Cardiac catheterization, urinary catheterization and intravenous therapy were the principal procedures leading to problems, with falls also a serious issue. Staying longer in hospital was associated with a higher risk of iatrogenic disease. Steel and colleagues stopped short of a direct assessment of preventability, stressing that their definition did not imply culpability. Nevertheless, by 1981, they were certainly willing to imply that many of the problems might be preventable. They called for monitoring of adverse occurrences, especially on medical wards, and educational programmes about iatrogenic disease. Thirty years on, iatrogenic disease and safety issues are still finding only a small corner in some medical and nursing curricula, but we are at least now recognizing incidents and adverse outcomes to a much greater extent.

Medical nemesis

'The medical profession has become a major threat to health.' This arresting sentence begins Ivan Illich's polemic 'Limits of medicine', subtitled 'Medical nemesis: the expropriation of health' (Illich, 1977). Nemesis represents divine vengeance on mortals who behave in ways that the gods regard as their own prerogative. Medicine, argued Illich, had sought to move beyond its proper boundaries and by doing so was causing harm. Illich's broader argument, expressed in a number of books, was that many institutionalized activities had counter productive effects. In 'Deschooling society' for instance, he argued that formal, institutionalized education robbed people of their own intellectual curiosity and abilities, just as medicine robbed people of their own capacities for self care and autonomous living. Illich emphasized that medical harm was not just an unfortunate side effect of medical treatment that would eventually be resolved by technological and pharmacological advances; the only solution was for people themselves to resist unnecessary medical intervention and the medicalization of life.

Illich described three forms of iatrogenic effects:

- *Clinical iatrogenesis* – the direct harm done to patients;
- *Social iatrogenesis* – the excessive use of medicine to solve problems of living which encouraged people to become consumers of medicine, rather than actively involved in shaping their own health and environment;
- *Cultural iatrogenesis* – a deep culturally mediated sapping of people's ability to deal with sickness and death. Ordinary suffering and the experience of life and death then become commodities, illnesses that required treatment, rather than life to be lived and experienced – the 'paralysis of healthy responses to illness and suffering' in Illich's memorable phrase.

In the early 21st century, some aspects of this critique carry less force. Far from trying to medicalize life, doctors are now in retreat from the demands and unreasonable expectations thrust upon them. However, Illich's first theme of clinical iatrogenesis has proved remarkably farsighted, though we might now see the causes of iatrogenic harm as different from those suggested by Illich. He assembled a powerful set of charges against medicine and the medical profession, encompassing a critique of the lack of evidence for high technology medicine, evidence of useless or unnecessary treatment and doctor inflicted injuries. After reviewing the extant studies on the adverse effects of drugs, accidents in hospital and the hazards of hospitalization, he concluded that:

The pain, dysfunction, disability, and anguish resulting from technical medical intervention now rival the morbidity due to traffic and industrial accidents and even war-related activities, and make the impact of medicine one of the most rapidly spreading epidemics of our time. Amongst murderous institutional torts, only modern malnutrition injures more people than iatrogenic disease in its various manifestations.
(ILLICH, 1977: P. 35)

Illich's inflammatory language, and wholesale attack on the enterprise of medicine, hardly endeared him to the medical and nursing professions. Writing in 1997, John Bunker, who carried out some of the first studies on potentially unnecessary surgery, wrote that at the time he considered Medical Nemesis to be an ill-informed and irresponsible attack on the medical profession (Bunker, 1997). Bunker argued that Illich's more subtle, and more important message, about the dangers of social and cultural iatrogenesis, was perhaps misunderstood at the time. Illich's belief in the healing powers of friendship, personal autonomy, social networks and relationships and the importance of these factors in a fulfilled and healthy life now seems particularly prescient. There is now, as there was not in the 1970s, a huge literature on the importance of psychological and social factors in health and an acceptance on all sides of the importance of personal responsibility for health.

Illich's particular contribution to the gradually growing literature on medical harm was in the ferocity of his argument and the challenge he posed to medicine and the medical profession. Others had recorded and written about the hazards of drugs and therapeutics, but Illich went much further to suggest that healthcare was actually a threat to health, comparable to that from traffic and industrial accidents. As we shall see in the next chapter, this claim, outrageous and inflammatory at the time, reappears in sober government documents towards the end of the 20th century.

References

Barr, D.P. (1956) Hazards of modern diagnosis and therapy – the price we pay. *Journal of the American Medical Association*, **159**, 1452–1456.

Bunker, J.P. (1997) Ivan Illich and the pursuit of health. *Journal of Health Services Research and Policy*, **2**, 56–59.

Chantler, C. (1999) The role and education of doctors in the delivery of healthcare. *The Lancet*, **353**, 1178–1181.

Illich, I. (1977) *Limits to Medicine. Medical Nemesis: The Expropriation of Health*, Pelican Books, London.

Jarvis, W.R. (1994) Handwashing – the Semmelweis lesson forgotten? *The Lancet*, **144**, 1311.

Moser, R.H. (1959) *Diseases of Medical Progress*, Chas. Thomas, Springfield IL.

Neuhauser, D. (2002) Ernest Amory Codman MD. *Quality & Safety in Health Care*, **11**(1), 104–105.

Porter, R. (1999) *The Greatest Benefit to Mankind. A Medical History of Humanity From Antiquity to the Present*, Fontana Press, London.

Schimmel, E.M. (1964) The hazards of hospitalisation. *The Annals of Internal Medicine*, **60**, 100–110.

Sharpe, V.A. and Faden, A.I. (1998) *Medical Harm. Historical, Conceptual and Ethical Dimensions of Iatrogenic Illness*, Cambridge University Press, Cambridge.

Steel, K., Gertman, P.M., Crescenzi, C. and Anderson, J. (1981) Iatrogenic illness on a general medical service at a university hospital. *New England Journal of Medicine*, **304** (11), 638–642.

Thomas, L. (1984) *The Youngest Science*, Oxford University Press, Oxford.

CHAPTER 2

The emergence of patient safety

Medical error and patient harm have been described and studied for well over a century. However, apart from a few isolated pioneers, the medical and nursing professions did not appear to recognize the extent and seriousness of the problem or, if they did, were not prepared to acknowledge it. One of the great achievements of the last ten years is that medical error and patient harm are now acknowledged and discussed publicly by healthcare professionals, politicians and the general public.

Before this, medical error was seldom acknowledged to patients, almost never mentioned in medical journals and not even considered by governments; research on safety in medicine was viewed as at best a fringe topic and at worst disreputable. The fact that thousands, probably millions, of people were being harmed unnecessarily and vast amounts of money were being wasted seemed to have escaped everyone's attention. From our current understanding this seems a curious state of affairs. It is as if an epidemic were raging across a country without anybody noticing or troubling to investigate.

In the 1980s, there was so little research available, that when reviewing the extant literature I suggested in the title of a paper that the lack of research attention given to medical accidents and medical negligence was itself negligent (Vincent, 1989). In 1990, the editor of the *British Medical Journal* argued for a study of the incidence of adverse events and was roundly criticized by the president of a medical royal college for drawing the attention of the mass media to medical error (Smith, 2000). In 1990, Medline, one of the main medical research databases, did not even have a subject heading for medical error. Since the mid-1990s, however, the number of papers on error and safety related topics has increased exponentially, with several hundred a year listed under medical error. In 2000, the *British Medical Journal* devoted an entire issue to the subject of medical error (Leape and Berwick, 2000), in a determined effort to move the subject to the mainstream of academic and clinical enquiry. Many other leading medical journals have now followed suit, with major articles and series on patient safety.

Patient Safety, 2nd edition. By Charles Vincent. Published 2010 by Blackwell Publishing Ltd.

How then did patient safety evolve and emerge to assume its present importance? Understanding patient safety will be easier if we see how it emerged as a distinctive set of ideas and initiatives in a particular historical context. Understanding the origins and influences on patient safety is critical to understanding its distinctive character and place in the general quality assurance and improvement armament, which we will consider in the next chapter. There have, of course, always been doctors and nurses who, in addition to being safety conscious in their personal practice, have also worked to improve the overall safety of care. However, the wider safety movement has also been driven and shaped by several other influences; these include the broader movement to improve the quality of care, reflections on the nature of error, high profile cases, lessons from psychology, human factors and high risk industries, litigation and pressure from patients, the public and governments.

Improving the quality of healthcare

Unless substantial progress had been made in the understanding and practice of quality improvement, it is highly unlikely that the tougher issues underlying patient safety would have emerged. Although Ernest Codman was one of the few clinicians to explicitly address error (in the context of surgery), there are many other examples of pioneering quality initiatives early in the 20th century. For instance, in 1928, the British Ministry of Health set up a committee to examine maternal morbidity and mortality, instigating confidential enquiries on 5800 cases (Kerr, 1932). This spurred Andrew Topping, a remarkable Medical Officer for Health, to set up his own programme, which became known as the Rochdale experiment. At that time, Rochdale, an industrial town in the English Midlands, had a maternal mortality of 9 deaths per 1000 deliveries. Topping instituted ante-natal clinics, meetings between midwives and family doctors, and established a puerperal fever ward and a specialist consultant post and backed it all by education and public meetings. Within five years mortality had reduced to 1.7 per 1000 (Oxley, Phillips and Young, 1935).

National reports on maternal mortality were produced intermittently in subsequent years, but progress was rather haphazard. Finally, the Confidential Enquiry into Maternal Deaths was established which, since 1952, has produced triennial reports on all maternal deaths and endeavoured to establish why they had occurred and how they might be prevented (Sharpe and Faden, 1998). Similar enquiries are now conducted into deaths after surgery, stillbirth, and homicide and suicide (Vincent, 1993).

By the early 1970s, it was clear that there were widespread variations in quality of care across different geographical areas; for instance, at that time in the United States, surgery might be routinely offered for a particular medical condition in one state but hardly ever in a neighbouring state with a similar population (Wennberg and Gittlesohn, 1973). Quality problems were inferred from these variations, but much of the imperative for examining variation, particularly in the United States, stemmed from economic considerations rather than the harm caused by unnecessary surgery. Attempts were also being made to improve the processes and organization of healthcare, drawing on the practice and methodology of quality assurance approaches in manufacturing industry, such as continuous quality improvement, total quality management, business process re-engineering and quality circles. Such methods had been particularly influential in Japan, sometimes credited for the emergence of high quality and reliability in the Japanese motor industry. These approaches combine a respect for and reliance on data as a basis for quality improvement, together with an attempt to harness the ideas and creativity of the workforce to create change, test the effects and sustain them (Langley *et al.*, 1996). Regulatory agencies and professional societies investigated and acted on complaints made about healthcare professionals although, in Britain at least, this seldom extended to assessment of clinical competence. Amazingly, it was only in 1995 that the General Medical Council was finally empowered, by act of parliament, to investigate the clinical abilities of doctors as well as their general conduct (HMG, 1995). Prior to that, sexual misdemeanours might bring down the wrath of the Council, but competence did not fall within their remit.

Doctors and other clinical staff were, as always, committed to providing high quality care to individual patients. However, the quality of the system overall was really someone else's business; they wanted to be left to get on with treating their patients. The basic assumption for many was that quality was a natural outcome of conscientious work by highly motivated clinicians, with quality problems being due to the occasional 'bad apple'. In 1984, Robert Maxwell (Maxwell, 1984) still had to argue that an honest concern about quality, however genuine, is not the same as methodical assessment based on reliable evidence. There was also little understanding that poor quality might not be due to bad apples, but inherent in the very structures and processes of the healthcare system itself.

Progress over the next decade in the United Kingdom has been well summarized by Kieran Walshe and Nigel Offen, in their description of their report of the background to the events of the Bristol Royal Infirmary Enquiry (2001):

Between 1984 and 1995 the place of quality improvement in the British NHS was transformed. At the start of that period . . . clinicians took part in a range of informal and quasi-educational activities aimed at improving the quality of practice, but there were few, if any, healthcare organizations who could claim to have a systematic approach to measuring or improving quality. Moreover many clinicians and professional organizations had a record of being disinterested, sceptical, or even actively hostile towards the idea that systematic or formal quality improvement activities had much to offer in healthcare.

10 years later much had changed. A raft of national and local quality initiatives . . . had generated a great deal of activity, virtually all healthcare organizations had established clinical audit or quality improvement systems and structures, and the culture had been changed substantially. It had become common to question clinical practices and to seek to

improve them, activities which might have been difficult or even impossible a decade earlier.
(WALSHE AND OFFEN, 2001: P. 251)

The developments described by Walshe and Offen in Britain were paralleled in other healthcare systems, although with different emphases and different timescales. This section can obviously only sketch a very rough outline of the evolution of quality assurance in healthcare. The main thrust should however be clear. In the 1980s and early 1990s, prior to the full emergence of patient safety, there was a massive growth in awareness of the importance of systematic quality improvement. Clinicians, managers and policy makers began to un-derstand that quality was not just another headline capturing government initiative to be endured while it was flavour of the month, but was here to stay. This was an essential support and background to the hard look at the damage done by healthcare that was to follow.

Learning from error

In 1983 Neil McIntyre, Professor of Medicine, and the philosopher Sir Karl Popper, published a paper 'The critical attitude in medicine: the need for a new ethics', which called for clinicians to actively seek out errors and use them to advance both their personal knowledge and medical knowledge generally. This paper is densely, almost unbelievably, rich in ideas and embraces ethics, philosophy of science, the doctor-patient relationship, attitudes to fallibility and uncertainty, professional regulation and methods for enhancing the quality of care. Summarizing all the arguments is not feasible, but two extracts illustrate some of the main themes:

To learn only from one's own mistakes would be a slow and painful process and unnecessarily costly to one's patients. Experiences need to be pooled so that doctors may also learn from the errors of others. This requires a willingness to admit one has erred and to discuss the factors that may have been responsible. It calls for a critical attitude to one's own work and that of others.

No species of fallibility is more important or less understood than fallibility in medical practice. The physician's propensity for damaging error is widely denied, perhaps because it is so intensely feared ... Physicians and surgeons often flinch from even identifying error in clinical practice, let alone recording it, presumably because they themselves hold ... that error arises either from their or their colleagues' ignorance or ineptitude. But errors need to recorded and analysed if we are to discover why they occurred and how they could have been prevented.
(McIntyre and Popper, 1983: p. 1919)

The call to learn from mistakes has close links with Popper's philosophy of science, in which he argued that scientific knowledge is inherently provisional and that progress in science depends, at least in part, on the recognition of flaws in accepted theories. Popper argues that while there is some truth in the traditional view that knowledge grows through the accumulation of facts, advances often come about through the recognition of error, by the overthrow of old knowledge and mistaken theories. In this view, error becomes something of value, a resource and clue to progress, both scientifically and clinically. Many famous scientists, such as Sir Peter Medawar, have been profoundly influenced by Popper in their approach to fundamental scientific problems, finding the emphasis on hypothesis and conjecture both creative and liberating (Medwar, 1969).

McIntyre and Popper (1983) argue that being an authority, in the sense of a wise and reliable fount of knowledge, is often seen as a professional ideal in both science and medicine. However, this idealized view of authority is both mistaken and dangerous. Authority tends to become important in its own right; an authority is not expected to err and, if he does, his errors tend to be covered up to uphold the idea of authority. So mistakes are hidden, and the consequence of this tendency may be worse than those of the mistake being hidden.

It is not only scientific authority that is questioned here, but professional authority of all kinds. In medicine this means that, while one should respect the knowledge and experience of senior clinicians, one should not regard them as 'authorities' in the sense of inevitably being correct. An environment, in which junior staff feel unable to question senior staff about their decisions and actions, is profoundly dangerous to patients. There are, of course, many obstacles to more open communication and the spirit of Karl Popper may be no help to the hapless junior doctor when their authoritarian consultant turns his baleful eye on them. Popper's view of error is however a constant reminder that error and uncertainty are no respecters of status.

Reminding oneself that one may be wrong and that an absolute sense of certainty can be highly misleading, is not something that comes easily to us. Gerd Gigerenzer has advised us to always remember what he terms 'Franklin's law', so called because of Benjamin Franklin's statement that nothing in life is certain except death and taxes (Gigerenzer, 2002). Franklin's law makes us mindful of fallibility and uncertainty, enabling us to constantly reappraise apparent certainties in the certainty that some of them will turn out to be wrong!

Tragedy and opportunities for change

The knowledgeable health reporter for the Boston Globe, Betsy Lehman, died from a drug overdose during chemotherapy. Willie King had the wrong leg amputated. Ben Kolb was eight years old when he died during 'minor' surgery during a drug mix-up. These horrific cases that made the headlines are just the tip of the iceberg. (Opening paragraph of the Institute of Medicine report, To err is human, Kohn, Corrigan and Donaldson, 1999.)

Certain 'celebrated' cases attain particular prominence and evoke complicated reactions. Cook, Woods and Miller (1998) describe some particularly sad cases in their introduction to the report 'A tale of two stories: contrasting views of patient safety' and make some important comments about the public perception of these cases:

The case of Willie King in Florida, in becoming the 'wrong leg case', captures our collective dread of wrong site surgery. The death of Libby Zion has come to represent not just the danger of drug-drug interaction but also the issues of work hours and supervision of residents – capturing symbolically our fear of medical care at the hands of overworked, tired or novice practitioners without adequate supervision. Celebrated cases such as these serve as markers in the discussion of the healthcare system and patient safety. As such, the reactions to these tragic losses become the obstacles and opportunities to enhance safety.
(COOK, WOODS AND MILLER 1998: P. 7)

Cook, Woods and Miller go on to argue that the public account of these stories is usually a gross over-simplification of what actually occurred, and that it is equally important to investigate run-of-the-mill cases and success stories in order to understand the complex, dynamic process of healthcare. Such disastrous cases however, came to symbolize fear of a more widespread failure of the healthcare system, provoking more general concerns about medical error. Perhaps it isn't just a question of finding a good, reliable doctor. Perhaps the system is unsafe? Such concerns are magnified a 100-fold when there is hard evidence of longstanding problems in a service and a series of tragic losses. This is well illustrated by the events that led to the UK Inquiry into infant cardiac surgery at the Bristol Royal Infirmary (Box 2.1).

BOX 2.1 Events leading up to the Bristol inquiry

In the late 1980s, some clinical staff at the Bristol Royal Infirmary began to raise concerns about the quality of paediatric cardiac surgery by two surgeons. In essence it was suggested that the results of paediatric cardiac surgery were less good than at other specialist units and that mortality was substantially higher than in comparable units. Between 1989 and 1994, there was a continuing conflict at the hospital about the issue between surgeons, anaesthetists, cardiologists and managers. Agreement was eventually reached that a specialist paediatric cardiac surgeon should be appointed and in the meantime that a moratorium on certain procedures should be observed. In January 1995, before the surgeon was appointed, a child called Joshua Loveday was scheduled for surgery against the advice of anaesthetists, some surgeons and the Department of Health. He died and this led to further surgery being halted, an external enquiry being commissioned and to extensive local and national media attention.

Parents of some of the children complained to the General Medical Council which, in 1997, examined the cases of 53 children, 29 of whom had died and 4 of whom suffered severe brain damage. Three doctors were found guilty of serious professional misconduct and two were struck off the medical register.

The Secretary of State for Health immediately established an Inquiry, costing £14 million, chaired by Professor Ian Kennedy. The Enquiry began in October 1998 and the report published in July 2001 made almost 200 recommendations.

(REPRODUCED FROM *QUALITY & SAFETY IN HEALTH CARE*, K WALSHE, N OFFEN. "A VERY PUBLIC FAILURE: LESSONS FOR QUALITY IMPROVEMENT IN HEALTHCARE ORGANIZA-TIONS FROM THE BRISTOL ROYAL INFIRMARY". **10**, NO. 4, [250–256], 2001, WITH PERMISSION FROM BMJ PUBLISHING GROUP LTD.)

The impact in the United Kingdom of the events at Bristol on healthcare professionals and the general public is hard to understate. The editor of the *British Medical Journal* wrote an editorial entitled 'All changed, changed utterly. British medicine will be transformed by the Bristol case' (Smith, 1998), in which he highlighted a number of important issues, but particularly its impact on the faith and trust which people have in their doctors. The subsequent Inquiry, led by Professor Sir Ian Kennedy, could have been recriminatory and divisive but, in fact, achieved the remarkable feat of bringing positive, forward looking change from disaster and tragedy.

The Inquiry report is massive and we can only make a few general points here about the relevance of the Bristol affair to patient safety. The tragedy for all concerned was undeniable, the media attention relentless and sustained. The fact that routine, although highly skilled and complex, healthcare could be substandard to the point of being dangerous, was abundantly clear. The impetus for open scrutiny of surgical performance, and indeed the outcomes of healthcare generally, was huge and the subject of error and human fallibility in healthcare was out in the open (Treasure, 1998).

The Inquiry was noteworthy, from the outset, in adopting a systems approach to analysing what had happened; poor performance and errors were seen as the product of systems that were not working well, as much as the result of any particular individual's conduct (*Learning from Bristol*, 1999). In practice, this meant that, whereas most Inquiries would have started by grilling the surgeons involved, Professor Kennedy's team began by examining the wider context and only gradually moved towards specific events and individuals. This approach revealed the role of contextual and system factors much more powerfully and demonstrated that the actions of individuals were influenced and constrained by the wider organization and environment. Bristol therefore came to exemplify wider problems within the NHS, and its conclusions were widely applicable. Recommendations were made on open and honest risk communication to patients, the manner of communication and support, the process of informed consent, the need for a proper response to tragic events, the vital role of team work, the monitoring of the quality of care, the role of regulation and a whole host of other factors.

Many other countries have had their Bristols. Canada, for instance, experienced a similar high profile tragedy in the paediatric cardiac service at Winnipeg. Jan Davies, the leading clinical advisor to that Inquiry, drew explicit parallels between Winnipeg and a major aviation disaster at Dryden (Davies, 2000), holding out the hope that both events would provoke enduring system wide changes.

Studying the safety of anaesthesia: engineering a solution

Whereas practitioners of quality improvement in healthcare tended to look to industrial process improvement as their model, patient safety researchers and practitioners have looked to high-risk industries, such as aviation, chemical and nuclear industries, which have an explicit focus on safety usually reinforced by a powerful external regulator. The industries have invested heavily in human factors, a hybrid discipline drawing on ergonomics, psychology and practical experience in safety critical industries. Many of the important developments in the psychology of error have their origins in studies of major accidents in these complex industries. Healthcare has drawn some important lessons from them, gaining a much more sophisticated understanding of the nature of error and accidents and a more thoughtful and constructive approach to error prevention and the management of error. These issues will be addressed in more detail in later chapters. For the moment we will simply set the scene and demonstrate the importance of this line of work to patient safety.

One of the true pioneers in this area is Jeffrey Cooper, who trained originally as a bioengineer. In 1972 he was employed by the Massachusetts General Hospital to work on developing machines for anaesthesiology researchers (Cooper *et al.*, 1978; Cooper, Newbower and Kitz, 1984; Gawande, 2002). Observing anaesthetists in the operating room he noticed how poorly anaesthetic machines were designed and how conducive they were to error. For example, a clockwise turn of a dial decreased the concentration of a powerful anaesthetic in some machines but increased the concentration in others – a real recipe for disaster. Cooper's work extended well beyond the more traditional approach to anaesthetic misadventure, in that he examined anaesthetic errors and incidents from an explicitly psychological perspective, exploring both the clinical aspects and the psychological and environmental sources of error such as inexperience, fatigue and stress.

Cooper's 1984 paper provides a remarkably sophisticated analysis of the many factors that contribute to errors and adverse outcomes and is the foundation of much later work on safety in anaesthesia. Contrary to the prevailing assumption that the initial stages of the anaesthesia were the most dangerous, Cooper discovered that most incidents occurred during the operation when the anaesthetist's vigilance was most likely to ebb. The most important problems involved errors in managing the patient's breathing, such as undetected disconnections and mistakes in managing the airway or the anaesthetic machine.

Cooper also discussed factors that might have contributed to an error, such as fatigue and inadequate experience.

Cooper (1994), reflecting on the impact of the studies, noted that they seem to have stirred the anaesthesia community into recognizing the frequency of human error. Cooper's work provoked much debate but little action, until Ellison Pierce was elected President of the American Society of Anaesthesiologists in 1982. The daughter of a friend had died under anaesthetic while having wisdom teeth extracted, and this case in particular galvanized Pierce to persuade the profession that it was possible to reduce the then 1 in 10 000 death rate from anaesthesia (Gawande, 2002) to the extremely low rate seen today. Anaesthesia. together with obstetrics, led the way in a systematic approach to the reduction of harm, foreshadowing the wider patient safety movement a decade later (Gaba, 2000).

Error in medicine

In 1994, the subject of error in medicine was, with some notable exceptions, largely confined to anaesthesia. A prescient and seminal paper (Leape, 1994), still widely cited, addressed the question of error in medicine head on and brought some entirely new perspectives to bear. Lucian Leape began by noting that a number of studies suggested that error rates in medicine were particularly high, that error was an emotionally fraught subject and that medicine had yet to seriously address error in the way that other safety critical industries had. He went on to argue that error prevention in medicine had characteristically followed what he called the 'perfectibility model'. If physicians and nurses were motivated and well trained, then they should not make mistakes; if they did, then punishment in the form of disapproval or discipline was the most effect remedy and counter to future mistakes. Leape summarized his argument by saying:

The professional cultures of medicine and nursing typically use blame to encourage proper performance. Errors are caused by a lack of sufficient attention or, worse, lack of caring enough to make sure you are correct.
(LEAPE, 1994: P. 1852)

Leape, drawing on the psychology of error and human performance, rejected this formulation on several counts. Many errors are often beyond the individual's conscious control; they are precipitated by a wide range of factors, which are often also beyond the individual's control; systems that rely on error-free performance are doomed to failure, as are reactive attempts to error prevention that rely on discipline and training. He went on to argue that if physicians, nurses, pharmacists and administrators were to succeed in reducing errors in hospital care, they would need to fundamentally change the way they think about errors (Leape, 1994).

Leape went on to outline some central tenets of cognitive psychology, in particular the work of Jens Rasmussen and James Reason (discussed in detail in Chapter 4). While Reason had made some forays into the question of error in medicine (Eagle, Davies and Reason, 1992; Reason, 1993), Lucian Leape's paper brought his work to the attention of healthcare professionals in a leading medical journal. Leape explicitly stated that the solutions to the problem of medical error did not primarily lie within medicine, but in the disciplines of psychology and human factors, and set out proposals for error reduction that acknowledged human limitations and fallibility and relied more on changing the conditions of work than on training.

Cooper and Leape are not the only authors to understand the importance of human factors and psychology to medical harm and medical error at an early stage. For instance, Marilyn Bogner's 1994 book 'Human error in medicine' contained many insightful and important chapters by David Woods, Richard Cook, Neville Moray and others; James Reason articulated his theory of accidents and discussed its application in medicine in *Medical Accidents* (Vincent, Ennis and Audley, 1993). Cooper and Leape were, however, particularly important influences and they illustrate the more general point that some of the defining characteristics of patient safety are its acceptance of the importance of psychology and the lessons to be learnt from other safety critical industries.

Litigation and risk management

Until relatively recently litigation was seen as a financial and legal problem, patients who sued were often seen as difficult or embittered and doctors who helped them as professionally and often personally suspect. Only gradually did those addressing the problem come to understand that litigation was a reflection of the much more serious underlying problem of harm to patients; for this reason litigation is part of the story of patient safety.

Litigation and medical malpractice crises have occurred on a regular basis for over 150 years, each time accompanied by worries about public trust in doctors and much associated commentary and soul searching, some of it rather hysterical in nature. Litigation in medicine dates back to the middle of the 19th century, when the relaxation of professional regulation and introduction of a free market in both medical and legal services, simultaneously fuelled a decline in standards in medicine, dissatisfaction from patients and the availability of lawyers to initiate proceedings. Between 1840 and 1860, the rate of malpractice cases increased 10-fold and medical journals, after more than 50 years of barely noticing malpractice, suddenly became all but obsessed with the problem (Mohr, 2000).

Since then there have been recurrent crises usually coinciding with rising malpractice premiums paid by doctors. By 1989, US malpractice premiums appeared to have reached a plateau, though that plateau was very high for some specialties (Hiatt *et al.*, 1989). Insurance premiums for Long Island neurosurgeons and obstetricians ranged from $160 000 to $200 000 per annum, although admittedly New York State premiums were amongst the highest in the United States and probably in the world. Since then however, premiums in many countries appear to have stabilized and even declined (Hiatt et al., 1989; Mohr, 2000).

An historical perspective on litigation tempers reaction to the latest media driven litigation crisis, but there is no doubt that litigation is a longstanding problem for healthcare. Some believe that doctors are under attack (occasionally true) and that healthcare is burdened by numerous frivolous lawsuits brought by greedy patients. In passing, we might usefully dispose of a few myths. First, patients, as we shall see, very seldom sue after adverse events. Second, the huge awards that hit the headlines for severely damaged babies are very rare. Compensation for being condemned to a life of pain and suffering after hospital injury is meagre or non-existent in most countries and much of the money expended is swallowed up in fees and administration. Third, where there is no actual negligence, patients hardly ever receive compensation; it is more common that patients who claim and should receive compensation are denied it (Studdert et al., 2006). Fourth, while compensation is important in some cases, patients often turn to litigation for entirely other reasons, being driven in despair to litigation through a failure to receive the apologies, explanations and support that they both deserve and need (Vincent, 2001a). Finally, consider the simple fact that patients or families who need money because they cannot work or have to look after a relative generally have no other option but to sue. Shamefully, few hospitals have a proactive policy of actively helping the patients they injure, although as we will see this is beginning to change. We, as payers of tax, fees or insurance, have in fact been remarkably tolerant of the failings of the healthcare system and litigation has by any standard been used very sparingly. We must remember however, that the process of litigation in serious cases can be traumatic for both patients and doctors, but this is a subject for later chapters.

Litigation, as a means of reparation for injured patients, is expensive and in many cases a rather inefficient means of compensating injured patients. The threat of litigation is also often cited as a deterrent to the open reporting and investigation of adverse events and as a major barrier to patient safety. However, for all this, litigation has undoubtedly been a powerful driver of patient safety. Litigation raised public and professional awareness of adverse outcomes, and ultimately led to the development of clinical risk management. In the United States, risk management has had a primarily legal and financial orientation, and risk managers are only now becoming involved in safety issues. In the United Kingdom and other countries however, risk management had a clinical orientation from its inception as well as a concern with legal and financial issues. The terminology varies from country to country but the aims of clinical risk management and patient safety are the same – to reduce or eliminate harm to patients (Vincent, 1995; Vincent, 2001b).

Litigation has had one other unexpected benefit. The rising rate of litigation in the 1980s led some to consider whether compensation might be offered on a no-fault basis, bypassing the expense and unpleasantness of the adversarial legal process. The Harvard Medical Practice Study (HMPS), still the most famous study in the field of patient safety, was originally established to assess the number of potentially compensable cases in New York State, not primarily as a study of the quality and safety of care (Hiatt *et al.*, 1989). However, its major legacy has been to reveal the scale of harm to patients. The study found that patients were unintentionally harmed by treatment in almost 4% of admissions in New York, and about 1% of patients were seriously harmed (e.g. resulting in death or permanent disability) (Brennan *et al.*, 1991; Leape *et al.*, 1991). These findings were later to receive massive publicity with the release of the Institute of Medicine report 'To Err is Human' in 1999.

Professional and government reports: patient safety hits the headlines

The US Institute of Medicine's 1999 report 'To err is human', is a stark, lucid and unarguable plea for action on patient safety at all levels of the healthcare system. Without doubt the publication of this report was the single most important spur to the development of patient safety, catapulting it into public and political awareness and galvanizing political and professional will at the highest levels in the United States.

President Clinton ordered a government wide study of the feasibility of implementing the report's recommendations. The Institute of Medicine called for a national effort to include establishment of a Centre for Patient Safety within the Agency for Healthcare Research and Quality, expanded reporting of adverse events and errors, and development of safety programmes by healthcare organizations, regulators and professional societies. However, as Lucian Leape recalls, one particular statistic provided a focus and impetus for change:

However, while the objective of the report, and the thrust of its recommendations, was to stimulate a national effort to improve patient safety, what initially grabbed public attention was the declaration that between 44 000 and 98 000 people die in US hospitals annually as a result of medical errors.
(LEAPE, 2000: P. 95)

'To err is human', the first of a series of reports on safety and quality from the Institute, was far more wide ranging than the headline figures suggest. A large number of studies of error and harm were reviewed; the causes of harm, the nature of safe and unsafe systems and the role of leadership and regulation were all examined, themes we will return to in later chapters. The principal aim of the report was to establish patient safety as a major requirement and activity of modern healthcare, by establishing national centres and programmes, expanding and improving reporting systems and driving safety in clinical practice through the involvement of clinicians, purchasers of healthcare, regulatory agencies and the public (Box 2.2).

BOX 2.2 To err is human: principal recommendations of the IOM report

- Congress should create a Centre for Patient Safety.
- A nationwide mandatory reporting system should be established.
- The development of voluntary reporting should be encouraged.
- Congress should pass legislation to extend peer review protection to patient safety data.
- Performance standards and expectations for healthcare organizations and healthcare professional should focus greater attention on patient safety.
- The Food and Drug Administration should increase attention to the safe use of drugs in both the pre- and post-marketing processes.
- Healthcare organizations and the professionals affiliated with them should make continually improved patient safety a declared and serious aim, by establishing patient safety programmes with defined executive responsibility.
- Healthcare organizations should implement proven medication safety practices.

(FROM KOHN, CORRIGAN AND DONALDSON, 1999)

An organization with a memory: learning from adverse events in the NHS

Since the publication of the Institute of Medicine report, many governments and professional organizations have released reports and official statements on patient safety. The British equivalent of the Institute of Medicine report was prepared by a group led by Professor Liam Donaldson, the UK Chief Medical Officer (Department of Health, 2000). Unlike the Institute of Medicine report, it emanated from government and was bravely authorized for release by the then Secretary of State for Health, Alan Milburn.

The report's primary emphasis was, as the title suggests, on learning. Reviewing the systems of learning from errors in the NHS, the report identified numerous weaknesses within the processes and contrasted this unfavourably with other high-risk industries (Table 2.1). Great stress was also laid on understanding the underlying causes of adverse events and on the potential parallels between healthcare and other environments, although the parallels between healthcare and other industries should not be overstated, as we will discuss later. The report argued that all human beings who work in complex systems are prone to similar errors and subject to similar pressures (Box 2.3). In comparison with 'To err is human', 'An Organization with a Memory' (Department of Health, 2000) has a much stronger focus on learning from other

Table 2.1 A new approach to responding to adverse events in the NHS

Past	Future
Fear of reprisals common	Generally blame free reporting
Individuals scapegoated	Individuals held to account where justified
Disparate adverse event databases	All databases co-ordinated
Staff do not always hear the outcome of an investigation	Regular feedback to frontline staff
Individual training dominant	Team-based training more common
Attention focuses on individual error	Systems approach to hazards and prevention
Short-term fixing of problems	Emphasis on sustained risk reduction
Many adverse events regarded as isolated 'one-offs'	Potential for replication of similar adverse events recognized
Lessons from adverse events seen as primarily for the team concerned	Recognition that lessons may be relevant to others
Individual learning	Team-based learning and developing of non-technical skills

Adapted from *An organisation with a memory*, 2000

BOX 2.3 Parallels between healthcare and aviation

Misinterpretation of Instruments

Aviation

Two aircraft came close to colliding over London, when an air traffic controller instructed the wrong pilot to descend. The two aircraft were circling waiting to land, but the aircraft were so close to each other on the controller's radar screen that their identity tags were difficult to read. The controller wanted the lower of the two aircraft to descend but mistakenly instructed the higher aircraft to do so. The aircraft were within approximately 400 feet of each other when the pilot of the higher aircraft spotted the danger and climbed to safety.

Healthcare

Cardiotocographs (CTGs) are used to monitor and display foetal heart rate during labour. They rely on ultrasonic detection of foetal heart movements. Reports to the Medical Devices Agency revealed that several incidents occurred where, despite the fact that the monitors were showing a heart trace, babies were delivered stillborn. In all probability, the CTG was recording the mother's heartbeat rather than that of the foetus. A safety notice issued in March 1998 advised users of CTG monitors to confirm that the CTG is displaying the foetal heart rate, to use monitors in accordance with manufacturers' instructions and not to place reliance on a single monitoring system.

Dangerous Omissions

Aviation
An aircraft of the Royal Flight was forced to make an emergency landing when the aircrew noticed that all four of the aircraft's engines were experiencing a significant drop in oil pressure. Before landing the pilot had to shut down two of the engines and a third as they taxied on the runway. Upon investigation, the cause of the problem was found to be that none of the engine oil seals had been replaced during routine maintenance and so when the engines were running they were all losing oil.

Healthcare
Two patients died in separate incidents when partially used containers of intravenous fluid were reconnected to administration sets. Both patients suffered fatal air embolisms (air bubbles in the bloodstream). A subsequent safety notice emphasized that partially used intravenous fluid containers should always be discarded because re-use increases the risk of both air embolism and infection.

(FROM AN ORGANIZATION WITH A MEMORY (2000): PP. 40–41 AND 43)

high-risk industries, systems thinking and the need for cultural change. The themes and progress on culture, teamwork, reporting and systems thinking highlighted in these reports will all be examined in later chapters. But first we need to examine the studies of the nature and scale of harm. Can it really be true that healthcare kills tens of thousands of people each year in the United States and, by implication, perhaps hundreds of thousands across the world?

References

Bogner, M.S. (1994) *Human Error in Medicine*, Lawrence Erlbaum, Hillsdale NJ.
Brennan, T.A., Leape, L.L., Laird, N.M. *et al.* (1991) Incidence of adverse events and negligence in hospitalized patients; results from the Harvard Medical Practice Study I. *New England Journal of Medicine*, **324**(6), 370–376.
Bristol Royal Infirmary (2001) Learning from Bristol: Report of the Public Inquiry in to Children's Heart Surgery at the Bristol Infirmary, The Stationery Office, London.
Cook, R.I., Woods, D.D. and Miller, C.A. (1998) *A Tale of Two Stories: Contrasting Views of Patient Safety*, US National Patient Safety Foundation.
Cooper, J.B., Newbower, R.S., Long, C.D. and McPeek, B. (1978) Preventable anesthesia mishaps: a study of human factors. *Anesthesiology*, **49**, 399–406.

Cooper, J.B., Newbower, R.S. and Kitz, R.J. (1984) An analysis of major errors and equipment failures in anesthesia management: considerations for prevention and detection. *Anesthesiology*, **60**, 34–42.

Cooper, J.B. (1994) Towards patient safety in anaesthesia. *Annals Academy of Medicine*, **23** (4), 552–557.

Davies, J.M. (2000) From Dryden to Winnipeg and all Points Beyond, in *Avebury Aviation Management, Vol. 1, Proceedings of the Fourth Australian Aviation Psychology Symposium (* B.N. Hayward and M.C. Lowe), Ashgate, Aldershot UK.

Department of Health (2000) *An Organisation with a Memory: Learning from Adverse Events in the NHS*, The Stationery Office, London.

Eagle, C.J., Davies, J.M. and Reason, J. (1992) Accident analysis of large-scale technological disasters applied to an anaesthetic complication. *Canadian Journal of Anaesthesia*, **39**(2), 118–122.

Gaba, D.M. (2000) Anaesthesiology as a model for patient safety in health care. *British Medical Journal*, **320**(7237), 785–788.

Gawande, A. (2002) *Complications: A Surgeons Notes on an Imperfect Science*, Picador, New York.

Gigerenzer, G. (2002) *Reckoning with Risk. Learning to Live with Uncertainty*, Penguin Books, London.

Her Majesty's Government (1995) Medical (Professional Performance) Act. The Stationery Office, London.

Hiatt, H.H., Barnes, B.A., Brennan, T.A. *et al.* (1989) A study of medical injury and medical malpractice: an overview. *New England Journal of Medicine*, **321**(7), 480–484.

Kerr, J.M. (1932) *Maternal Mortality and Morbidity*, E & S Livingstone, Edinburgh.

Kohn, L., Corrigan, J. and Donaldson, M.E. (1999) *To Err is Human*, National Academy Press, Washington DC.

Langley, G.J., Nolan, K.M., Nolan, T.W. *et al.* (1996) *The Improvement Guide: A Practical Approach to Enhancing Organizational Performance*, Jossey-Bass Publishers, San Francisco CA.

Leape, L.L., Brennan, T.A., Laird, N. *et al.* (1991) The nature of adverse events in hospitalized patients. Results of the Harvard Medical Practice Study II. *The New England Journal of Medicine*, **324**(6), 377–384.

Leape, L.L. (1994) Error in medicine. *Journal of the American Medical Association*, **272**(23), 1851–1857.

Leape, L.L. and Berwick, D.M. (2000) Safe healthcare: are we up to it? *British Medical Journal*, **320**(7237), 725–726.

Leape, L.L. (2000) Institute of Medicine medical error figures are not exaggerated. *Journal of the American Medical Association*, **284**(1), 95–97

Maxwell, R. (1984) Quality assessment in health. *British Medical Journal*, **288**, 1470–1472.

McIntyre, N. and Popper, K. (1983) The critical attitude in medicine: the need for a new ethics. *British Medical Journal*, **287**, 1919–1923.

Medwar, P. (1969) *The Art of the Soluble. Creativity and Originality in Science*, Pelican Books, London.

Mohr, J.C. (2000) American medical malpractice litigation in historical perspective. *Journal of the American Medical Association*, **283**(13), 1731–1737.

Oxley, W.H.F., Philips, M.H. and Young, J. (1935) Maternal mortality in Rochdale. *British Medical Journal*, **1**, 304–307.

Reason, J.T. (1993) The human factor in medical accidents, in *Medical Accidents* (eds C. Vincent, M. Ennis and R.J. Audley), Oxford University Press, Oxford, pp. 1–16.

Sharpe, V.A. and Faden, A.I. (1998) *Medical Harm. Historical, Conceptual and Ethical Dimensions of Iatrogenic Illness*, Cambridge University Press, Cambridge.

Smith, R. (1998) All changed, utterly changed. *British Medical Journal*, **316**(7149), 1917–1918.

Smith, R. (2000) Facing up to medical error. *British Medical Journal*, **320**, 320, doi: 10.1136/bmj.320.7237.0.

Studdert, D.M., Mello, M.M., Gawande, A.A. *et al.* (2006) Claims, errors, and compensation payments in medical malpractice litigation. *The New England Journal of Medicine*, **354**(19), 2024–2033.

Treasure, T. (1998) Lessons from the Bristol case. More openness – on risks and an individual surgeons' performance. *British Medical Journal*, **316**, 1685–1686.

Vincent, C.A. (1989) Research into medical accidents: a case of negligence? *British Medical Journal*, **299**, 1150–1153.

Vincent, C.A. (1993) The study of errors and accidents in medicine, in *Medical Accidents* (eds C.A. Vincent and M. Ennis), Oxford University Press, Oxford.

Vincent, C.A., Ennis, M. and Audley, R.J. (1993) *Medical Accidents*, Oxford University Press, Oxford.

Vincent, C.A. (1995) *Clinical Risk Management*, 1st edn, British Medical Journal Publications, London.

Vincent, C.A. (2001a) Caring for patients harmed by treatment, in *Clinical Risk Management: Enhancing Patient Safety*, 2nd edn (ed. C.A. Vincent), BMJ Books, London, pp. 461–479.

Vincent, C.A. (2001b) *Clinical Risk Management*, 2nd edn, BMJ Books, London.

Walshe, K. and Offen, N. (2001) A very public failure: lessons for quality improvement in healthcare organisations from the Bristol Royal Infirmary. *Quality and Safety in Health Care*, **10**(4), 250–256.

Wennberg, J. and Gittlesohn, A. (1973) Small area variations in health care delivery. *Science*, **182**(117), 1102–1108.

CHAPTER 3
Integrating safety and quality

Patient safety is our top priority. You can now hear this from government ministers, chief executives, speakers on conference platforms and from many applicants during job interviews. This primary emphasis on safety is very welcome but the statement, though it may be sincere, is not strictly correct as I heard from an oil executive:

Safety is not our top priority. Our top priority is getting oil out of the ground. However, when safety and productivity conflict, then safety takes priority.

Similarly, in healthcare, safety is not the overriding priority. Delivering healthcare to patients is the priority but, just as in the oil industry, safety should almost always take priority over other objectives when there is a clash. The reality is that safety is one of a number of competing objectives but, being less tangible and sometimes less valued than a balance sheet or activity summary, it is easily marginalized and forgotten in the press of events. In practice, a Chief Executive balances costs, safety, efficiency, access to care, patient satisfaction and a variety of other objectives. A nurse in charge of a ward juggles safety with the need for a rapid throughput of patients. A clinician may discuss a risky but potentially curative procedure with a patient who also in their turn has to balance safety against other objectives. In all these examples, safety is being balanced against some other aspect of the quality of care all within the context of cost and resource limitations. In this chapter we first define and discuss patient safety, then examine safety within the broader context of other dimensions of quality of care.

Defining patient safety

Patient safety can, at its simplest, be defined as:

The avoidance, prevention and amelioration of adverse outcomes or injuries stemming from the process of healthcare.
(VINCENT, 2006)

Patient Safety, 2nd edition. By Charles Vincent. Published 2010 by Blackwell Publishing Ltd.

This definition goes some way to differentiate patient safety from more general concerns about the quality of healthcare; the focus is on the 'dark side of quality' (Vincent, 1997), care that is actually harmful rather than just not of a good standard. Healthcare is, in many cases at least, inherently hazardous and the definition implicitly acknowledges this. The definition also refers to the amelioration of adverse outcomes or injuries, which broadens the definition beyond traditional safety concerns towards an area that would, in many industries, be called disaster management. In healthcare, amelioration firstly refers to the need for rapid medical intervention to deal with the immediate crisis, but also to the need to care for injured patients and to support the staff involved.

The short definition given above however, does not really capture the defining characteristics of patient safety and its associated conceptual background. The US National Patient Safety Foundation sought to do this when setting out a research agenda for patient safety (Box 3.1). They pointed particularly to the fact that traditional quality initiatives had not fully addressed error and harm, that safety resides in systems as well as people, and that safety has to be actively pursued and promoted. Simply trying to avoid damage is not enough; rather one must reduce errors of all kinds and pursue high reliability as an essential component of high quality care.

BOX 3.1 Defining characteristics of patient safety

Patient safety is concerned primarily with the avoidance, prevention and amelioration of adverse outcomes or injuries stemming from healthcare itself. It should address events that span the continuum of 'errors' and 'deviations' to accidents.

Safety emerges from the interaction of the components of the system. It is more than the absence of adverse outcomes and it is more than avoidance of identifiable 'preventable' errors or occurrences. Safety does not reside in a person, device or department. Improving safety depends on learning how safety emerges from the interaction of components.

Patient safety is related to 'quality of care', but the two concepts are not synonymous. Safety is an important subset of quality. To date, activities to manage quality have not focused sufficiently on patient safety issues.

(© [2000] NATIONAL PATIENT SAFETY FOUNDATION. REPRINTED WITH PERMISSION OF NPSF. ALL RIGHTS RESERVED)

Patient safety – reducing harm or reducing error?

Patient safety is sometimes equated with preventing error. This seems innocent enough, but is a potentially limiting assumption. There is no question that an understanding of error is fundamental to patient safety; however, there are differences of view as to whether the focus of patient safety research and practice should be on error or on harm. Formulating an objective of a specific programme purely in terms of error reduction makes sense when, for instance, your aim is simply to reduce failures in a clinical process in the reasonable belief that this will increase overall reliability, efficiency and safety. However, when we consider the overall aim of patient safety, there are a number of reasons for keeping harm in the forefront of our minds.

The first reason is very simple. Harm is what patients care most about. We will all put up with errors in our care, to some extent at least, as long as we do not come to harm.

Second, consider all the myriad forms of harm that can come from healthcare: complications of surgery, infection from unsafe injections, infection from over crowded hospitals, adverse drug reactions, overdoses from badly designed infusion pumps and so on. Should we assume that all these are necessarily due to error? If we equate patient safety with error reduction, we run the risk of not addressing any form of harm which is either not due to error, or only partly due to error.

Third, many errors do not lead to harm and, indeed, may be necessary to the learning and maintenance of safety. Surgeons for instance, may make quite a number of minor errors during a procedure, none of which really compromise the safety of the patient or the final outcome of the operation (Joice, Hanna and Cuschieri, 1998). As Hofer, Kerr and Hayward (2000) have argued, identifying errors does not equate to identifying them as causes of harm. They imagine a hypothetical study of a series of blood transfusion reactions, which reveals errors in the process of care in 60% of patients with reactions. This finding should certainly alert us to the possibility that errors are causing harm. However, they go on to argue:

Now, suppose that in transfusions in which no reaction occurred there was also an error rate of 60%. Can we argue that the errors caused the adverse event? Can we infer that by engineering out the errors, transfusion reactions would be eliminated? It is clear we cannot.
(HOFER, KERR AND HAYWARD, 2000)

This difficulty of linking errors to harm is an instance of the more general problem of linking process measures to outcome (Lilford *et al.*, 2004) and is not particular to patient safety. We may in fact attempt to reduce harm without considering error at all. In their paper 'Patient safety efforts should focus on medical injuries', Peter Layde and colleagues (2002) describe the well established public health approach to reduction of injuries, which is rooted in efforts to control infectious disease. The injury prevention model sets out the host factors that predispose to injury, which are essentially those pertaining to the patient (being old or otherwise vulnerable for instance), the agent factors (the various hazards of drugs and interventions) and the social, physical and environmental aspects of the environment.

Two particular points emerge from this brief summary. First, it is possible to think about injury reduction without even mentioning the term error. Second, while sophisticated models of the causes of injury can be built, problems can sometimes be circumvented simply by intervening at a critical point in the causal chain:

While numerous factors undoubtedly contributed to fatal childhood falls in New York City, including personality characteristics and behavioural characteristics of the children and their caretakers, the New York City Health Department proposed a classic injury prevention strategy – installation of window barriers.
(LAYDE *ET AL.*, 2002)

What is quality?

Let's start with the big picture, the coverage of healthcare across organizations and countries. The World Health Organization defines effective health coverage as the probability of an individual receiving health gain if needed, which is influenced by a range of clinical, economic, political and other factors. In this framework, quality of care is defined as the proportion of potential health gain actually delivered by a healthcare organization for its set of patients. The essential idea is that quality reflects the gap between what can be achieved and what actually happens. When the gap is small, quality is good; when the gap is large, quality is poor. Potential health gain may not be achieved due to a variety of quality problems, including inequity of provision, lack of access to care, and inefficient and unsafe, perhaps harmful, healthcare.

The quality gap has been nicely expressed by Donabedian in a simple diagram, which depicts the course of an untreated or partially treated disease, against the course of a disease when the patient receives correct and timely treatment. I have added an additional curve to depict a situation in which the patient is actually made worse by their treatment, essentially to underline

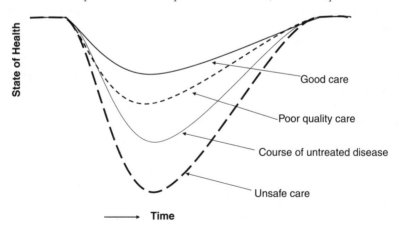

Figure 3.1 Trajectories of Healthcare and Disease (Adapted from Donabedian, 2003).

the safety dimension. This is, of course, a highly idealized picture; in reality a typical patient's course, on whatever index it might be plotted, is an uneven path towards recovery in which good treatment is intermingled with quality and safety problems. However, the quality gap is both real and substantial, in fact a chasm according to the Institute of Medicine (2001).

The quality chasm

Elizabeth McGlynn and colleagues carried out a study of 6712 adults in the United States, by examining their medical records and conducting telephone interviews (McGlynn et al., 2003). Whereas most studies of the quality of care delivered have focused on a particular disease or a particular type of treatment, they wanted to make a general assessment of the quality of care delivered to adult Americans with significant health problems. Quality of care indicators were developed for a range of both acute and chronic conditions, which reflected the standard care that should have been delivered according to national guidelines (Table 3.1).

Incredibly, even in the United States with its legendarily high health costs, albeit mainly spent on 80% of the population, patients received only 55% of recommended care overall. Both overuse of care, unnecessary tests and treatment, and underuse were assessed, but underuse of healthcare was the more frequent problem. The extent of underuse varied considerably between different medical conditions, ranging from almost 80% of correct care provided for senile cataract and breast cancer, down to below 25% for atrial fibrillation, hip fracture and alcohol dependence (Table 3.2). While the researchers acknowledge that more care could have been given than was recorded or remembered by patients, previous studies suggest that this would at most add a few percentage points to the indicator scores. They concluded soberly that:

Our results indicate that on average Americans receive about half of recommended medical care processes.... These deficits, which pose serious threats to the health and well-being of the US public, persist despite initiatives by both the federal government and private healthcare delivery systems to improve care.
(MCGLYNN ET AL., 2003)

McGlynn and her colleagues argue that these findings have important implications for the general health of the population implying, in a sense, avoidable harm. For example, only 24% of the diabetics in the study had regular blood tests, a requirement for close blood glucose control and the avoidance of complications. People with hypertension received 65% of the recommended care; uncontrolled hypertension increases risk for heart disease, stroke and death. Naturally, we cannot assess the implications for individual patients, many of whom may not have been affected, but the overall picture is alarming to say the least. Recent studies on children reveal a similar picture (Mangione-Smith et al., 2007).

Table 3.1 Selected quality indicators and conditions

Condition (Number of Indicators)	Description of Selected Indicator	Type of Care	Mode	Problem with Quality
Asthma (25)	Long acting agents for patients with frequent use of short acting beta antagonists	Chronic	Medication	Underuse
Colorectal cancer (12)	Appropriate surgical treatment	Chronic	Surgery	Underuse
Congestive heart failure (36)	Ejection fraction assessed before medical therapy	Chronic	Laboratory testing or radiography	Underuse
Coronary artery disease (37)	Avoidance of nifedipine for patients with an acute myocardial infarction	Chronic	Medication	Overuse
Hip fracture (9)	Prophylactic antibiotics given on day of surgery	Acute	Medication	Underuse
Headache (21)	Use of appropriate medication for patients with acute migraine	Acute	Medication	Overuse
Hypertension (27)	Change in treatment when blood pressure is persistently under controlled	Chronic	Medication	Underuse
Preventive care (38)	Screening for cervical cancer	Preventive	Laboratory testing or radiography	Underuse

Adapted from McGlynn *et al.* (2003)

As this particular study is set in the United States, it is difficult to predict whether the results would be similar in different kinds of health system. In a publicly funded and more tightly controlled system, such as the British NHS, one might expect a closer adherence to procedure and protocol; on the other hand, most US physicians have financial incentives to investigate and treat, so one might expect higher rates of intervention.

The relationship between safety and quality

Avedis Donabedian, the great theorist of healthcare quality, made the now classic distinction between the structure, process and outcome of healthcare, which was fundamental to understanding that quality depended on the relationship between many components and that process and outcome could be separately assessed (Donabedian, 1968). Donabedian (1968) also emphasized that quality of care encompassed not only technical excellence of the care but also the manner and humanity with which it was delivered, a commonplace distinction nowadays but not in the 1960s. This is not to say that clinicians were not caring and compassionate, only that this was not viewed as a component of quality of care, still less that these subtle, human features of healthcare might be measured. Maxwell (1984) took this idea further, identifying six core dimensions of quality: technical excellence, social acceptability, humanity, cost, equity and relevance to need.

Safety does not feature at all in Maxwell's list of quality dimensions, although it is certainly related to technical excellence and acceptability. Why is this? It seems the most basic requirement of any public or privately delivered service where risk is involved. If we travel by road or train, if we fly, stay in hotels, or live near nuclear power plants, we want above all to be safe. It is easy now, with the benefit of hindsight, to see that safety is an essential part of quality, but at that time the language of error and harm had not entered healthcare discourse. By 1999 however, The Institute of Medicine report 'To Err is Human' put safety to the forefront, describing it as the first dimension of quality (Kohn, Corrigan and Donaldson, 1999).

The relationship between safety and quality of care has been variously expressed, presenting safety as a dimension of quality or, in contrast, on a broad continuum. Many people are content to describe the relationship between safety and quality as a continuum, with safety issues simply being the 'hard edge' of more general quality concerns. However, this does little more than sidestep the issue, and tends to suggest that safety and quality concerns are necessarily complementary. The quality of healthcare has been described in a number of different ways by various authors (Donabedian, 1968; Maxwell, 1984; Langley *et al.*, 1996 – all from Boaden), but the most important aspects, including safety, are well captured by the six dimensions that provide the foundation of the Institute of Medicine's 'Crossing the Quality Chasm' report (Box 3.2). Making sense of all this is not straightforward. However, it does become clearer when we start to examine specific instances of unsafe or poor quality care.

BOX 3.2 Six specific aims for improvement

Safe – avoiding injuries to patients from the care that is intended to help them;

Effective – providing services based on scientific knowledge to all who could benefit and refraining from providing services to those not likely to benefit (avoiding underuse and overuse);

Patient-centred – providing care that is respectful of and responsive to individual patient preferences, needs and values and ensuring that patient values guide all clinical decisions;

Timely – reducing waits and sometimes harmful delays for both those who receive and those who give care;

Efficient – avoiding waste, in particular waste of equipment, supplies, ideas and energy;

Equitable – providing care that does not vary in quality because of personal characteristics such as gender, ethnicity, geographic location and socio-economic status;

(REPRINTED WITH PERMISSION FROM THE NATIONAL ACADEMIES PRESS, © 2001, NATIONAL ACADEMY OF SCIENCES.)

BOX 3.3 Ms Martinez

Ms Martinez, a divorced working mother in her early 50s with two children in junior high school, had to choose a new family doctor. After receiving some recommendations from a neighbour, she called several of the offices to sign up. The first two she called were not accepting new patients. Although she knew nothing about the practice she finally found, she assumed it would be adequate. Ms Martinez delayed calling her new doctor's office for several months. When she called for an appointment, she was told that the first available non-urgent appointment was in two months; she hoped she would not run out of her blood pressure medication in the interim.

When she went for her first appointment, she was asked to complete a patient history form in the waiting room. She had difficulty remembering dates and significant past events and doses of her medications. After waiting for an hour, she met with Dr McGonagle and had a physical exam. Although her breast exam appeared to be normal, Dr McGonagle noted that she was due for a mammogram.

Ms Martinez called a site listed in her provider directory and was given an appointment for a mammogram in six weeks. The staff suggested that she arrange to have her old films mailed to her. Somehow, the films were never sent, and distracted by other concerns, she forgot to follow up.

A week after the mammogram, she received a call from Dr McGonagle's office notifying her of an abnormal finding and saying that she should make an appointment with a surgeon for a biopsy. The first available appointment with the surgeon was nine weeks later. By now, she was very anxious. She hated even to think about having cancer in her body, especially because an older sister had died of the disease. For weeks she did not sleep, wondering what would happen to her children if she were debilitated or to her job if she had to have surgery and lengthy treatment.

After numerous calls, she was finally able to track down her old mammograms. It turned out that a possible abnormal finding had been circled the previous year, but neither she nor her primary care physician had ever been notified.

Finally, Ms Martinez had her appointment with the surgeon, and his office scheduled her for a biopsy. The biopsy showed that she had a fairly unusual form of cancer, and there was concern that it might have spread to her lymph nodes. She felt terrified, angry, sad and helpless all at once, but needed to decide what kind of surgery to have. It was a difficult decision because only one small trial comparing lumpectomy and mastectomy for this type of breast cancer had been conducted. She finally decided on a mastectomy.

Before she could have surgery, Ms Martinez needed to have bone and abdominal scans to rule out metastases to her bones or liver. When she arrived at the hospital for surgery however, some of this important laboratory information was missing. The staff called and hours later finally tracked down the results of her scans, but for a while it looked as though she would have to reschedule the surgery.

During her mastectomy, several positive lymph nodes were found. This meant she had to see the surgeon, an oncologist and a radiologist, as well as her primary care physician, to decide on the next steps. At last it was decided that she would have radiation therapy and chemotherapy. She was given the phone number for the American Cancer Society. Before six months had gone by, Ms Martinez found another lump, this time under her arm. Cancer had spread to her lung as well. She was given more radiation, then more chemotherapy. Wherever she went for care, the walls were drab, the chairs uncomfortable, and sometimes she would wait hours for a scheduled appointment.

(REPRINTED WITH PERMISSION FROM THE NATIONAL ACADEMIES PRESS, © 2001, NATIONAL ACADEMY OF SCIENCES.)

The Institute of Medicine report 'Crossing the Quality Chasm' (Institute of Medicine, 2001) provides a composite story of Ms Martinez, a working mother in her 50s. Two routine mammograms showed abnormal findings, but she was not notified of the first. Most of the clinicians she saw were thoughtful and caring people but, overall, the healthcare system let her down badly. Long delays between appointments, missing laboratory information, poor communication and a host of other problems reduced her chances of survival. Her anxiety and suffering was made very much worse by the dangers and inefficiencies of the healthcare system. She suffered preventable, long-lasting disability – and could have lost her life. The report points out that Ms Martinez' care failed on several counts:

- First, it was not safe. Neither she nor her previous primary care doctor had been notified of an abnormal finding on her earlier mammogram. As a result, at least a year elapsed before the abnormality was addressed. Ms Martinez was never confident that those directing her care had all the information about her that was needed. She was repeatedly required to tell her story, which became longer and more complex as time passed.

- Second, her care was not effective. Much of her care did not follow best practice; treatments tried and proven futile in one admission would be recommended in the next as if they were fresh ideas.
- Third, her care was not timely. There were continual, repeated, delays between tests and follow-up care.
- Fourth, her care was not patient-centred. She had little assistance or information to help her understand the implications of choices about her surgery, radiation therapy or chemotherapy.
- Finally, her care was not efficient because much of its complexity and expense came from treating a tumour at a later stage than should have occurred.

The first point to emerge from this example is that there is no sharp dividing line between safety and more general quality concerns. Ms Martinez did not suffer harm in the sense that she was injured by a drug or complication of surgery, but she did certainly suffer preventable harm from the many lapses and deficiencies in her care, which allowed the disease to progress to a much greater extent. However, there were a variety of other problems with her care, in terms of efficiency, timeliness and patient centredness which we would hesitate to describe as safety issues, though they may have contributed to the preventable harm. The various problems also made Ms Martinez 'feel unsafe', which is important in its own right, although not usually considered under the heading of patient safety. More generally, patient experience of safety and quality, which may be strongly influenced by communication, caring and staff attitudes, may not accord well with more technical assessments of process and outcome. This does not mean that one of these perspectives is 'correct', simply that quality has many facets.

When does a quality issue become a safety issue?

We can see then that safety is one dimension of broader quality concerns though, I would argue, the most critical and defining for patients. What then leads to an issue being badged as a safety issue rather than a quality issue? The most dramatic examples tend to be of rare incidents, such as the death following an injection of Vincristine discussed later. On an individual level, these are some of the most tragic failures one could imagine. However, at a population level, the harm from failure, for example, to give thrombolytics or to carry out routine investigations, may be much greater. Consider this summary of a study of 9356 patients with suspected angina pectoris (Hemingway *et al.*, 2008):

The authors determined the appropriateness of angiography in 9356 patients with suspected angina pectoris ... and measured outcomes at 3 years. More than half of the patients who had appropriate indications for angiography did not have the procedure. Not undergoing coronary angiography when indicated was associated with a 2.5-fold worse composite outcome (cardiac death, myocardial infarction and acute coronary syndrome).

(REPRODUCED FROM *ANNALS OF INTERNAL MEDICINE*, DAVID P. FAXON. "ASSESSING APPROPRIATENESS OF CORONARY ANGIOGRAPHY: ANOTHER STEP IN IMPROVING QUALITY". VOL. 149, PP.276–278, AUG 2008, WITH PERMISSION FROM AMERICAN COLLEGE OF PHYSICIANS)

Quality of care was poor for many of these patients; care was not timely or appropriate. Furthermore, poor quality care was associated with harm, not in the sense that it directly caused harm but in the sense that some patients came to harm because of deficiencies in their care. This would, in most of the major studies of adverse events (see next chapter) have been regarded as a preventable adverse event, although the link between the poor care and the outcome would have had to have been assessed in each case. The more general point though is that poor quality care and unsafe care are, in this instance at least, one and the same thing.

Brown, Hofer Johal and colleagues (2008) have argued that failures of different kinds will be viewed differently, as safety issues or more general quality issues, according to the strength of causation and the immediacy of harm. Essentially, events that cause definite harm and are clearly related to specific lapses of problems in the process of care, are more likely to be described as safety issues. Table 3.2 gives some examples of different kinds of failure and outcomes to illustrate this point. The first two examples, an adverse drug event and a surgical complication, are more likely to be described as safety issues and, incidentally, are more likely to attract the term 'error'. The failure to vaccinate again could be naturally thought of as a safety issue, in that harm is likely to result. There is a sense in which harm befell the patients in the other two examples (where both patients suffered a myocardial infarction) and there were certainly lapses in their care; however, the lack of a clear link between the lapses and the harm tends to push these examples into more general quality of care concerns.

Table 3.2 Safety and quality, causality and immediacy

	Failure	Causality	Immediacy
Safety ↑	Intrathecal administration of vincristine/ potassium chloride resulting in death	High	High
	Severing of the common bile duct in cholecystectomy	High	High
	Failure to vaccinate, resulting in the person developing the disease the vaccination was intended to prevent	High	Low
	Failure to give thrombolytics in myocardial infarction. Patient dies in hospital of further myocardial infarction	Low	High
↓ Quality	Failure to prescribe beta-blockers after discharge from hospital following myocardial infarction. Patient has a further MI at a later date	Low	Low

Reproduced from *Quality & Safety in Health Care*, C Brown, T Hofer, A Johal et al. "An epistemology of patient safety research: a framework for study design and interpretation. Part 3. End points and measurement". **17**, no. 3, [158–162], 2008, with permission from BMJ Publishing Group Ltd.

The emergence of concerns about safety in healthcare also, I believe, marks a shift in social attitudes and assessments of what is an acceptable level of risk. We saw in the last chapter that in the 1950s many hazards of healthcare were recognized, at least by some, but largely viewed as the inevitable consequences of medical intervention. Gradually, certain types of incidents and harms have come to seem both unacceptable and deemed to be potentially preventable. The clearest example in recent times is healthcare associated infection, which was not exactly tolerated but viewed an unfortunate side effect of healthcare. With increased understanding of both underlying processes, mechanisms of transmission and methods of prevention, coupled with major public and regulatory pressure, such infections are becoming unacceptable to both patients and professionals. By this I do not mean that all such infections can be prevented, simply that they are no longer to be tolerated as they once were. The list of 'never events' (Chapter 6), such as wrong site surgery or suicide of a patient while in hospital, put forward in various countries, is similarly a willingness to say that certain types of failure cannot be tolerated. Safety is in this sense, an aspiration to better care, and the labelling of an issue as a safety issue is a strongly motivational, perhaps emotional, plea that such outcomes cannot and should not be tolerated.

What has safety brought to quality?

The attention given to patient safety did, I think it is fair to say, annoy some of those who had worked in quality improvement for decades. Certainly, one can detect a note of irritation in some of the papers pointing out that some safety concepts and the 'new understanding' were simply a reworking of longstanding quality improvement ideas. If safety is a core dimension of quality, did we need to invent patient safety at all? Timothy Hofer, Eve Kerr and Rodney Hayward pose the essential question in a paper written in 2000, critiquing the concept of medical error:

How does the search to identify error differ from the widespread efforts over the past 15–20 years to monitor, profile and improve the quality of care? Does the elimination of error provide us with a way to substantially hasten improvement in healthcare?
(HOFER, KERR AND HAYWARD, 2000)

Healthcare, as with many other industries, is notorious for coming up with new initiatives which, on closer inspection, turn out to be remarkably similar to the old initiatives but with a new label. Some of the core ideas and concepts of patient safety could certainly be identified in earlier writings from the quality pioneers, though often in rather embryonic form. Safety however, did enrich the quality movement by bringing new force, new ideas and new approaches to bear on the shared quest to improve healthcare. Most importantly, we began to realize that patients were suffering much more than had previously been thought and were being let down by the healthcare system. Some of the main contributions of safety are:

- Showing clearly that healthcare can be positively dangerous to patients;
- Drawing attention to the impact and aftermath of error and harm;
- Facing the issue of medical error squarely and addressing the nature and causes of error;
- Bringing a much stronger focus on human performance;
- Bringing a much stronger focus on ergonomics and psychological issues;
- Using a wider range of industrial models for safety and quality, particularly from high risk industries;
- Bringing new tools and techniques to healthcare improvement.

Don Berwick has perhaps done more than anyone in the world in his decades-long quest to improve the quality of care. He is deeply imbued with the knowledge and practice of quality and has sought lessons and experience from many different quarters. Yet in 2001 the emergence of patient safety still brought him some new insights:

In the field of safety, I continue to regard myself as a novice. This is not false humility; it's a true confession. I came relatively new to this field of safety four years ago. . . . I continue to discover that things I thought to be true simply are not. And things that I learned and then thought to be true aren't true either. This continuing evolution in my own understanding has affected the way I talk about safety. Here is a series of lessons that have caused me to change the way I think about safety.
(BERWICK, 2002)

Don Berwick is a safety novice in the same way that the American golfing legend Tiger Woods would be a novice if he decided to take up tennis; you might feel he had just a bit of an edge on other neophyte tennis players. But the lessons he drew show us some of the perspectives from the safety world that have proved instructive in the broader attempt to improve quality (Box 3.4).

BOX 3.4 Patient safety – lessons from a novice

Lesson 1 – I thought: The problem is errors.
I learned: The problem is harm.

If we believe our battle is against errors, we will lose. The problem is harm. Errors are inevitable; they will always be there... I would like to see the vocabulary of patient safety focus more on the question, 'How can we keep patients from being hurt in our hands?' and less on 'How can we keep errors from happening?'

Lesson 2 – I thought: Rules create safety.
I learned: Rules and breaking the rules create safety.

Safety is a continually emerging property of a complex system – it's more like driving a car than baking a cake... Breaking the rules is the adaptive response of an intelligent workforce involved at the sharp end of health-care. In the violation of the rules, it is the next level of information about what to do to make a person safe. Rules should be more like instructions for driving a car – allowing the driver to adapt to current circumstances – than a point-by-point recipe for baking a cake. Overspecification is a problem in safety.

Lesson 3 – I thought: Reporting is necessary to track problems and progress.
I learned: Stories are necessary to gain knowledge.

We're hooked on reporting now. Reporting for measurement contains almost no information. What we need are *stories*. Reporting that loses the story is mostly a waste. We need to harvest the knowledge. We need firesides, not spreadsheets.

The question 'How many?' isn't powerful enough. The question should be 'What happened?'

Lesson 4 – I thought: Technology is the mainstay of safety.
I learned: Conversation is the mainstay of safety.

Every technology – even those for improving safety – has hazards. The world of technology has to be a world with dykes around it, or it will hurt us. Building technology for safety is crucial, but it must be supported by conversation – a human mechanism for getting control back. Technology without collective mindfulness will make things worse, not better.

Lesson 5 – I thought: Healthcare is mostly the same as other high-hazard industries.
I learned: Healthcare differs a lot from other high-hazard industries.

There is so much to learn from other industries. But there are crucial, important differences between healthcare and other fields. The simple-minded adoption of safety practices from other industries is problematic because the range of risk levels in healthcare is extremely wide. No single answer can possibly do. It's important to know which level you're working on.

Lesson 6 – I thought: What's important happens before the injury.
I learned: What happens after the injury is equally important.

Part of our safety culture has got to focus on the healing side. We have to heal both people who are hurt – the injured person and the person who caused the injury. We need to get some energy back on the healing side of the table. The most important barrier may be skills – especially the ability to apologize. Some doctors are unwilling or unable to say how sorry they are. Apology begins the process of re-affiliation with the patient.

(ADAPTED FROM BERWICK, 2002)

Safety and quality research

Patient safety, and indeed safety in many other industries, has relied exten-sively on the detailed analysis and understanding of accidents and incidents. The analysis of individual cases in system terms (Chapter 7) can be enormously productive in terms of showing the wider influences on safety and quality, providing important hypotheses for further investigation and because of the additional cultural and educational value, both of which may be safety relevant. Stories may, in addition to their analytic potential, be genuinely important vehicles of safety culture and understanding within organizations. A second defining feature has been the reliance on the concept of error. Both of these features have aroused some suspicion amongst people more accustomed to standard epidemiological approaches and the associated methodological armament of population based approaches and randomized controlled trials.

We do not need to jettison case studies, which have a long and honourable history in medicine, or the subtleties of psychological analysis and the insights of other disciplines. Patient safety has not however, as we will argue later, addressed measurement sufficiently; this is now coming home to roost and seriously impeding progress. Safety and quality interventions have not, in many cases, been evaluated in the same way as drugs and other major interventions (and nor, we might add, have most healthcare management or policy initiatives). Safety initiatives do not necessarily require complex evaluation and in some instances randomized trials are neither feasible nor desirable; there have, after all, been few randomized controlled trials in aviation but the planes remain in the air. Nevertheless, patient safety needs to reconnect with standard scientific methodology and epidemiological approaches and give measurement and epidemiology equal weight to understanding and analysis.

References

Berwick, D.M. (2002) Patient safety: lessons from a novice. *Advances in Neonatal Care*, **2**(3), 121–122.

Brown, C., Hofer, T., Johal, A. *et al.* (2008) An epistemology of patient safety research: a framework for study design and interpretation. Part 1: Conceptualising and developing interventions. *Quality and Safety in Health Care*, **17**(3), 158–162.

Donabedian, A. (2003) *An Introduction to Quality Assurance in Health Care*, Oxford University Press, Oxford.

Donabedian, A. (1968) Promoting quality through evaluating the process of patient care. *Medical Care*, **6**(3), 181–202.

Faxon, D.P. (2008) Assessing appropriateness of coronary angiography: another step in improving quality. *Annals of Internal Medicine*, **149**(4), 276–278.

Hemingway, H., Chen, R., Junghans, C. *et al.* (2008) Appropriateness criteria for coronary angiography in angina: reliability and validity. *Annals of Internal Medicine*, **149**(4), 221–231.

Hofer, T.P., Kerr, E.A. and Hayward, R.A. (2000) What is an error? *Effective Clinical Practice*, **3**(6), 261–269.

Institute of Medicine (2001) *Crossing the Qualitfry Chasm. A New Health System for the 21st Century*, National Academy Press, Washington DC.

Joice, P., Hanna, G.B. and Cuschieri, A. (1998) Errors enacted during endoscopic surgery – a human realiability analysis. *Applied Ergonomics*, **29**(6), 409–414.

Kohn, L., Corrigan, J. and Donaldson, M.E. (1999) *To Err is Human*, National Academy Press, Washington DC.

Langley, G.J., Nolan, K.M., Nolan, T.W. et al. (1996) *The Improvement Guide: A Practical Approach to Enhancing Organizational Performance*, Jossey-Bass Publishers, San Francisco CA.

Layde, P.M., Maas, L.A., Teret, S.P. *et al.* (2002) Patient Safety Efforts Should Focus on Medical Injuries. *JAMA: The Journal of the American Medical Association*, **287**(15), 1993–1997.

Lilford, R., Mohammed, M.A., Spiegelhalter, D. and Thomson, R. (2004) Use and misuse of process and outcome data in managing performance of acute medical care: avoiding institutional stigma. *Lancet*, **363**(9415), 1147–1154.

Mangione-Smith, R., DeCristofaro, A.H., Setodji, C.M. *et al.* (2007) The quality of ambulatory care delivered to children in the United States. *The New England Journal of Medicine*, **357**(15), 1515–1523.

Maxwell, R. (1984) Quality assessment in health. *British Medical Journal*, **288**(6428), 1470–1472.

McGlynn, E.A., Asch, S.M., Adams, J. *et al.* (2003) The quality of health care delivered to adults in the United States. *New England Journal of Medicine*, **348**(26), 2635–2645.

United States National Patient Safety Foundation (2000) Agenda for research and development in patient safety. http:/www.npsf.org/pdf/r/researchagenda.pdf.

Vincent, C. (2006) *Patient Safety*, Elsevier Churchill Livingstone, Edinburgh.

Vincent, C.A. (1997) Risk, safety and the dark side of quality. *British Medical Journal*, **314**(7097), 1775–1776.

The Hazards of Healthcare

CHAPTER 4

The nature and scale of error and harm

How safe is healthcare? How often do errors occur? Are the high profile cases rare isolated accidents in an otherwise safe system or are they, in the time honoured phrase, just the tip of the iceberg? These apparently straightforward questions are, for various reasons, not easy to answer. Defining error and harm is not as simple as it might seem; different types of study illuminate different aspects of the problem and comparing findings from different settings is not always feasible. We can however, gain an understanding of the overall scale of the problem and the challenges we face. As we shall see, while rates of error and harm vary in different settings, there is now substantial evidence of very high rates of error in many contexts and considerable evidence of harm to patients. First though, we must consider the main methods available for studying error and harm as, without this, it will be very difficult to make sense of the findings.

Studying errors and adverse events

There are a number of methods of studying errors and adverse events, each of which has evolved over time and been adapted to different contexts. Each of the methods has particular strengths and advantages, and also weaknesses and limitations. Well, what's the best method, you might reasonably ask? The answer is, as so often in research, that it depends on what you are trying to do and what questions you are trying to answer. Some methods are useful for identifying how often adverse events occur, others are stronger on why they happen; some are warning systems, rather than methods of counting, and so on. Failing to understand that different methods have different purposes has led to considerable confusion and much fruitless debate over the years. For instance, the major retrospective record reviews have sometimes been criticized for not providing data on human factors and other issues not identified in medical records. In fact, such studies are not intended to provide such information. Their primary purpose is to assess the nature and scale of harm, although recent review techniques also suggest that valuable information on cause and prevention can be extracted. In all cases, the methodology of a study

Patient Safety, 2nd edition. By Charles Vincent. Published 2010 by Blackwell Publishing Ltd.

will depend on the questions being addressed, the resources available and the context of the study.

Methods of study

Thomas and Petersen (2003) classified methods of studying errors and adverse events into eight broad groups and reviewed the respective advantages and disadvantages of each method. In their paper, they use the term error to include terms such as mistakes, close calls, near misses and factors that contribute to error. In a later chapter we will discuss the difficulties of defining and classifying errors, but in this section the term error is used as a catch-all for any incident that does not involve patient harm. The terms 'near miss' and 'close call' are seldom clearly defined but broadly speaking refer to incidents in which harm was only narrowly avoided; this includes both incidents which never developed to the point of actually harming a patient and those in which prompt action averted disaster.

Tables 4.1 and 4.2 summarize the main types of studies of errors and adverse events, and their respective advantages and limitations. Thomas and Petersen's original source version has been separated into two separate tables and the content has been adjusted; in particular, a section on case analysis has been added. Case analyses, usually referred to as root cause analysis or systems analysis, share some of the features of morbidity and mortality meetings, but are generally more focused and follow a particular method of analysis (Vincent, 2003) (Chapter 8).

Methods differ in several respects. Some methods are orientated towards detecting incidence (how many) of errors and adverse events (Table 3.1), while others address their causes and contributory factors (why things go wrong) (Table 3.2). The various methods rely on different sources of data: medical records, observations, claims data, voluntary reports and so on. Some focus on single cases or small numbers of cases with particular characteristics, such as claims, while others attempt to randomly sample a defined population. Thomas and Petersen suggest that the methods can be placed along a continuum with active clinical surveillance of specific types of adverse event (e.g. surgical complications) being the ideal method for assessing incidence, and methods such as case analysis and morbidity and mortality meetings being more orientated towards causes. There is no perfect way of estimating the incidence of adverse events or of errors. For various reasons, all of them give a partial picture. Record review is comprehensive and systematic, but by definition is restricted to matters noted in the medical record. Reporting systems are strongly dependent on the willingness of staff to report and are a very imperfect reflection of the underlying rate of errors or adverse events (though they have other uses).

Hindsight bias

Hindsight bias is mentioned several times in the table. What is hindsight bias? The term derives from the psychological literature and in particular from

Table 4.1 Methods of measuring errors and adverse

Study Method	Advantages	Disadvantages
Administrative data analysis	Uses readily available data	May rely upon incomplete and inaccurate data
	Inexpensive	The data are divorced from clinical context
Record review/chart review	Uses readily available data	Judgements about adverse events not reliable
	Commonly used	Medical records are incomplete Hindsight bias
Review of electronic medical record	Inexpensive after initial investment	Susceptible to programming and/or data entry errors
	Monitors in real time	Expensive to implement
	Integrates multiple data sources	
Observation of patient care	Potentially accurate and precise	Time consuming and expensive
	Provides data otherwise unavailable	Difficult to train reliable observers
	Detects more active errors than other methods	Potential concerns about confidentiality
		Possible to be overwhelmed with information
Active clinical surveillance	Potentially accurate and precise for adverse events	Time consuming and expensive

Adapted from Thomas and Petersen, 2003

experimental studies showing that people exaggerate in retrospect what they knew before an incident occurred – the 'knew it all along' effect. After a disaster, with the benefit of hindsight, it all looks so simple and the 'expert' reviewing the case wonders why the clinician involved couldn't see the obvious connections. Looking back, the situation actually faced by the clinician is inevitably grossly simplified. We cannot capture the multiple pathways open to the clinician at the time or the unfolding story of a clinical encounter. Still less can we capture the pressures and distractions that may have been affecting clinical judgement, such as fatigue, hunger and having to deal with several other patients with complex conditions.

Hindsight bias has another facet, perhaps better termed outcome bias, which is particularly relevant in healthcare. When an outcome is bad, those looking back are much more likely to be critical of care that has been given and more likely to detect errors. For instance, Caplan, Posner and Cheney (1991) asked two groups of physicians to review sets of notes. The sets of notes were identical

Table 4.2 Methods of understanding errors and adverse

Study Method	Advantages	Disadvantages
Morbidity and mortality conferences and autopsy	Can suggest contributory factors	Hindsight bias
	Familiar to health care providers	Reporting bias
		Focused on diagnostic errors Infrequently used
Case analysis/Root cause analysis	Can suggest contributory	Hindsight bias
	Structured systems approach	Tends to focus on severe events
	Includes recent data from interviews	Insufficiently standardized in practice
Claims analysis	Provides multiple perspectives (patients, providers, lawyers)	Hindsight bias
		Reporting bias
		Non-standardized source of data
Error reporting systems	Provide multiple perspectives over time	Reporting bias
	Can be a part of routine operations	Hindsight bias

Adapted from Thomas and Petersen, 2003

except that for one group the outcomes were satisfactory, and for the other group the outcome was poor for the patient. Much stronger criticisms were made of the care of the group who believed outcomes were poor, even though the care described was exactly the same. So, we simplify things in retrospect and tend to be more critical when the outcome is bad.

Studying adverse events using case record review

Retrospective reviews of medical records aim to assess the nature, incidence and economic impact of adverse events and to provide some information on their causes. Adverse events are defined as an unintended injury caused by medical management rather than the disease process that results in some definite injury or, at the very least, spent on additional days in hospital (Box 4.1). Definitions are critical in patient safety and one has to be constantly aware of differences in terminology. For instance, a study by Andrews *et al.* (1997) in the United States showed a 17.7% rate of serious adverse events in a surgical unit, much higher than most other studies. However, their definition of adverse event was different from that usually employed and they used observation rather than record review, as most other studies do. These are not flaws; the study is a good one. The point is that one has to be careful about definitions when interpreting findings and comparing studies.

BOX 4.1 Defining adverse events

An adverse event is an unintended injury caused by medical management rather than by the disease process and which is sufficiently serious to lead to prolongation of hospitalization or to temporary or permanent impairment or disability to the patient at time of discharge or both:

- Medical management includes both the actions of an individual member of staff or the overall healthcare system.
- Medical management includes acts of omission (e.g. failure to diagnose or treat) and commission (e.g. incorrect treatment).
- Causation of adverse event by medical management is judged on a 6-point scale, where 1 indicates *'virtually no evidence for causation'* and 6 indicates *'virtually certain evidence for causation'*. Only adverse events with a score of 4 or higher, requiring evidence that causation is more likely than not, are reported in the results.
- Adverse events may or may not be preventable, a separate judgement from that of causation. Preventability was also judged on a 6-point scale, with only those adverse events scoring 4 or higher being considered preventable.
- Injury may result from intervention or from failure to intervene. Injuries that come about from failure to arrest the disease process are also included, provided that standard care would clearly have prevented the injury.
- The injury has to be unintended, since injury can occur deliberately and with good reason (e.g. amputation).
- Adverse events include recognized complications, which will be judged as leading to harm but being of low preventability.

(FROM BRENNAN *ET AL.*, 1991)

The basic record review process is as follows. In phase I, nurses or experienced record clerks are trained to identify case records that satisfy one or more of 18 well-defined screening criteria – such as death, transfer to a special care unit or re-admission to hospital within 12 months. These have been shown to be associated with an increased likelihood of an adverse event (Neale and Woloshynowych, 2003). In phase II, trained doctors analyse positively screened records in detail to determine whether or not they contain evidence of an adverse event using a standard set of questions. The basic method has been followed in all the major national studies, though modifications of the review form and data capture have been developed (Woloshynowych, Neale and Vincent, 2003). In France, Phillipe Michel used prospective review, in the sense that record review is carried out close to the time of discharge on a previously defined set of patients and, in some cases, combined with interviews with staff (Michel *et al.*, 2004).

The classic, pioneering study in this area is the Harvard Medical Practice Study, still hugely influential and much debated 20 years after it was carried out (Box 4.2). Similar studies have been conducted in Australia (Wilson *et al.*, 1995), Utah and Colorado (Gawande *et al.*, 1999), United Kingdom (Vincent, Neale and Woloshynowych, 2001), Denmark (Schioler *et al.*, 2001), New Zealand (Davis *et al.*, 2002), Canada (Baker *et al.*, 2004) France (Michel *et al.*, 2007) and other countries. The results of these studies are summarized in Table 4.3 and constitute, as Peter Davis expresses it, a new public health risk:

Of the top 20 risk factors that account for nearly three-quarters of all deaths annually, adverse in-hospital events come in at number 11 above air pollution, alcohol and drugs, violence and road traffic injury.
(DAVIS, 2004)

BOX 4.2 The Harvard medical practice study

The Harvard Medical Practice Study reviewed patient records of 30, 121 randomly chosen hospitalizations from 51 randomly chosen acute care, non-psychiatric hospitals in New York State in 1984. The goal was to better understand the epidemiology of patient injury and to inform efforts to reform systems of patient compensation. The focus was therefore on injuries that might eventually lead to legal action. Minor errors and those causing only minor discomfort or inconvenience were not addressed.

Adverse events occurred in 3.7% of hospitalizations and 27.6% were due to negligence (defined as care that fell below the standard expected of physicians in that community, and which might therefore lead to legal action). Almost half of adverse (47.7%) events were associated with an operation. The most common non-operative adverse events were adverse drug events, followed by diagnostic mishaps, therapeutic mishaps, procedure related events and others. Permanent disability resulted from 6.5% of adverse events and 13.6% involved the death of a patient. Extrapolations from this data suggested that approximately 100 000 deaths each year were associated with adverse events. Later analyses indicated that 69.6% of adverse events were potentially preventable.

(FROM BRENNAN *ET AL.*, 1991; LEAPE *ET AL.*, 1991)

Rates of adverse events in most recent studies lie between 8 and 12%, a range now accepted as being typical of advanced healthcare systems (de Vries *et al.*, 2008). The rate per patient is always slightly higher, as some patients suffer more than one event, and about half of adverse events are generally judged to be preventable. US rates are much lower, Australia seemingly much higher.

Table 4.3 Adverse events in acute hospitals in ten countries

Study	Authors	Date of admissions	Number of hospital admissions	Adverse event rate (% admissions)
Harvard Medical Practice Study (HMPS)	Brennan et al., 1991; Leape et al., 1991	1984	30 195	3.7
Utah-Colorado Study (UTCOS)	Thomas et al., 2000b	1992	14 052	2.9
Quality in Australian Health Care Study (QAHCS)	Wilson et al., 1995	1992	14 179	16.6
United Kingdom	Vincent, et al., 2001	1999	1014	10.8
Denmark	Schioler et al., 2001	1998	1097	9.0
New Zealand	Davis et al., 2002	1998	6579	11.2
Canada	Baker et al., 2004	????	3745	7.5
France	Michel et al., 2007	2004	8754	6.6% per 1000 d admission
United Kingdom	Sari et al., 2007	2004	1006	8.7
Spain	Aranaz-Andres et al., 2008	2005	5624	8.4
The Netherlands	Zegers et al., 2009	2006	7926	5.7
Sweden	Soop et al., 2009	2006	1967	12.3

The lower US rates might reflect better quality care, but most probably reflect the narrower focus on negligent injury rather than the broader quality improvement focus of most other studies (Thomas *et al.*, 2000a). Eric Thomas and colleagues also found, in a careful comparison of specific types of adverse events, that Australian reviewers reported many more minor expected or anticipated complications, such as wound infection, skin injury and urinary tract infection. These are adverse events by the strict definition of the term, but were not included by the American reviewers, who were focusing on more serious injuries (Thomas *et al.*, 2000a).

Examples of adverse events from the first British study are shown in Box 4.3. Some, such as the reaction to anaesthetic, are not serious for the patient but are classed as an adverse event because there was an increased stay in hospital of one day; it was probably not preventable in that it would have been hard to predict such an idiosyncratic reaction. Many adverse events, about 70% in most studies, do not have serious consequences for the patient; the effects of minor events may be more economic, in the sense of wasted time and resources, than clinical. Others however, as the remaining examples show, cause considerable unnecessary suffering and extended time in hospital.

BOX 4.3 Examples of adverse events of varying severity

An 18-year-old girl was admitted as a day surgery case for examination of ears under anaesthetic. During recovery the patient suffered three fits related to the anaesthetic and required intravenous medication to control fits and an extended stay for overnight observation.

A 65-year-old lady was admitted to hospital for repair of a strangulated incisional hernia. Post-operatively the wound site failed to heal. The patient was sent home with a discharging and offensive wound. She returned three days later with a gaping and infected wound, which required cleansing and re-suturing under a general anaesthetic, antibiotics and an extended hospital stay of 15 days.

A 24-year-old woman with spina bifida presented to the emergency department feeling unwell. Her ankles were swollen and she was noted to have recently had a urinary tract infection. She was treated with antibiotics and discharged home. A week later she was admitted to hospital with very swollen lower limbs, high blood pressure and raised central venous pressure. A diagnosis of hypertensive congestive cardiac failure was made, delayed a week because of an incomplete initial assessment in the emergency department.

A 53-year-old man with a history of stroke, MRSA infection, leg ulcers and heart failure was admitted for treatment of venous ulceration and cellulitis of both legs. Post-operatively the patient had a urinary catheter in place; incorrect management of the catheter resulted in necrosis of the tip of the penis. He underwent a supra-pubic catheterization and developed an infection. The patient's hospital stay was extended by 26 days.

(FROM VINCENT, NEALE AND WOLOSHYNOWYCH, 2001; NEALE, WOLOSHYNOWYCH AND VINCENT, 2001)

The impact and cost of adverse events

As the examples show, many patients suffer increased pain and disability from serious adverse events. They often also suffer psychological trauma and may experience failures in their treatment as a terrible betrayal of trust. Staff may experience shame, guilt and depression after making a mistake, with litigation and complaints imposing an additional burden (Vincent, 1997). These profoundly important aspects of patient safety, generally given far too little attention, are considered in Chapters 8 and 9.

The financial cost of adverse events, in terms of additional treatment and extra days in hospital, are considerable and vastly greater than the costs of litigation. One of the most consistent findings from the record reviews is that, on average, a patient suffering an adverse event stays an extra six to eight days in hospital. An extra few days in hospital is, clinically speaking, an unremarkable event and it is not necessarily particularly traumatic or unpleasant for the patient. However, when the sums are done and the findings extrapolated nationally the costs are staggering. In Britain, the cost of preventable adverse events is £1 billion per annum in lost bed days alone (Vincent, Neale and Woloshynowych, 2001). The wider costs of lost working time, disability benefits and the wider economic consequences would be greater still. The Institute of Medicine report (1999) was able to estimate that in the United States total annual national costs (lost income, lost household production, disability, healthcare costs) were between $17 billion and $29 billion for preventable adverse events and about double that for all adverse events; healthcare costs accounted for over one half of the total costs incurred. Even when using the lower estimates, the total national costs associated with adverse events and preventable adverse events represent approximately 4% and 2%, respectively of national health expenditure (Kohn, Corrigan and Donaldson, 1999).

Costs of direct hospital care, essentially additional time in hospital, have recently been estimated from the Dutch adverse events study finding that about 3% of all bed days and 1% of the total health budget could be attributed to preventable adverse events. The real overall costs are probably a good deal higher, as this estimate does not include additional treatments and investigations or any of the associated societal costs discussed above. Remember also that these estimates are confined to the hospital sector; we have no idea of the additional costs of adverse events in primary care or mental health.

Complications and adverse events in surgery

A significant percentage of adverse events are associated with a surgical procedure. For instance, in the Utah Colorado Medical Practice Study, the annual incidence rate of adverse events amongst hospitalized patients who received an operation was 3%, of which half were preventable. Some operations, such as extremity bypass graft, abdominal aortic aneurysm repair and colon resection, were at particularly high risk of preventable adverse events (Thomas *et al.*, 2000b; Thomas and Brennan, 2001).

In the United Kingdom, complication rates for some of the major operations are 20–25% with an acceptable mortality of 5–10% (Vincent *et al.*, 2004). However, at least 30–50% of major complications occurring in patients undergoing general surgical procedures are thought to be avoidable. In Canada, Wanzel *et al.* (2002) prospectively monitored the presence and documentation of complications for all 192 patients admitted over a two month period to a general surgical ward. 75 patients (39%) of the patients suffered a total of 144 complications, 2 of which were fatal, 10 life threatening and 90 of moderate severity. Almost all the complications were documented in the patient's notes but only 20% were reviewed at the weekly morbidity and mortality rounds; about one-fifth of complications were due, in part, to error. Many adverse events classified as operative are, on closer examination, found to be due to problems in ward management rather than intra-operative care. For instance Neale, Woloshynowych and Vincent (2001) identified preventable pressure sores, chest infections, falls and poor care of urethral catheters in their study of adverse events, together with a variety of problems with the administration of drugs and intravenous fluids.

Deaths from adverse events: can we believe the findings of retrospective record review?

Retrospective review of medical records, like any other research method, has its limitations and the findings of the studies have to be interpreted with due regard to the methodological limitations. Adverse events that are not recorded in the notes, or at least cannot be discerned from the notes, will not be detected and therefore record review probably provides a lower estimate of the actual scale of harm. The process of record review also necessarily relies on implicit clinical judgement, and agreement between reviewers, particularly on judgements of preventability, have often only been moderate (Neale and Woloshynowych, 2003). Great efforts have been made to strengthen the accuracy and reproducibility of these judgments by training, by the use of structured data collection, by duplicate review with re-review and by resolution of disagreements; however, even with training the reliability of such judgments is only moderate. Nevertheless, following a series of careful studies, Kieran Walshe concluded that the recognition of adverse events by record review had moderate to good face, content and construct validity with respect to quality of care in a hospital setting (Walshe, 2000).

These and other methodological issues have come to the fore in debates about the number of deaths due to adverse events, particularly after the headline capturing claims that up to 98 000 Americans were dying each year from adverse events in hospital. The methodological arguments are too complex to summarize in their entirety here, but it is important to note that the figures have been challenged, and to give a flavour of the arguments. For instance, one research team argued, following estimates of the death rates in hospital at the time of the study, that the patients who reportedly died from adverse events in the Harvard study were already severely ill and likely to die anyway (McDonald, Weiner and Hui, 2000). In a further challenge to the figures, Hayward and Hofer (2001) compared the findings with their own review of the standard of care of patients who died in hospital while having active, as opposed to palliative, care. They found that only 0.5% of patients would have lived longer than three months, even if they had all had optimal care. So, yes, there were some deaths which were perhaps preventable, but the great majority of these people were already very ill and would have died anyway.

In a reply to McDonald and colleagues, Lucian Leape (2000) noted that some people seemed to have the impression that many of the deaths that had been attributed to adverse events were minor incidents in the care of people who were severely ill and likely to die anyway. He pointed out that terminally ill patients had been excluded from the study, but agreed that there were a small group of patients (14% of deaths attributed to adverse events) who had been severely ill; for these patients the adverse event had tipped the balance. However, for the remaining 86%, the deficiencies in the care they received were a major factor leading to the death:

Examples include a cerebrovascular accident in a patient with atrial flutter who was not treated with anticoagulants, overwhelming sepsis . . . in a patient with signs of intestinal obstruction that was untreated for 24 hours, and brain damage from hypotension due to blood loss from unrecognized rupture of the spleen.
(LEAPE, 2000)

The issue of the incidence of adverse events in patients who died and their preventability has been addressed more recently in a major study in The Netherlands (Zegers *et al.,* 2009). The records of 7926 patients were reviewed across 21 hospitals: 3943 admissions of discharged patients and 3983 admissions of hospital patients who died in 2004. A large sub-sample of deceased hospital patients was included to determine the incidence of potentially preventable deaths more precisely compared to previous international studies. Of these patients, 663 experienced a total of 744 adverse events, with 10% of patients suffering two or more adverse events. For deceased patients, the incidence of adverse events was 10.7%, and a rate of 5.2% for preventable adverse events. The incidence of adverse events was significantly higher therefore than for living patients. About half of the patients with preventable adverse events had a life expectancy of more than one year; the exact contribution of the adverse event to the death is not clear but the implication is that life was shortened by some months for these people. The authors estimate that in 2004 around 1735 deaths (95%CI 1482–2032) in Dutch hospitals were potentially preventable. We should note that the terminology is slightly confusing here, in that the adverse events described here are not the death itself, but serious problems in patients' care that led to harm which in turn hastened death. We should also remember that an adverse event near the end of life should not only be assessed by the extent to which death was hastened; contracting *Clostrium difficile* or sustaining a major adverse drug reaction in one's final days may turn a potentially relatively peaceful passing into a nightmare of pain and suffering.

Hospital acquired infection

The power of the major adverse event studies is that they reveal the overall scale of harm to patients and also, to some extent, the nature and causes of harm. In the following sections we will examine two of the major types of harm, healthcare nosocomial infection and adverse drug events. We will then address a further important question of who is most vulnerable to harm.

Nosocomial infection, or healthcare associated infection (HCAI), is the commonest complication affecting hospitalized patients. In the Harvard Medical Practice Study, a single type of hospital acquired infection, surgical wound infection, was the second largest category of adverse events (Burke, 2003). Currently 5–10% of patients admitted to hospital in Britain and the United States acquire one of more infections; millions of people each year are affected. In a massive survey of over 75 000 patients in 2006, Smyth *et al.* found a prevalence rate of 7.59% in the United Kingdom (Smyth *et al.*, 2008). In the United States, 90 000 deaths a year are attributed to these infections, which add an estimated $5 billion to the costs of care. Intensive care units sustain even higher rates, approximately 30% of patients being affected, with an impact on both morbidity and mortality (Vincent, 2003).

Four types account for about 80% of nosocomial infections: urinary tract infections, often associated with catheter use; bloodstream infections, often due to intravascular devices, surgical site infection and pneumonia. Each of these four types may arise in more than one way and may be due to one or more different bacterial species. Intravenous lines are a particular potent source of infection, and the chance of infection is increased the longer the line remains in place. This is particularly disturbing as lines inserted into patients are often not being used. In one study, a third of patients in a general hospital setting had intravenous lines or catheters inserted; one-third of the lines were not in active use; 20% of the cannulas inserted were never used at all and overall 5% of the lines in use led to an unpleasant complication (Baker, Tweedale and Ellis, 2002). Not all infections are necessarily preventable by any means, with overcrowding and understaffing being important contributory factors (Clements *et al.*, 2008). However, there is a consensus that many could be avoided by interventions such as the proper use of prophylactic antibiotics before surgery and hand hygiene campaigns amongst staff. Despite many studies, and massive campaigns, there is still widespread failure to adhere to basic standards of hand hygiene and it is hugely difficult to bring about change.

Infection control has for decades been seen as a public health problem and tackled by specialist doctors and infection control nurses, rather than linked with general quality improvement work. The emergence of the patient safety movement has energized and supported infection control, leading to those involved widening their remit to monitor antibiotic use as well as infection and to associate themselves with the broader drive to make healthcare safer (Burke, 2003). Patient safety in turn may be able to learn much from the techniques of infection control, particularly in the methods of surveillance, rapid response to problems and epidemiological analyses. Infection control requires, amongst other things, careful specification of the types of infection coupled with both a rapid response to outbreaks and systematic, routine surveillance and monitoring.

Injection safety in developing countries

atient safety, in the form described in this book, has primarily developed in advanced, relatively well resourced healthcare systems. However, the safety of healthcare is of huge concern in poorer countries where infections are the leading cause of mortality. Deaths and morbidity from disease dominate, but the risks of infection from healthcare itself are terrifying. To get a sense of the scale of problems facing developing healthcare systems, we will look briefly at the question of injection safety, drawing on a comprehensive review by Yvan Hutin and colleagues (Hutin, Hauri and Armstrong, 2003). This review is one of a number of safety related programmes established by the World Health Organization, concerning such matters as the safety of blood products, chemical safety, vaccine and immunization safety, drug safety and medical device safety.

During the 20th century, injection use has increased tremendously, and injections are now probably the commonest healthcare procedure. Many injections given to provide treatment in developing countries are in fact unnecessary, as oral drug treatment would be equally or more effective. The belief in the power of injections, as opposed to pills, is one reason for the continuation of this practice. The dangers come from the reuse of syringes without sterilization, with syringes often just being rinsed in water between injections. This should not be seen as simply due to poor training or low standards; in a poor country everything is reused, simply because there is no alternative. Although lack of knowledge and poor standards play a part, the danger is hugely compounded by the basic lack of resources and the need to reuse any item of equipment if at all possible.

A huge proportion of injections are given unsafely and the numbers of people affected are staggering (Figure 4.1). In some countries in Southeast Asia, as many as 75% of injections are unsafe, leading to massive risk of hepatitis, HIV infection and other blood borne pathogens. Hutin and colleagues call for the risks of unsafe injections to be highlighted in all HIV programmes, better management of sharps waste and the increased use of single use syringes which are unusable after the first injection has been given. They suggest that donors funding programmes of drug delivery should ensure that they include the cost of these syringes, or they may do more harm than good. WHO programmes, particularly in Burkina Faso, have demonstrated that major change can be achieved.

The extent of harm to patients from healthcare systems in the developing world is largely unknown, but the potential for error and harm in fragile, underfunded systems is proportionately greater still. The poor state of infrastructure and equipment, unreliable supply and quality of drugs, shortcomings in waste management and infection control and severe underfinancing of essential operating costs make the probability of error and harm much greater

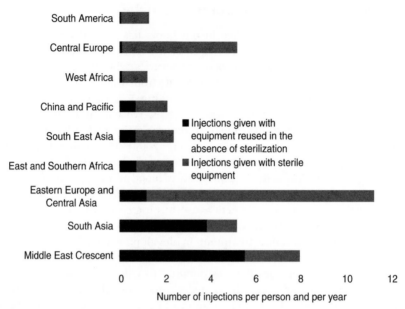

Injections Given with Sterile and Reused Equipment Worldwide

Figure 4.1 Injections given with sterile and reused equipment worldwide (Reproduced from British Medical Journal, Yvan J F Hutin, Anja M Hauri, Gregory L Armstrong. "Use of injections in healthcare settings worldwide, 2000: literature review and regional estimates". **327**, no. 7423, [1075], 2003, with permission from BMJ Publishing Group Ltd.).

than in industrialized countries. We might think that aiming for safety in healthcare is the prerogative of rich countries and advanced healthcare systems, that safety is a luxury poor people cannot afford. In fact, the reverse may be true. When you have few resources, it is all the more important that you do not cause harm or waste those resources with poor quality care. Those living in poverty with little healthcare available can least afford unsafe care.

Studies of medication errors and adverse drug events

Studies of medical error have been conducted in many areas of clinical practice encompassing, for instance, diagnostic errors, studies of autopsies, histopathology, interpretation of X-rays and other areas as well as an extensive literature on medical decision making and decision-making biases of various kinds (Leape, 1994; Croskerry, 2002). Studies of error are one way of examining the process of care and assess whether it is meeting certain specified standards. Are diagnostic X-rays being read correctly? Are drugs being prescribed and administered correctly? Studies of errors therefore have a different orientation to studies of adverse events, which are focused on the outcomes of care. The most extensively studied area, which we will use as an exemplar of error studies, is medication error.

Medication errors

Medication errors may occur at any stage of the process of prescribing, preparation of the order, and administration to the patient. Examples of the basic types of medication errors include prescribing errors, omitting to give the drug, giving the wrong drug, giving too much or too little of the drug, failing to order the drug, preparing it incorrectly and giving it by the wrong route or the wrong rate of administration. With so many small steps in the chain from prescribing to the patient receiving the drug, there is plenty of scope for error. Studies of medication error have sometimes addressed the whole sequence of medication, from prescribing to administration, but mostly focused on one particular area. Writing in 1994, Lucian Leape summarized current knowledge of medication error by stating that studies suggested that they occurred in 2–14% of patients admitted to hospital (Leape, 1994). Since then, many hospitals in the United States, and to a lesser extent elsewhere, have introduced computerized order entry systems greatly reducing the possibilities of some types of error, particularly as they often incorporate warning systems and flags of possible contraindications and allergic reactions.

Most hospitals worldwide however, are still using written orders and interpretation. Bryony Dean and colleagues examined the rate of clinically meaningful prescribing error in one British hospital still using written orders, using pharmacists to prospectively check prescription details of a sample of patients over a four-week period (Dean *et al.*, 2002). About 36 200 orders were written, 1.5% of which contained a prescribing error, a quarter of which were potentially serious. For instance, an elderly patient was prescribed 5 times the intended 10 mg dose of diazepam, when the order was written up as 10 ml (equivalent to 50 mg). These figures equated to about 150 prescribing errors per week in that hospital, and about 35 serious errors. Dean and colleagues commented that a medication order was written about every 20 seconds during the daytime, so the rate of error did not seem that high. However, annually hundreds of patients were experiencing potentially serious errors. While the annual rate of medication error in Britain is unknown, as in every other country, published findings show no sign of any reduction in medication errors over time (Vincent *et al.*, 2008).

Intravenous drug administration, requiring some technical skill and the use of equipment, offers additional hazards and possibilities for error over oral medication. Taxis and Barber (2003) observed 430 intravenous drug doses and found that almost half involved an error, either of the preparation of the drug or its administration. Some examples of more serious errors are shown in Box 4.4. Most preparation errors were associated with multiple step preparations – for example, drugs that required reconstitution with a solvent and addition of a dilutent. Typical errors were preparing the wrong dose or selecting the wrong solvent. The more complex the procedure, the more chance of error occurring, a theme we will return to in later chapters.

BOX 4.4 Examples of potentially serious intravenous drug errors

The whole content of a vial containing 125 000 international units of heparin was prepared as a continuous infusion, resulting in a 5 times overdose to a patient on a general medical ward in a teaching hospital.

Comment: Haemorrhage is one of the serious, potentially life threatening complication of an overdose of heparin.

A nurse injected 750 mg vancomycin into an infusion bag of 0.9% sodium chloride (already connected to the patient's cannula) without mixing the solution. The patient probably received a concentrated solution of vancomycin as a bolus.

Comment: Rapid infusions of vancomycin carry the risk of reactions, such as severe hypotension (including shock and cardiac arrest) and flushing of the upper body.

An intensive care patient's continuous infusion of adrenaline (epinephrine) was interrupted for about 10 minutes as the new infusion had not been prepared in advance.

Comment: This patient's blood pressure dropped to a dangerously low level. A bolus dose of adrenaline was given to stabilize him until the adrenaline infusion was restarted.

(REPRODUCED FROM BRITISH MEDICAL JOURNAL, KATJA TAXIS, NICK BARBER. "ETHNOGRAPHIC STUDY OF INCIDENCE AND SEVERITY OF INTRAVENOUS DRUG ERRORS". **326**, NO. 7391, [684], 2003, WITH PERMISSION FROM BMJ PUBLISHING GROUP LTD.)

Medication error rates are not always so high. In some settings, perhaps those with more routine use of specific drugs or those where a highly proceduralized approach is possible, rates are lower. For instance, in one study the rate of major errors in 30 000 cytotoxic preparations was only 0.19% (Limat *et al.*, 2001). This rate is impressively low, but still might equate to substantial numbers of patients being affected each year across a hospital and still more across a country.

Adverse drug events

Studies of medication errors, as we have seen, assess whether a drug was prescribed and administered correctly; there may or may not have been any actual or potential harm to the patient. Studies of adverse drug events, in contrast, focus on the harm, which may or may not have been caused by an error. For instance, if a patient suffers an allergic reaction which could not have been predicted then this is unfortunate, but not an error. If their medical record specifies the allergy and they are still given the drug, then it certainly can be classed as an error, although investigation may reveal a quite complex net of causes.

In a review of 10 studies from 4 different countries, Kanjanarat and colleagues (Kanjanarrat *et al.*, 2004) found that the median rate of ADEs in hospitalized patients was 1.8%, with about a third being judged preventable. Examples of frequent ADEs were overdoses of antihypertensive drugs leading to bradycardia or hypertension, penicillin prescribed with a known history of allergic reactions to the drug, warfarin overdoses and inadequate monitoring leading to haemorrhages and opiod overdose or underdose associated with respiratory depression and poor pain control respectively. The underuse of a drug is a slightly wider than usual definition of ADE, but there is no doubt that the erroneous underuse of a drug for pain does cause avoidable suffering.

Evidence is accumulating that many adverse drug events occur outside hospital, often then leading to hospital admission. For instance, in Boston, Tejal Gandhi and colleagues reviewed 661 outpatients on a variety of drug regimens in a careful study that involved both record review and telephone interviews with the patients over a three-month period (Gandhi *et al.*, 2003). Incredibly, almost a quarter of these people were assessed as suffering adverse drug reactions and about 6% of the patients were suffering serious reactions. Serious adverse drug reactions included bradycardia, hypotension and gastrointestinal bleeding, many of which were clearly preventable.

Other consequences were less serious, in that they did not present immediate threats to life, but were certainly serious for the patient. For instance, one patient suffered prolonged sexual dysfunction after his doctor failed to stop a selective serotonin uptake inhibitor; another had continued sleep disturbance due to taking an anti-depressant that his doctor was not aware of. Such reactions represent prolonged, avoidable suffering over many months, to say nothing of the waste of time and resources. If these findings were replicated across the United States, the cost implications would be staggering.

Many patients experiencing drug related problems outside hospital, end up in hospital because of them; treatment aimed at keeping people well has the opposite effect and puts them into hospital. In a review of 15 studies, Winterstein *et al.* (2002) found an average of 4.3% of all hospital admissions were drug related, concluding that drug related morbidity is a significant healthcare problem and that much of it is preventable. Use of the following groups of drugs is the most likely to lead to drug-related admissions: antibiotics, anticoagulants, beta-blockers, digoxin, diuretics, hypoglycaemics and non-steroidal anti-inflammatories (Howard *et al.*, 2003; Wiffen *et al.*, 2002).

Vulnerability to harm: the old and the frail

Most people in hospital are old. In Britain for instance, patients over 65, mostly with multiple long-term conditions, account for about 60% of admissions and 70% of bed days; many of these people are also physically frail and may have some degree of cognitive impairment (Oliver, 2008). Curiously, relatively little attention has been paid to patient safety in older people, although they are particularly vulnerable to healthcare error and harm (Tsilimingras, Rosen and

Berlowitz, 2003; Long, 2010). Dramatic, usually sudden deaths of younger people are the cause celebres of patient safety, being more memorable and seemingly more important, than the slow decline of an elderly person from dehydration, drug errors and neglect. My colleague, Susy Long, reviewed all the major adverse event studies to see whether the rate of adverse events for older people was different from other age groups:

In all the major adverse event studies for which it was possible to extract evidence regarding the elderly, there is incontrovertible evidence that elderly people experience more adverse events than younger people. . . . As would be expected, the elderly tend to experience more of certain types of adverse events than their younger counterparts in hospital, such as falls, hospital acquired infections and drug errors rather than complications related to invasive procedures.
(LONG, 2010)

Is this just ageism? Are older people receiving worse treatment because they are regarded as 'crumblies', bed blockers' and so on? Are societal attitudes towards older people permeating healthcare and influencing the care they receive. 'Acopia' for instance continues to be used in medical records on occasions, in preference to a proper wide ranging assessment of clinical and functional problems leading to an 'ageist therapeutic nihilism' (Oliver, 2008). This is a very complex question, as it concerns not only the attitudes of clinical staff and others, but also the provision of services, decisions about resource and so on. Health services are not sufficiently orientated towards the care of older people with multiple conditions, although they should be as the elderly are their main customers. Medicine for older people is also particularly complex and challenging, requiring an ability to juggle the treatment of multiple conditions while also considering a range of psychological, family and social issues; given this, it is odd that one of the most challenging specialties has low prestige amongst medical trainees (Gawande and Rockwood, 2006).

Although attitudes, culture and delivery of healthcare all influence the quality of care provided, older people are also vulnerable to harm for solid physiological reasons. First, they are more likely to suffer from multiple conditions, receive multiple treatments and to stay longer in hospital. A longer stay increases the risk of all the complications of hospitalization. Second, the frailty of older people means that they have a reduced physiological reserve and are more strongly affected by, say, an adverse drug event than their younger counterparts and take much longer to recover. Third, once weakened they become vulnerable to a downward spiral in which, for example, a fall weakens them, an infection sets in, followed by delirium which makes feeding difficult, in turn leading to malnutrition and increasing frailty; such a scenario once entrenched is very hard to reverse (Long, 2010).

Older people suffer from a range of geriatric syndromes ('geriatric giants') when in hospital, complicating the treatment of other underlying conditions and worsening their overall quality of life. These syndromes include delirium,

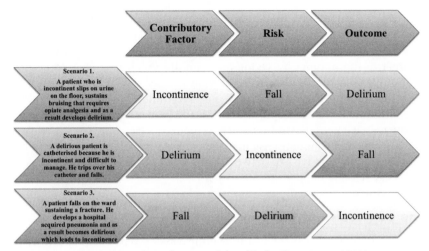

Figure 4.2 Downward spirals in the care of the elderly (from Long, 2010).

depression, pressure sores, incontinence, dehydration and malnutrition. These conditions can affect anyone, but the older people are much more vulnerable to them. These syndromes seldom occur in isolation (Figure 4.2). All too often, once the older patient has recovered sufficiently to leave hospital, the combined effect of these geriatric syndromes will have lead to (often irreversible) functional decline, loss of independence and possibly institutionalization. Conversely, active and effective management of these conditions at an early stage can produce rapid improvement on several fronts (Long, 2010).

Many acute admissions to hospital of older people are primarily caused by one of these syndromes, often overlaid on pre-existing medical conditions; however, each of the syndromes can also develop in hospital as an entirely new problem. If this occurs, the occurrence of these syndromes should be considered an adverse event, because they are largely preventable and are associated with increased morbidity and mortality (Inouye *et al.*, 1999). We will briefly consider the onset of delirium to illustrate this.

Delirium is a condition characterized by acute confusion and interference with consciousness and cognitive function. About 30% of elderly inpatients suffer with delirium during their hospital stay. Delirium may be precipitated by any one, or more often a combination, of the following: illness itself (e.g. sepsis), specific treatments of illnesses (e.g. drugs) and preventable underlying conditions such as constipation. Patients who are admitted to hospital with delirium are at risk of their delirium going unrecognized, being misdiagnosed or inadequately managed. Strategies to prevent or treat delirium take a number of forms, some addressing underlying metabolism and others being more concerned with cognitive orientation and good nursing care. A widely quoted study by Inouye *et al.* (1999) demonstrates that the incidence of delirium can be drastically reduced by careful implementation of known strategies. They targeted six known risk factors for delirium: cognitive impairment, sleep deprivation, immobility, visual impairment, hearing impairment and dehydration, with simple, but carefully monitored strategies, and drastically reduced the incidence of delirium in an elderly unit, from 15 to 9%. We might summarize the findings by saying that you are much less likely to become delirious if your care is directed to helping you see what you're doing, hear what's happening, move around, get some sleep, and have enough to drink, in an environment where people talk to you and let you know what's going on.

The management of delirium, once recognized, essentially consists of good nursing care and commonsense management. As we will see so often in this book, there is a massive gap between what everyone knows should be done and what actually happens to the patient.

The vulnerability of the very young

At the beginning of life, neonates and young babies can be as vulnerable as the very old. We cannot at present assess the real scale of harm and misadventure, but studies are appearing which suggest that the safety of neonates and young children should be of serious concern. We will briefly review three illustrative studies, which between them track the progress of very young children with serious infections such as meningitis, through the healthcare system.

Meningococcal disease remains the most common infectious cause of death in children in many developed countries. Most patients present to their nearest emergency department and many deteriorate so rapidly that death from shock and multiorgan failure often occurs before transfer to a specialist paediatric intensive care unit (PICU). The speed with which the diagnosis is made, antibiotics administered, and the associated shock and multiorgan failure treated is a major determinant of outcome (Ninis *et al.*, 2005). Nelly Ninis and colleagues compared the care given to children who died and those who survived, to see sub-optimal management played any part in reducing the chance of survival. The results showed that three factors greatly reduced the chances of survival: failure to be looked after by a paediatrician, failure of sufficient supervision of senior staff and failure of staff to administer fluids adequately and correctly. Their conclusions and reflections of the causes of these problems are highly instructive:

In children there are age related differences in normal values for blood pressure, heart rate, and respiratory rate, which were often not appreciated by medical teams. Many children had extreme increases in pulse rate and respiratory rate without apparently attracting the attention of the medical team . . . . Often this seemed to be due to their care being undertaken mainly by doctors trained to recognise serious illness in adults – emergency teams, intensive care specialists, and anaesthetists – who documented but did not seem to appreciate the importance of signs of serious illness. We found that children being looked after by doctors without paediatric training were at increased risk of dying. Lack of supervision by a consultant was also an independent risk factor for death. Unsupervised junior doctors managing sick children may lack the experience to recognise

the speed of disease progression, the need for paediatric intensive care, and the need for inotrope therapy.
(REPRODUCED FROM BRITISH MEDICAL JOURNAL, NELLY NINIS, CLAIRE PHILLIPS, LINDA BAILEY ET AL. "THE ROLE OF HEALTHCARE DELIVERY IN THE OUTCOME OF MENINGOCOC-CAL DISEASE IN CHILDREN: CASE-CONTROL STUDY OF FATAL AND NON-FATAL CASES". **330**, NO. 7506, [1475], 2005, WITH PERMISSION FROM BMJ PUBLISHING GROUP LTD.)

Serious infectious disease in young children may therefore not be recognized or, if recognized, not treated with sufficient urgency. This was confirmed more recently by David Inwald and colleagues (2009), in a study of children arriving in PICUs in a state of shock. A state of shock requires urgent and aggressive treatment with fluids and vasoactive drugs, with each hour of delay greatly increasing the risk of death. Yet, 62% of children with shock admitted to PICU had not been treated appropriately according to standard guidelines.

Once admitted to PICU, these children are of course much more likely to receive the treatment they need, but they then face other hazards recently mapped in a number of studies. In The Netherlands, Snijders and colleagues reviewed 4846 incident reports from 3859 admissions to neonatal intensive care units, the first speciality based study of locally reported incidents in these units. Medication and equipment problems dominated the reports though diagnostic issues, which are not usually well reported, were also frequent (Table 4.4). Significant patient harm was described in 70 of these reports (~2% of admissions):

Two of these incidents may have contributed to the death of a patient (a 10-fold morphine overdose in a premature, unstable patient; and dysfunctional cerebral function monitoring that delayed treatment of seizures). Another five incidents were expected to result in permanent major harm: 3-day delay in test results for congenital hypothyroid disorder, defective ventilator resulting in severe metabolic acidosis, arterial line occlusion resulting in foot necrosis, burns due to chlorhexidene, and skin necrosis after subcutaneous infusion of packed cell.
(SNIJDERS *ET AL.*, 2009)

Further confirmation of the hazards of neonatal care in particular is provided in a comprehensive study by Isabelle Ligi and colleagues in a French neonatal ICU of events which 'compromised the safety' of the patient. A form was included in the records of each baby and a physician visited the ward twice a week to capture any additional incidents not reported by staff. A total of 388 patients were studied over a total of 10 436 days, with 267 iatrogenic events being recorded in 116 patients. Nosocomial infections and respiratory events were the most serious, with cutaneous injuries and medication errors being more frequent but generally less consequential. Patients with very low birthweights were, not surprisingly, at particular risk of adverse events, as they require more invasive procedures, longer admissions and substantial physiological support. The rate of reported events is quite low, with one occurring about every 40 days for each patient. However, as the neonates stayed for about a month on average, each is likely to experience some kind

Table 4.4 Incidents in neonatal intensive care

Incident type	Description	Frequency
Mechanical ventilation lines/cannulas/ other material/equipment	Wrong settings	260
	Unplanned removal	147
	Wrong usage	92
	Loosening	79
	Subcutaneous infusion	74
	Dysfunctional machine	75
	Wrong connection	64
	Material damage	43
	Unavailable	33
	Occlusion	29
	Prolonged indwelling time	17
	Other	471
	Combination of descriptions	65
Medication/nutrition/blood products	Wrong dose	463
	Wrong infusion care	214
	Wrong time	143
	Incomplete administration	126
	Wrong concentration	105
	Wrong product	102
	Wrong route of administration	52
	Product out of date	50
	Patient misidentification	47
	Other	563
	Combination of descriptions	102
Diagnostic procedures	Exam not performed	140
	Unnecessary exam	61
	Delayed results	46
	Material not received	26
	Wrong time	21
	Wrong test requested	15
	Patient misidentification	12
	Wrong test performed	8
	Other	219
	Combination of descriptions	38
Other incident/combination of incidents		196
Total incidents with descriptions		4198

of event which compromises their safety (Ligi *et al.*, 2008). The true rate of incidents is also, as we will see in the next chapter, almost certainly much higher than the reported rate, so these young children may well face a higher level of hazard than reflected in these figures.

References

Andrews, L.B., Stocking, C., Krizek, T. *et al.* (1997) An alternative strategy for studying adverse events in medical care. *Lancet*, **349**, 309–313.

Aranaz-Andres, J.M., Aibar-Remon, C., Vitaller-Murillo, J. *et al.* and the ENEAS work group (2008) Incidence of adverse events related to healthcare in Spain: results of the Spanish National Study of Adverse Events. *Journal of Epidemiology and Community Health*, **62**(12), 1022–1029.

Baker, G.R., Norton, P.G., Flintoff, V. *et al.* (2004) The Canadian adverse events study: the incidence of adverse events among hospital patients in Canada. *Canadian Medical Association Journal*, **170**(11), 1678–1686.

Baker, N., Tweedale, C. and Ellis, C.J. (2002) Adverse events with medical devices may go unreported. *British Medical Journal*, **325**(7369), 905.

Brennan, T.A., Leape, L.L., Laird, N.M. *et al.* (1991) Incidence of adverse events and negligence in hospitalized patients. *New England Journal of Medicine*, **324**(6), 370–376.

Burke, J.P. (2003) Infection control – a problem for patient safety. *The New England Journal of Medicine*, **348**(7), 651.

Caplan, R.A., Posner, K.L. and Cheney, F.W. (1991) Effect of outcome on physicians' judgements of appropriateness of care. *Journal of the American Medical Association*, **265**, 1957–1960.

Clements, A., Halton, K., Graves, N. *et al.* (2008) Overcrowding and understaffing in modern health-care systems: key determinants in meticillin-resistant *Staphylococcus aureus* transmission. *Lancet Infectious Diseases*, **8**(7), 427–434.

Croskerry, P. (2002) Achieving quality in clinical decision making: cognitive strategies and detection of bias. *Academic Emergency Medicine*, **9**(11), 1184–1204.

Davis, P., Lay-Yee, R., Briant, R. *et al.* (2002) Adverse events in New Zealand public hospitals I: occurrence and impact. *New Zealand Medical Journal*, **115** (1167), U271.

Davis, P. (2004) Health care as a risk factor. *Canadian Medical Association Journal*, **170**(11), 1688–1689.

de Vries, E.N., Ramrattan, M.A., Smorenburg, S.M. *et al.* (2008) The incidence and nature of in-hospital adverse events: a systematic review. *Quality and Safety in Health Care*, **17**(3), 216–223.

Dean, B., Schachter, M., Vincent, C. and Barber, N. (2002) Prescribing errors in hospital inpatients: their incidence and clinical significance. *Quality and Safety in Health Care*, **11** (4), 340–344.

Gandhi, T.K., Weingart, S.N., Borus, J. *et al.* (2003) Adverse drug events in ambulatory care. *New England Journal of Medicine*, **348**(16), 1556–1564.

Gawande, A. and Rockwood, K. (2006) The way we age now. New York 30th, April.

Gawande, A., Thomas, E.J., Zinner, M.J. and Brennan, T.A. (1999) The incidence and nature of surgical adverse events in Utah and Colorado in 1992. *Surgery*, **126**(1), 66–75.

Hayward, R.A. and Hofer, T.P. (2001) Estimating hospital deaths due to medical errors. *Journal of the American Medical Association*, **286**(4), 415–420.

Howard, R.L., Avery, A.J., Howard, P.D. and Partridge, M. (2003) Investigation into the reasons for preventable drug related admissions to a medical admissions unit: observational study. *Quality and Safety in Healthcare*, **12**(4), 280–285.

Hutin, Y.J.F., Hauri, A.M. and Armstrong, G.L. (2003) Use of injections in healthcare settings worldwide, 2000: literature review and regional estimates. *British Medical Journal*, **327**(7423), 1075.

Inouye, S.K., Bogardus, S.T. Jr., Charpentier, P.A. *et al.* (1999) A multicomponent intervention to prevent delirium in hospitalized older patients. *The New England Journal of Medicine*, **340**(9), 669–676.

Inwald, D.P., Tasker, R.C., Peters, M.J. *et al.* and on behalf of the Paediatric Intensive Care Society Study Group (PICS-SG) (2009) Emergency management of children with severe sepsis in the United Kingdom: the results of the Paediatric Intensive Care Society sepsis audit. *Archives of Disease in Childhood*, **94**(5), 348–353.

Kanjanarrat, P., Winterstein, A.G., Johns, T.E. *et al.* (2004) Nature of preventable adverse drug events in hospitals: a literature review. *American Journal of Health System Pharmacy*, **60**, 1750–1759.

Kohn, L., Corrigan, J. and Donaldson, M.E. (1999) *To Err is Human*, National Academy Press, Washington DC.

Leape, L.L. (2000) Institute of Medicine medical error figures are not exaggerated. *Journal of the American Medical Association*, **284**(1), 95–97.

Leape, L.L., Brennan, T.A., Laird, N. *et al.* (1991) The nature of adverse events in hospitalized patients. Results of the Harvard Medical Practice Study II. *The New England Journal of Medicine*, **324**(6), 377–384.

Leape, L.L. (1994) Error in medicine. *Journal of the American Medical Association*, **272**(23), 1851–1857.

Ligi, I., Arnaud, F., Jouve, E. *et al.* (2008) Iatrogenic events in admitted neonates: a prospective cohort study. *The Lancet*, **371**(9610), 404–410.

Limat, S., Drouhin, J.P., Demesmay, K. *et al.* (2001) Incidence and risk factors of preparation errors in a centralized cytotoxic preparation unit. *Pharmacy World and Science*, **23**(3), 102–106.

Long, S. (2010) Adverse events in the care of the elderly (Unpublished PhD thesis).

McDonald, C.J., Weiner, M. and Hui, S.L. (2000) Deaths due to medical errors are exaggerated in Institute of Medicine report. *Journal of the American Medical Association*, **24**(1).

Michel, P., Quenon, J.L., Djihoud, A. *et al.* (2007) French national survey of inpatient adverse events prospectively assessed with ward staff. *Quality and Safety in Health Care*, **16**(5), 369–377.

Michel, P., Quenon, J.L., de Sarasqueta, A.M. and Scemama, O. (2004) Comparison of three methods for estimating rates of adverse events and rates of preventable adverse events in acute care hospitals. *British Medical Journal*, **328**(7433), 199.

Neale, G., Woloshynowych, M. and Vincent, C.A. (2001) Exploring the causes of adverse events in NHS hospital practice. *Journal of the Royal Society of Medicine*, **94**(7), 322–330.

Neale, G. and Woloshynowych, M. (2003) Retrospective case record review: a blunt instrument that needs sharpening. *Quality and Safety in Health Care*, **12**(1), 2–3.

Ninis, N., Phillips, C., Bailey, L. *et al.* (2005) The role of healthcare delivery in the outcome of meningococcal disease in children: case-control study of fatal and non-fatal cases. *British Medical Journal*, **330**(7506), 1475.

Oliver, D. (2008) 'Acopia' and 'social admission' are not diagnoses: why older people deserve better. *Journal of the Royal Society of Medicine*, **101**(4), 168–174.

Sari, A.B.-A., Sheldon, T.A., Cracknell, A. and Turnbull, A. (2007) Sensitivity of routine system for reporting patient safety incidents in an NHS hospital: retrospective patient case note review. *British Medical Journal*, **334**(7584), 79.

Schioler, T., Lipczak, H., Pedersen, B.L. *et al.* (2001) Danish adverse event study. [Incidence of adverse events in hospitals. A retrospective study of medical records]. *Ugeskr Laeger*, **163**(1), 1585–1586.

Smyth, E.T., McIlvenny, G., Enstone, J.E. *et al.* (2008) Four country healthcare associated infection prevalence survey 2006: overview of the results. *Journal of Hospital Infection*, **69**(3), 230–248.

Snijders, C., van Lingen, R.A., Klip, H. *et al.* and on behalf of the NEOSAFE study group (2009) Specialty-based, voluntary incident reporting in neonatal intensive care: description of 4846 incident reports. *Archives of Disease in Childhood – Fetal and Neonatal Edition*, **94**(3), F210–F215.

Soop, M., Fryksmark, U., Koster, M. and Haglund, B. (2009) The incidence of adverse events in Swedish hospitals: a retrospective medical record review study. *International Journal for Quality in Health Care*, **21**(4), 285–291.

Taxis, K. and Barber, N. (2003) Ethnographic study of incidence and severity of intravenous drug errors. *British Medical Journal*, **326**(7391), 684.

Thomas, E.J., Studdert, D.M., Runciman, W.B. *et al.* (2000a) A comparison of iatrogenic injury studies in Australia and the USA 1: context, methods, casemix, population, patient and hospital characteristics. *International Journal for Quality in Health Care*, **12**(5), 371–378.

Thomas, E.J., Studdert, D.M., Burstin, H.R. *et al.* (2000b) Incidence and types of adverse events and negligent care in Utah and Colorado. *Medical Care*, **38**(3), 261–271.

Thomas, E.J. and Brennan, T. (2001) Errors and adverse events in medicine: an overview, in *Clinical Risk Management. Enhancing Patient Safety*, 2nd edn (ed. C.A. Vincent), BMJ Publications, London, pp. 31–44.

Thomas, E.J. and Petersen, L.A. (2003) Measuring errors and adverse events in healthcare. *Journal of General Internal Medicine*, **18**(1), 61–67.

Tsilimingras, D., Rosen, A.K. and Berlowitz, D.R. (2003) Patient safety in geriatrics: A call for action. *Journals of Gerontology Series A – Biological Sciences and Medical Sciences*, **58**(9), 813–819.

Vincent, C., Neale, G. and Woloshynowych, M. (2001) Adverse events in British hospitals: preliminary retrospective record review. *British Medical Journal*, **322**(7285), 517–519.

Vincent, C. (2003) Understanding and responding to adverse events. *New England Journal of Medicine*, **348**(11), 1051–1056.

Vincent, C., Moorthy, K., Sarker, S.K. *et al.* (2004) Systems approaches to surgical quality and safety: from concept to measurement. *Annals of Surgery*, **239**, 475–482.

Vincent, C.A. (1997) Risk, safety and the dark side of quality. *British Medical Journal*, **314**, 1775–1776.

Vincent, C., Aylin, P., Franklin, B.D. *et al.* (2008) Is healthcare getting safer? *British Medical Journal*, **337**(nov 13), a2426.

Vincent, J.L. (2003) Nosocomial infections in adult intensive care units. *Lancet*, **361**(9374), 2068–2077.

Walshe, K. (2000) Adverse events in healthcare: issues in measurement. *Quality in Health Care*, **9**(1), 47–52.

Wanzel, K.R., Hamstra, S.J., Anastakis, D.J. *et al.* (2002) Effect of visual-spatial ability on learning of spatially-complex surgical skills. *The Lancet*, **359**(9302), 230–231.

Wiffen, P., Gill, M., Edwards, J. and Moore, A. (2002) Adverse drug reactions in hospital patients. A systematic review of the prospective and retrospective studies. Bandolier Extra. 22-11-2004.

Wilson, R.M., Runciman, W.B., Gibber, R.W. *et al.* (1995) The Quality in Australian Health Care Study. *Medical Journal of Australia*, **163**, 458–471.

Winterstein, A.G., Sauer, B.C., Hepler, C.D. and Poole, C. (2002) Preventable drug-related hospital admissions. *The Annals Of Pharmacotherapy*, **36**(7–8), 1238–1248.

Woloshynowych, M., Neale, G. and Vincent, C. (2003) Case record review of adverse events: a new approach. *Quality and Safety in Health Care*, **12**(6), 411–415.

Zegers, M., de Bruijne, M.C., Wagner, C. *et al.* (2009) Adverse events and potentially preventable deaths in Dutch hospitals: results of a retrospective patient record review study. *Quality and Safety in Health Care*, **18**(4), 297–302.

CHAPTER 5

Reporting and learning systems

Reporting: A word with many shades of meaning and associations, which range from the innocuous to the sinister. The school report, dreaded by many of us, prepared by an authority which, depending on your school days, might be benevolent, indifferent or malign. In the darker reaches of its meaning, reporting has overtones of Big Brother, treachery and betrayal. Yet, reporting is also communication; positive, informative and necessary. The reporting of events around the world in the news, the reports produced by organizations and governments to inform (or to obscure) and the simple telling of stories and recounting of events. The many types of reporting in healthcare have associations with all these meanings, which leads to much confusion and considerable suspicion of attempts to encourage reporting of errors, clinical incidents and safety issues.

Reporting in patient safety is, ideally, the communication of safety relevant information. However, patient safety reporting is often confused, or at least tainted, with other forms of reporting and there are circumstances in which different forms of reporting may simultaneously be invoked. Confused? It's hardly surprising. Reporting systems in most healthcare systems lack cohesion and integration; there is frequent duplication of function; multiple systems in operation within any one institution; and many different activities are lumped together under the general term reporting. As a first step, we will examine some of the different types of reporting as a necessary prelude to examining safety reporting systems.

Varieties of healthcare reporting systems

Every healthcare system uses reporting systems of various kinds, which have different purposes. To illustrate the principal types, we will examine reporting systems in the British National Health Service (NHS) and some of the problems of the existing abundance of poorly integrated systems. As a national system, the NHS should, in principle be able to develop a more rational system than, say, the United States with its hugely heterogeneous system of public and privately

Patient Safety, 2nd edition. By Charles Vincent. Published 2010 by Blackwell Publishing Ltd.

funded healthcare providers. However, reporting systems have mushroomed and, with the new interest in patient safety, no professional speciality or organization is complete without a reporting system (Box 5.1) The agencies listed in the table have many responsibilities and in most cases receiving reports of one kind or another is only a small part of their function. Nevertheless, for the NHS to respond, or even remember, the agencies who might require reports is, to say the least, burdensome.

BOX 5.1 Some of the authorities requiring reports in the British National Health Service

Chief medical Officer
Coroner
Counter-fraud and Security Agency
Environmental Health Agency
General Dental Council
General Medical Council
Health and Safety Executive
Health Professions Council
Health Protection Agency
Care Quality Commission
Medicines Healthcare Products Regulatory Agency
National Clinical Assessment Authority
National Patient Safety Agency
NHS Estates
NHS Information Authority
NHS Litigation Authority
Nursing and Midwifery Council
Police
Prison Health Service
Purchasing and Supply Agency
Royal Pharmaceutical Society
Royal College of Nursing
Sterilization and Embryology Authority
Strategic Health Authorities.

Investigation of serious incidents is a core function of some of the agencies, such as the Coroner or the police. Where circumstances are unusual or suspicious, perhaps criminal, the Coroner may carry out an investigation, although the depth and sophistication of the investigation of healthcare incidents is variable. Investigations may also be carried out by Health Authorities or regulatory agencies such as the Care Quality Commission. The Health and Safety Executive in the United Kingdom also acts as a regulator on safety matters, although their focus is on the safety of staff, buildings and equipment. Doctors in the United Kingdom have a duty to report any colleague, who is endangering patients, to the General Medical Council, and other professions have similar responsibilities. A small number of clinicians are indeed a danger, sometimes through recklessness or criminality, but more often because of lapsing skills, ill health or personal problems. Healthcare organizations are often slow to act on such problems, and slow to report, from loyalty to colleagues and an often misplaced confidence that 'things will sort themselves out'.

Learning and improvement may emerge from any reporting system, as an ancillary to the main function. In this book however, we are primarily concerned with systems that have learning as their principal focus. An early, and important, example is the UK Yellow Card system, which was set up in 1964 following the thalidomide tragedy, to provide a system for early detection of emerging drug safety hazards. Since the scheme was set up, over 600 000 reports of suspected adverse drug reactions have been received from patients, doctors and pharmaceutical companies, who have a legal obligation to report suspected serious side effects. The Yellow Card system has, for instance, provided the first evidence that warfarin can interact with cranberry juice by lessening its benefits and that the smoking cessation medicine Zyban can cause seizures (MHRA, 2009). Many countries operate similar systems for adverse effects of drugs, problems with medical devices, the safety of blood products and other issues.

The increasing attention paid to patient safety has led to the establishment of many new reporting and learning systems, most notably in Britain, the Reporting and Learning System (RLS) established by the National Patient Safety Agency. This has brought more co-ordination of information about safety issues and harm and wider dissemination of the lessons from serious incidents, such as deaths from spinal injections. Local risk management systems may also have a learning focus, but still primarily act as warnings of impending complaints and litigation, functions which often sit uneasily with patient safety initiatives. Before describing these systems however, we will examine reporting systems outside healthcare to see how incident reporting and analysis is approached and what lessons have been learned over the years.

Aviation, aerospace and nuclear reporting and learning systems

Safety reporting systems in healthcare have drawn their inspiration from similar systems in other industries, particularly aviation and the nuclear industry. Reporting systems in aviation are now well developed and provide important safety related feedback, although this has not always been the case. Captain Mike Holton describes the situation which led to the establishment of the British Airways safety information system (BASIS), a state of affairs which may be strangely familiar to many clinicians and managers in healthcare:

In 1989 British Airways possessed 47 four-drawer filing cabinets full of the results of past investigations. Most of this paperwork had only historic value. An army of personnel

would have been required if the files were to be comprehensively examined for trends or to produce useful analyses.
(DOH, 2000)

In the last 20 years though, there have been major advances in the way safety issues are reported and monitored. The Aviation Safety System (Box 4.2) operates internationally, linking regulatory oversight with company information systems. The system has five principal components, which combine to provide a means of detecting, analysing and acting on actual incidents and 'near misses' or other errors, along with proactive identification of issues which have the potential to pose a safety risk if left unchecked. These systems can respond very rapidly when the occasion demands (Table 5.1).

The comparisons between healthcare and aviation are often over-stated, but the experience of large-scale reporting systems in aviation have proved extremely instructive. While the content of reports in aviation and healthcare will obviously be very different, there is much common ground in respect of the

Table 5.1 Components of the aviation safety system

Component	Function and mechanism
Accident and serious incident investigations	Governed by the International Convention on International Civil Aviation (ICAO), Accident/Incident Data Reporting Programme (ADREP). ADREP includes provision for the international dissemination of investigation reports
The Mandatory Occurrence Reporting Scheme (MORS)	Provides a mechanism for notifying and reporting a range of adverse occurrences regardless of whether they result in an accident. MORS feeds into a database at national level for trend analysis and feedback to the industry.
The Confidential Human Factors Incident Reporting Programme (CHIRP)	Administered by an independent body and which provides sensitive follow-up and feedback on reports of human errors that have been rendered anonymous.
Company safety information systems	An example is British Airways' BASIS system, which record all levels of safety-related incidents. Information is shared on a peer basis within systems, and staff report with an explicit reassurance that no individual will be pursued for an honest mistake
Operational monitoring systems	Proactively monitor crew competency through regular checks and review Flight Data Recorder information from every flight. There is management/union agreement on handling of any incidents or failures detected in this way.

From *An Organization with a Memory* (DOH, 2000: p. 44)

principles of reporting and the culture, attitudes and behaviour that must be fostered if they are to be trusted and effective. Most industrial reporting systems have a broad remit in that reporting of near misses, general safety issues and anything that worries the pilots or operators is encouraged (Barach and Small, 2000). All the reporting systems give feedback in the form of regular reports on recent incidents and, crucially, actions taken to enhance safety; they may also give feedback to individuals who make reports. Near miss reporting is vital, as such incidents give warnings of potential catastrophes and enable proactive, preventative approaches to safety, while also bringing a constant reminder of the ever present dangers in industries which, by any standard, are already very safe.

As we can see from Figure 5.1, NASA is absolutely explicit that every member of staff has a responsibility to report a safety issue, but equally explicit about the responsibility of the person receiving the report to do something about it; every member of staff is empowered to go higher up the chain until they get a response. If you work in healthcare, ask yourself how this compares with your own working environment; most healthcare organizations are still a long way from the openness espoused by NASA.

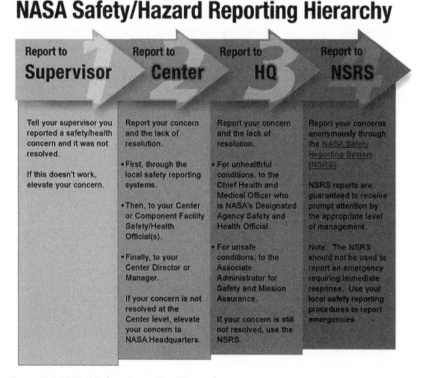

NASA Safety/Hazard Reporting Hierarchy

Report to **Supervisor**	Report to **Center**	Report to **HQ**	Report to **NSRS**
Tell your supervisor you reported a safety/health concern and it was not resolved. If this doesn't work, elevate your concern.	Report your concern and the lack of resolution. • First, through the local safety reporting systems. • Then, to your Center or Component Facility Safety/Health Official(s). • Finally, to your Center Director or Manager. If your concern is not resolved at the Center level, elevate your concern to NASA Headquarters.	Report your concern and the lack of resolution. • For unhealthful conditions, to the Chief Health and Medical Officer who is NASA's Designated Agency Safety and Health Official. • For unsafe conditions, to the Associate Administrator for Safety and Mission Assurance. If your concern is still not resolved, use the NSRS.	Report your concerns anonymously through the NASA Safety Reporting System (NSRS). NSRS reports are guaranteed to receive prompt attention by the appropriate level of management. Note: The NSRS should not be used to report an emergency requiring immediate response. Use your local safety reporting procedures to report emergencies.

Figure 5.1 NASA Safety Reporting Hierarchy.

Mandatory or voluntary?

Some of the reporting systems are mandatory, in that reporting is compulsory, but many operate on a voluntary basis. This may seem odd when the lives of so many people are at stake. Surely, people should be compelled to report incidents? Charles Billings, who designed, tested and managed the Aviation Safety Reporting System over a period of 20 years, takes the view that however you start, reporting always becomes voluntary in the end. This may be because of inertia on the part of the reporters, constraints such as shortage of time or because the staff decide that this particular incident falls outside the requirements because it is unusual in some respect or because of the fine print in the manual (Billings, 1998). This is not simply cynicism. The point is that reporting systems, whether mandatory or voluntary, only really work if the people reporting are committed to the system. If they can see it is worthwhile, they will report; if not, then there are always reasons why this or that incident does not need to be reported.

The Institute of Medicine report for instance, recommended that a nation-wide mandatory reporting system be established for adverse events that involve death or serious harm. This is intended to parallel the mandatory system for reporting serious aviation accidents, which runs alongside the voluntary reporting of incidents where no harm is done. Mandatory reporting to a regulatory body has other objectives beyond learning. Such systems demonstrate the accountability of organizations for serious incidents, offer a minimum level of protection to the public, and assurance that serious incidents are fully investigated. Most important, such bodies have the power to impose changes across healthcare organizations where necessary.

Confidentiality and anonymity

Confidentiality is common to all aviation and other industrial reporting systems and some care is taken, even in systems run by regulators, to separate reporting systems from disciplinary and performance management functions (Barach and Small, 2000). Very few of the systems offer anonymous reporting though, which would seem to be an easy way of ensuring confidentiality. Why is this? Professionalism and accountability play a part. A professional ethic demands that pilots report safety critical issues, not only because they are obliged to but because it is seen as important and a core professional responsibility; seen from this perspective, anonymity is not required, though the reports may be anonymized once the full story has been elicited. Anonymity of the reporter in any case carries a major disadvantage, which is that those running the system cannot go back for further information to clarify the story. Almost all systems encourage the reporting of a narrative, a story of what happened. Reporting that is restricted to basic factual details, as is often the case in healthcare, is not that useful, as it reveals little about the causes of the incident. The narrative, the pilot's reflections and the subsequent review by an expert, often a retired pilot, bring a richness to reporting data that is its real value.

Counting, classification and getting the story

In healthcare, many risk managers submit monthly reports of numbers of incidents to various committees, clinicians and managers. Billings suggests (Box 5.2) that this, by itself, is largely a waste of time, because reporting systems never capture the actual rate of incidents on the ground and it is as well to understand that from the start. The monthly graphs of incident counts produced by healthcare risk managers are largely uninformative, except as an index of the willingness of staff to report. Does that mean reporting is of no value? Not at all. It has a difference purpose, which is to alert people to the existence of a problem.

BOX 5.2 Understanding incident reports: lessons from aviation

Counting incident reports is a waste of time. Why? Because incident reporting is inherently voluntary. Because the population from which the sample is drawn is unknown and therefore cannot be characterized, and because you lose too much information and gain too little in the process of condensing and indexing these reports unless you do what we were fortunate enough to do blindly, and that is to keep all the narratives.

Incident reports are unique and not easily classified or pigeonholed. Generalizations may be possible in retrospect, given enough detailed data and enough understanding of data. But this requires understanding the details of the task, the context, the environment and its constraints, which can only be appreciated by those with relevant expertise. This is why you have to have experts looking at the reports. Simply constructing taxonomies is grossly insufficient.

Too many people have thought that incident reporting was the core and primary component of what was needed. These people thought that simply from the act of collecting incidents, solutions and fixes would be generated *sui generis* and that this would enhance safety. Although much is unclear about incident reporting systems, this one fact is quite clear: incident reporting is only one component of what you need.

Much effort is also devoted in healthcare to defining the incidents that should be reported and devising classification systems to capture them. Such classifications can be useful in providing broad brush descriptions of the major types of incidents. However, Billings cautions us that the real meaning of the incidents is apparent only in the narrative and will never be captured by classification alone. To make real sense of an incident, you must have the story and, furthermore, the story must be interpreted by someone who knows the work and knows the context. The implication of this is that if healthcare incident reports are to be of real value, they need to be reviewed by clinicians and, ideally, also by people who can tease out the human factors and organizational issues. One of the main problems that healthcare faces is that the number of reported incidents is so vast in mature systems that only a minority of incidents can be reviewed by those with relevant expertise.

Reporting systems in healthcare

Reporting systems operate at different levels within the healthcare system. Some systems are generic, in that they accept incidents of all types, while others are speciality specific. Some operate primarily at local level (risk management systems in hospitals), others at regional or national level. Sophisticated systems have also been established to investigate and understand a variety of specific issues, such as transfusion problems or safety in intensive care. The nature and purpose of these systems can only be fully understood by appreciating what level they operate on, who the audience is and how feedback and action are managed. In many cases, little thought is given to this so that national systems are dealing with issues that are best addressed locally and vice versa, resulting in huge frustration and duplication of effort. We will review some reporting systems to illustrate how the different kinds of systems operate and what their respective purposes are, and consider the issue of feedback in more detail later in the chapter.

Local reporting systems

The development of risk management in the United States, Europe and elsewhere led to the establishment of local incident reporting systems in hospitals. Typically there is a standard incident form, asking for basic clinical details and a brief narrative describing the incident. Staff are asked to report any incident which concerns them or might endanger a patient; in practice, serious incidents are followed by an urgent telephone call to the risk manager. In more sophisticated systems where staff within a unit may routinely monitor a designated list of incidents, staff are free to report other issues that do not fall into these categories (Table 5.2). Notice that the incidents to be reported are not necessarily errors; harm to the patient may be unavoidable or have natural causes (e.g. very low birthweight). All incidents however, are 'flags' of possible problems and vehicles for reflection on clinical practice.

Local systems are ideally used as part of an overall safety and quality improvement strategy but in practice may be dominated by managing claims and complaints. Early warning of potential claims through incident reporting allows healthcare organizations to investigate the problem rapidly, collect witness statements whilst recollection is fresh, secure the relevant medical records and reduce legal costs. Risk managers, at least the more proactive ones, also play a key role in communicating with injured patients, attending to their needs and maintaining a relationship with them at a time when they may, understandably, be distressed and angry. Incident reports also allow the organization to manage any subsequent media coverage in a proactive manner instead of being caught on the back foot. Many hospitals operate a claims and

Table 5.2 Examples of designated clinical incidents to be reported

Obstetrics	Mental health
Neonatal deaths and stillbirths	Overdose taken by inpatient on unit or while on leave
Apgar score < 4 at 5 min	Deliberate self-harm by patient
Subdural haematoma	Discovery of an object in patient's possession that could be used for self-harm
Unanticipated admission to Special Care Baby Unit	Discharge against medical advice by a patient not detoxing from alcohol or drugs
Major abnormality first detected at birth	Absconding from unit
Fracture or paralysis	Fire-setting in unit
Shoulder dystocia	Unexpected or sudden death of patient
Meconium aspiration	Serious physical assault or aggression
Maternal deaths	Discovery of illicit drugs/alcohol on unit
Transfer to intensive care	Injury of unknown origin
Convulsions	Drug error
Major anaesthetic problems	
Postpartum Haemorrhage > 1 litre	
30 min delay in Caesarean section	
Soft tissue injury, third-degree tear	
Ruptured uterus, bladder injury	
Drug errors	

incidents review committee, ideally led by the medical director or other board-level figure, which monitors litigation and also has the authority to institute changes in clinical practice where necessary. There is, however, sometimes a conflict between the risk management function and the broader patient safety function; responding to crises and major incidents can absorb all staff time so that little attention is given to longer-term programmes that might prevent the incidents in the first place.

Specialty reporting systems

Many different clinical specialities, particularly anaesthesia, have established reporting systems to assist them in improving clinical practice. These systems are designed to provide information on specific clinical issues which can be shared within the professional group. As an example, we will look at the Johns Hopkins Intensive Care Reporting System (ICU-SRS, Wu, Pronovost and Morlock, 2002) in the United States.

ICU-SRS is a Web-based safety reporting system which incorporates a framework of contributory factors developed for the analysis of clinical incidents. The Web-based form elicits a narrative description of the incident, contextual information about the patient and staff, factors that contribute to incidents and measures that might be taken to prevent similar incidents in the future. Staff use check boxes to describe information relating to the incident, such as patient demographics, location of the incident, degree of harm, and system factors that may have contributed to or prevented the incident, or mitigated the resulting harm. ICU-SRS is seen as a complement to other measurement and surveillance systems and as only one component of ICU safety and quality monitoring. Several methods of feedback are included to encourage staff to report, learn from mistakes and implement safety improvement efforts. Study teams and front line staff learn about the types of incidents that are occurring in ICUs and recommendations for improving safety through the case discussions, one-page case bulletin board summary, and the quarterly newsletter. In the first year of operation, ICU-SRS received 854 reports from the 30 participating units. Most incidents did not lead to harm, although 21% led to physical injury, and 14% were anticipated to increase length of stay. The analysis focused on understanding system factors:

In the first year of reporting we have found that training and education is a major factor contributing to incidents. Included under this category are knowledge, skills, supervision, seeking help, and failure to follow established protocol. The latter factor was most often checked because the provider was too inexperienced to know about the protocol. Team factors also contributed to incidents, particularly written and verbal communication among team members as well as the structure of a well-working team.

(REPRINTED FROM *JOURNAL OF THE AMERICAN MEDICAL INFORMATICS ASSOCIATION*, CHRISTINE G. HOLZMUELLER, PETER J. PRONOVOST, FERN DICKMAN, DAVID A. THOMPSON, ALBERT W. WU, LISA H. LUBOMSKI, MAUREEN FAHEY, DONALD M. STEINWACHS, LILLY ENGINEER, ALI JAFFREY, LAURA L. MORLOCK AND TODD DORMAN. "CREATING THE WEB-BASED INTENSIVE CARE UNIT SAFETY REPORTING SYSTEM". **12**, NO.2, [130–139], 2005, WITH PERMISSION FROM ELSEVIER)

The issues revealed by the analysis provided the basis for further investigations of the underlying problems and methods to address them. For instance, the units are now experimenting with a 'check back' system in which important messages are repeated back to ensure correct communication; this simple, resource neutral solution is proving very effective. Feedback from single incidents consists of powerful stories acting as a constant reminder of critical issues

National and other large-scale systems

National and other large-scale systems are expensive to run and have the disadvantage of being primarily reliant on the written reports, perhaps supplemented by telephone checking. On the positive side their sheer scale gives a wealth of data, and their particular power is in picking up events that may be rare at a local level, with patterns of incident only appearing at national level. The British National Patient Safety Agency's Reporting and Learning System is as yet the only truly national system, but the Veterans Affairs system in the United States is very wide ranging as is the Australian AIMS system, the grandfather of all large-scale systems in healthcare.

Australian incident monitoring system (AIMS)

The pioneer of large-scale reporting systems in healthcare is undoubtedly Bill Runciman, who founded the AIMS, which has been implemented in several Australian states (Runciman, 2002). AIMS provides a mechanism for reporting healthcare incidents of any kind using a single, standard form, either paper or Web-based. A classification has been established which allows information from various sources (such as coroners' recommendations, complaints, claims and incident reports) to be entered into the system (Runciman *et al.*, 2006). There are prompting questions on the type of incidents and the possible contributory factors they might consider. Management action taken on the incident is also recorded, though this is not a requirement of the report. AIMS has led to an impressive number of publications, well over 100 in peer-reviewed academic and medical journals, with a steady stream of new results and warnings about safety issues.

BOX 5.3 Examples of lessons learnt from AIMS

- Development of national standards and guidelines governing aspects of clinical practice, including equipment use and further monitoring of specific issues;
- Use of reported incident data to clarify and support problems identified with clinical equipment, leading to recall and modification of affected devices;
- Newsletters, publications and advice at national level, feedback of improvement actions and evidence of action occurs at local level;
- Increased consistency and identification of incident reporting and investigation, including prioritization and prevention of adverse events and near misses;
- Increased knowledge of the epidemiology of drug errors in anaesthesia and a greater understanding of the factors that can minimize errors.

(TAKEN FROM ABEYSEKERA *ET AL.*, 2005; BECKMANN *ET AL.*, 1996; RUNCIMAN, 1993, 2002; YONG AND KLUGER, 2003)

Bill Runciman has reflected thoughtfully about the value of large-scale systems, understanding that size does not necessarily equate to value; analysing incident reports from 100 000 falls for instance, probably gives much the same information as analysing 100 reports. However, Runciman makes the important point that many serious incidents do not occur sufficiently frequently at local level to give any sense of their overall importance or to permit meaningful analysis at local level. In addition, many important issues have not been recorded in the academic literature and reside only in these large systems (Runciman, 2002).

The UK national patient safety agency reporting and learning system

The United Kingdom launched the first truly national RLS in 2004. Incidents collected in local risk management systems are forwarded to the RLS and analyses of different types of incidents undertaken, alongside a variety of other national initiatives. Almost all NHS organizations report incidents, indeed are required to by the regulator, but 25 (6%) of the relevant organizations were still not reporting any incidents by 2009; it is not clear whether this is due to inefficiency, objections to the national system or wholesale denial of safety problems. Patients are able to report directly to the national system, although little information is available on how many incidents are reported by this route; the issue of patient reporting is discussed further in Chapter 15.

The technical and analytic challenges of such a system are considerable, as it deals with simply staggering numbers of incidents. Between 1 October 2008 and 31 December 2008, 268 997 incidents were reported in England, suggesting that over a million incidents are likely to be collected in 2009. By early 2009, the database contained over 3 million incidents in total, most of which, of necessity, have not been subject to any formal analysis.

As with AIMS, the power of such a system lies in the possibility of examining comparatively rare incidents and integrating them with other sources of data to provide a more complete picture of a problem (Scobie *et al.*, 2006). For instance, the NPSA identified a number of hazards associated with patients with tracheotomies transferred from an intensive care unit to a general ward. They identified 36 cases from their own system. From other sources they discovered that there had been 45 cases of litigation involving tracheotomy in the preceding 10 years, including seven deaths, all in the context of rising rates of tracheotomy generally and a worrying trend for these patients to be cared for outside surgical and anaesthetic specialties. Information about this issue was fed back to the NHS via the NPSAs *Patient Safety Bulletin* in July 2005. This is a good example of a national system integrating information that would have gone unnoticed at a local level.

Do healthcare reporting systems reflect the underlying rate of incidents?

Reporting systems in healthcare were established in response to the scale of harm revealed by case record review studies. The studies had shown the underlying problem; reporting systems were meant to provide information about adverse events on an ongoing basis. Do reporting systems actually capture adverse events successfully? A number of studies have now examined this issue, coming to broadly similar conclusions (Stanhope *et al.*, 1999; Sari *et al.*, 2007; Blais *et al.*, 2008). As an example, we will consider the study by Sari *et al.*, who carried out a classical case record review and compared the findings with locally reported incidents. They examined both incidents and adverse events, essentially potential and actual harm and concluded:

We found that 23% of hospital admissions in eight specialties were associated with patient safety incidents and 11% with adverse events. This is similar to rates found in studies using similar methods in the United Kingdom and internationally. The routine reporting system as implemented in this large hospital missed most patient safety incidents that were identified by case note review and detected only 5% of those incidents that resulted in patient harm. This suggests that the routine reporting system considerably under-reports the scale and severity of patient safety incidents.

(REPRODUCED FROM BRITISH MEDICAL JOURNAL, ALI BABA-AKBARI SARI, TREVOR A SHELDON, ALISON CRACKNELL ET AL. "SENSITIVITY OF ROUTINE SYSTEM FOR REPORTING PATIENT SAFETY INCIDENTS IN AN NHS HOSPITAL: RETROSPECTIVE PATIENT CASE NOTE REVIEW". **334**, NO. 7584, [79], 2007, WITH PERMISSION FROM BMJ PUBLISHING GROUP LTD.)

Their conclusion is cautiously expressed, no doubt because of the large investment in reporting systems in the United Kingdom. However, it is clear from this and other studies that incident reporting systems are very poor at detecting adverse events (Vincent, 2007). As a measure of harm, voluntary reporting systems are useless, detecting only 1 in 20 adverse events in Sari's study. Other studies have reported slightly better findings, but most studies have found that reporting systems only detect 7–15% of adverse events (Blais *et al.*, 2008). The most optimistic finding of adverse event detection was carried out by my colleague, Nicola Stanhope, who examined the reliability of adverse incident reporting systems in two obstetric units, which each had dedicated risk managers who were also trained midwives (Stanhope *et al.*, 1999). A retrospective review of the obstetric notes, 500 deliveries in all, identified 196 incidents. Staff had reported 23% of these and the risk managers identified a further 22% by carrying out their own additional investigations. A figure of 23% is probably an absolute ceiling, and would require a dedicated risk manager in every hospital unit constantly reminding staff of the need to report. Definitely not practical on a large scale.

Using multiple information systems

At a local level there is a great deal of confusion about the relationship between errors, adverse events and incidents that are reported. Risk managers, knowing that about 10% of patients admitted to hospital suffer adverse events, sometimes assess the success of their reporting systems on the basis of whether the number of reports they have equates to 10% of admissions. If it does, so the logic goes, they are capturing all the relevant incidents. This approach is seriously misguided. All adverse events by definition involve patient harm or additional time in hospital; in contrast, most reported incidents do not involve harm, but concern more general safety issues such as equipment problems. Some incidents will also be adverse events, but most will not. To compound the problem, the extent and nature of what is reported varies widely however, according to the incidents in question, the nature of the reporting system, the culture of the institution, how easy it is to report, the incentives or disincentives and other factors.

In practice risk management departments have multiple sources of data which potentially shed light on adverse events, with claims and major complaints tending to get the most attention. especially if an inquest is involved. Helen Hogan and colleagues examined 6 different sources of data routinely collected in a hospital, and also reviewed a sample of 220 case records, finding 40 (18.8%) adverse events (Hogan *et al.*, 2008). Extrapolating over a year, case record review of all admissions would have yielded about 8700 incidents, of which 4900 would have been adverse events. During the same period, 484 incidents were reported, 462 incidents could be detected from administrative data using standard codes, there were 221 complaints, 176 health and safety incidents, 21 inquests and 10 claims. As before, systematic record review reveals many more incidents and adverse events than any other source. Most importantly, there was very little overlap between these different data sources; the great majority of incidents only emerged from one source, showing that hospitals need to find ways of integrating these various sources of data if risks and hazards are to be effectively prioritized (Olsen *et al.*, 2007).

Barriers to reporting

As we have seen, errors, adverse events and incidents of all kinds are common, but reporting rates are low. Why is this? Admittedly it may not be necessary to report all incidents, or even the majority of them, but a higher flow of information on safety issues would undoubtedly assist the identification of potential problems. In an early study, Nicola Stanhope and colleagues (Stanhope *et al.*, 1999) examined this question in a survey of obstetricians and midwives. Even with a list of designated incidents, staff made their own assessments about whether to report; incidents might not be reported because the staff judged that the event was not preventable, that practice was of a good standard, or because there was no possibility of a complaint or claim, none of which are valid reasons for not reporting.

BOX 5.4 Reasons for not reporting incidents

- I do not know how to report incidents.
- I do not know which incidents should be reported.
- The circumstances or outcome of the case often make reporting unnecessary.
- It increases workload.
- Junior staff are often unfairly blamed for adverse incidents.
- When the ward is busy, I forget to make a report.
- I am worried about litigation.
- My colleagues may be unsupportive.

- As long as staff learn from incidents, it is unnecessary to discuss them further.
- I am worried about disciplinary action.
- I do not want the case discussed in meetings.
- I don't know whose responsibility it is to make a report.
- Incident reporting makes little contribution to the quality of care.

(*CLINICAL RISK*, FIRTH COZENS, REDFERN & MOSS. "CONFRONTING ERRORS IN PATIENT CARE". **10**:184–190, 1994. REPRODUCED WITH PERMISSION OF THE ROYAL SOCIETY OF MEDICINE PRESS)

BOX 5.5 Encouraging incident reporting and learning

- Systems and mechanisms to make error-reporting easy and fast;
- Clarifying the meaning of reportable error and incidents;
- Time for multidisciplinary discussion of individual and accumulated error;
- Feedback to individuals and the reporting community;
- A working assumption that those who report should be thanked, rather than automatically blamed if something has gone wrong;
- Providing support and understanding for those who have made errors;
- Treating error and incidents consistently across organizations and professional groups;
- Appropriate discretion in terms of nursing procedures and policy;
- Providing training for clinicians on the management of risk and safety;
- Having 'shop floor' staff on safety policy committees;
- Ensuring reporting is followed by appropriate action.

(*CLINICAL RISK*, FIRTH COZENS, REDFERN & MOSS. "CONFRONTING ERRORS IN PATIENT CARE". **10**:184–190, 1994. REPRODUCED WITH PERMISSION OF THE ROYAL SOCIETY OF MEDICINE PRESS)

Many of the reasons for not reporting are grounded in fear and guilt: fear of embarrassment, punishment by oneself or others, and fear of litigation (Leape, 1999; Robinson *et al.*, 2002). Junior staff feel these problems particularly acutely and it is clear that if incident reporting is going to be effective, whether at local or national level, considerable effort must be expended in reassuring staff that the purpose is enhancing safety, not blame or discipline. Other studies have found a variety of other barriers to reporting; a lack of feedback, and a belief that nothing will be done in response to reporting are major concerns (Firth-Cozens, 2002):

These things go on for months and months before anything is done ... This creates a feeling of apathy, that there is no point in filling in a needle-stick injury form, or a blood splash form.

I've worked in three different ITUs and this (confusion of different dose infusion pumps) has happened in all three ... I've suggested several times that they shouldn't be stored right next to each other but they're still stored together. And the error still happens.

(*CLINICAL RISK*, FIRTH COZENS, REDFERN & MOSS. "CONFRONTING ERRORS IN PATIENT CARE". **10**:184–190, 1994. REPRODUCED WITH PERMISSION OF THE ROYAL SOCIETY OF MEDICINE PRESS)

An observation common to almost all studies examining incident reporting is that doctors report only a fraction of the incidents reported by nurses. Most of the reasons for not reporting, already discussed, would seem to apply equally to all professions, so presumably other factors are at work. Smith *et al.* (2006) carried out 130 hours of observation of anaesthetic practice, observing 109 minor events; none threatened the patient directly, but some were direct violations of anaesthetic practice. None, however, were reported.

During the same period, 28 incidents were discussed at departmental meetings, five of which were viewed by the anaesthetic community as 'critical incidents' and, as such, needing discussion and presenting opportunities for learning and a reminder of hazards. Only 1 of the 28 were reported in the hospital information system, even though all anaesthetists seemed to be aware of the official definition of an incident provided by their own professional association as being one which 'could have led to harm'. The critical incidents, many of which certainly met the criteria for formal reporting, included:

- Tracheal tube severed by surgeon's osteotome during maxillary osteotomy;
- Diabetic patient brought to theatre with insulin infusion running but no dextrose;
- Postoperative fits in epileptic patient who had received propofol and alfentanil for general anaesthesia;
- Leaking thiopental syringe during rapid sequence induction for emergency Caesarian section – leak in pre-prepared syringe made up in pharmacy department.

  Smith and colleagues comment:

We interpret this as support for our notion that expertise in anaesthesia brings with it the authority to define the boundaries between routine and critical but also between acceptable and unacceptable practice. However, we suggest that such variability in what is considered critical, reportable and acceptable is a product of the culture of medicine. In other safety-critical industries, professional experience and judgement are not allowed to dictate reporting behaviour. In aviation, for instance, all pilots, regardless of rank or experience, are expected and required to describe and report even the most subtle and minor events, not just those deemed critical or serious by individual pilots.

(REPRINTED WITH PERMISSION FROM *BRITISH JOURNAL OF ANAESTHESIA*, A. F. SMITH, ET. AL. "ADVERSE EVENTS IN ANAESTHETIC PRACTICE: QUALITATIVE STUDY OF DEFINITION, DISCUSSION AND REPORTING". [715–721], 2006, OXFORD UNIVERSITY PRESS)

Feedback and action

Charles Billings presciently warned us that too many people thought that simply setting up an incident reporting system would magically lead to solutions to safety problems. When reporting systems were first established, all the effort went into acquiring the information; even now very little effort is devoted to analysis and even less to acting on the information. With the wisdom of hindsight I now believe that we addressed the reporting issue from the wrong end; rather than worrying about how to acquire data we should have first thought about what we would do with it when we got it. When I am now asked about setting up reporting systems, my first response is to ask how the information will be fed back and how action will be taken if a system is established.

We have already seen some examples of successful action and feedback in this chapter, in the form of responses to staff, safety improvement and publication and dissemination by various means. However, with the help of research carried out by my colleague Jonathan Benn and others (Benn *et al.*, 2009), we can go further and actually map the feedback networks. This research involved interviews with experts on reporting systems from a wide range of industries, including healthcare, and a very comprehensive literature review. It was clear that timely and effective feedback was critical to the success and utility of any system and, furthermore, that lack of feedback was one of the prime reasons for staff disillusionment with reporting. We should note, however, a critical difference between healthcare and most other industries, which is that other industries tend to receive hundreds of reports a year, even at a national level. In contrast, a single healthcare organization can be receiving thousands of reports, which severely limits the possibility of feedback to individuals.

Feedback and action can happen at multiple levels in an organization and different time points, and with a different purpose (Table 5.3 and Figure 5.2). The bounce back and rapid response ensures that staff remain engaged and understand that their reports are being taken seriously. However, it is impossible to analyse all reports in detail and for common incidents is largely pointless; better to analyse a small number of reports in depth than carry out a cursory analysis of a large number, which often produces little more than a few bar charts. Once analysis has been carried out though, there are various ways in which action can be taken. Some issues are only of concern in a particular unit, faulty equipment for instance or a system of handover within that unit. Others need action across an organization if, for instance, staffing levels are shown to be inadequate. Feedback that is restricted to a local system or speciality is attractive because it can be rapid and because it is being shared within a community of experts who understand the significance of the incident and the lessons it conveys. However, some safety issues, such as the design of equipment or drug packaging, cannot easily be addressed by any single organization and need action at a regional or national level.

All these routes are encapsulated in the diagram which, amongst other things, shows that a reporting system is not quite the simple, cost effective safety system it might seem. Properly construed, a reporting system should be seen as a 'reporting, analysis, learning, feedback and action' system. It is probably fair to say that few healthcare systems have achieved this on any level, but mapping the process in this way offers the chance of thinking about the entire system from the beginning and planning a rational strategy. This does

Table 5.3 Types of feedback

Mode	Type	Content and Examples
A: Bounce back	Information to reporter	• Acknowledge report filed (e.g. automated response) • Debrief reporter (e.g. telephone debriefing) • Provide advice from safety experts (feedback on issue type) • Outline issue process (and decision to escalate)
B: Rapid response	Action within local work systems	• Measures taken against immediate threats to safety or serious issues that have been marked for fast-tracking • Temporary fixes/workarounds until in-depth investigation process can complete (withdraw equipment; monitor procedure; alert staff)
C: Raise risk awareness	Information to all front line personnel	• Safety awareness publications (posted/on-line bulletins and alerts on specific issues; periodic newsletters with example cases and summary statistics) • Highlight vulnerabilities and promote correct procedures
D: Inform staff of actions taken	Information to reporter and wider reporting community	• Report back to reporter on issue progress and actions resulting from their report • Widely publicize corrective actions taken to resolve safety issue to encourage reporting (e.g. using visible leadership support)
E: Improve work systems safety	Action within local work systems	• Specific actions and implementation plans for permanent improvements to work systems to address contributory factors evident within reported incidents. • Changes to tools/equipment/working environment, standard working procedures, training programmes, and so on • Evaluate/monitor effectiveness of solutions and iterate.

Reproduced from Quality & Safety in Health Care, J Benn, M Koutantji, L Wallace et al. "Feedback from incident reporting: information and action to improve patient safety". **18**, no. 1, [11–21], 2009, with permission from BMJ Publishing Group Ltd.

not, I would emphasize, necessarily mean setting up some vast and complicated system. The lesson is to give equal weight to the different components at whatever level you are working; at the moment, in contrast, almost all healthcare reporting systems expend the majority of their effort on collection to the detriment of all the other aspects.

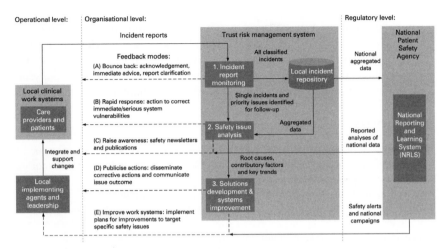

Figure 5.2 Framework for Safety Action and Information Feedback from Incident Reporting (SAIFIR) (Reproduced from Quality & Safety in Health Care, J Benn, M Koutantji, L Wallace et al. "Feedback from incident reporting: information and action to improve patient safety". **18**, no. 1, [11–21], 2009, with permission from BMJ Publishing Group Ltd.).

Reporting, surveillance and beyond

Reporting, whether voluntary or mandatory, is an attractive option because it is a relatively inexpensive method of detection. Nevertheless, as a data source it is unreliable, erratic and could never qualify as a measure of errors or adverse events, however defined. Reflecting on the enthusiasm for reporting, and the vast amounts of money poured into it (Vincent, 2007), it is hard to see why reporting systems were given such a dominant role in the drive to improve patient safety. In no other area of medicine could voluntary reporting ever be regarded as a substitute for systematic data collection. One reason is that it seemed as if aviation and other industries were using reporting to establish rates of serious incidents. In fact, aviation had already established the epidemiology of harm, in the form of comprehensive accident databases; reporting was always a supplement to systematic data collection, a complementary activity providing warnings and additional safety information.

Reporting will always be important, but has been overemphasized as a means of enhancing safety. The fact that only a small proportion of incidents are reported is not, in my view, critically important. As long as the system receives sufficient reports to identify the main safety issues, the absolute number of reports is not critical. Reporting systems also serve an important function in raising awareness and generating a culture of safety as well as providing data. However, the results of reporting are often misunderstood in that they are mistakenly held to be a true reflection of the underlying rate of errors and adverse events. In the future we should see information on error and harm collected from a wider range of sources, and hopefully move towards active surveillance of salient events. Incident reporting is crucial, but is only one component of the whole safety process. Incident reports in themselves are primarily flags and warnings of a problem area, but then they must be analysed and understood, which are the subject of two later chapters.

References

Abeysekera, A., Bergman, I.J., Kluger, M.T. and Short, T.G. (2005) Drug error in anaesthetic practice: a review of 896 reports from the Australian Incident Monitoring Study database. *Anaesthesia*, **60**(3), 220–227.

Barach, P. and Small, S.D. (2000) Reporting and preventing mdeical mishaps: lessons from non-medical near miss reporting systems. *British Medical Journal*, **320**, 759–763.

Beckmann, U., West, L.F., Groombridge, G.J. *et al.* (1996) The Australian Incident Monitoring Study in Intensive Care: AIMS-ICU. The development and evaluation of an incident reporting system in intensive care. *Anaesthesia and Intensive Care*, **24**(3), 314–319.

Benn, J., Koutantji, M., Wallace, L. *et al.* (2009) Feedback from incident reporting: information and action to improve patient safety. *Quality and Safety in Health Care*, **18** (1),11–21.

Billings, C. (1998) Incident reporting systems in medicine and experience with the aviation reporting system, in *A Tale of Two Stories: Contrasting Views of Patient Safety* (eds R.I. Cook, D.D. Woods and C.A. Miller), US National Patient Safety Foundation, pp. 52–61.

Blais, R., Bruno, D., Bartlett, G.and Tamblyn, R. (2008) Can we use incident reports to detect hospital adverse events? *Journal of Patient Safety*, **4**(1), 9–12.

Department of Health (2000) *An Organisation with a Memory: Learning from Adverse Events in the NHS*, The Stationery Office, London.

Firth-Cozens, J. (2002) Barriers to incident reporting. *Quality and Safety in Health Care*, **11** (1),7.

Firth-Cozens, J., Redfern, N. and Moss, F. (2004) Confronting errors in patient care: the experiences of doctors and nurses. *Clinical Risk*, **10**, 184–190.

Hogan, H., Olsen, S., Scobie, S. *et al.* (2008) What can we learn about patient safety from information sources within an acute hospital: a step on the ladder of integrated risk management? *Quality and Safety in Health Care*, **17**(3), 209–215.

Holzmueller, C.G., Pronovost, P.J., Dickman, F. *et al.* (2005) Creating the web-based intensive care unit safety reporting system. *Journal of the American Medical Informatics Association*, **12**(2), 130–139.

Leape, L.L. (1999) Why should we report adverse incidents? *Journal of Evaluation in Clinical Practice*, **5**(1), 1–4.

Medicines and Healthcare Products Regulatory Agency (2009) *Yellow Card Scheme First Anniversary for Patient Reporting – Reports from the Public Up 50%*, Medicines and Healthcare Products Regulatory Agency, London.

Olsen, S., Neale, G., Schwab, K. *et al.* (2007) Hospital staff should use more than one method to detect adverse events and potential adverse events: incident reporting, pharmacist surveillance and local real-time record review may all have a place. *Quality and Safety in Health Care*, **16**(1), 40–44.

Robinson, A.R., Hohmann, K.B., RIfkin, J.I. *et al.* (2002) Physician and public opinions on quality of healthcare and the problem of medical errors. *Archives of Internal Medicine*, **162**(19), 2186–2190.

Runciman, W.B., Webb, R.K., Lee, R. and Holland, R., (1993) System failures: an analysis of 2000 incident reports. *Anaesthesia and Intensive Care*, **21**, 684–695.

Runciman, W.B. (2002) Lessons from the Australian Patient Safety Foundation: setting up a national patient safety surveillance system – is this the right model? *Quality and Safety in Health Care*, **11**(3), 246–251.

Runciman, W.B., Williamson, J.A.H., Deakin, A. *et al.* (2006) An integrated framework for safety, quality and risk management: an information and incident management system based on a universal patient safety classification. *Quality and Safety in Health Care*, **15**(suppl_1), i82–i90.

Sari, A.B.-A., Sheldon, T.A., Cracknell, A. and Turnbull, A. (2007) Sensitivity of routine system for reporting patient safety incidents in an NHS hospital: retrospective patient case note review. *British Medical Journal*, **334**(7584), 79.

Scobie, S., Thomson, R., McNeil, J.J. and Phillips, P.A. (2006) Measurement of the safety and quality of healthcare. *Medical Journal of Australia*, **184**(10 Suppl), S51–S55.

Smith, A.F., Goodwin, D., Mort, M. and Pope, C. (2006) Adverse events in anaesthetic practice: qualitative study of definition, discussion and reporting. *British Journal of Anaesthesia*, **96**(6), 715–721.

Stanhope, N., Crowley-Murphy, M., Vincent, C. *et al.* (1999) An evaluation of adverse incident reporting. *Journal of Evaluation in Clinical Practice*, **5**(1), 5–12.

Vincent, C. (2007) Incident reporting and patient safety. *British Medical Journal*, **334** (7584), 51.

Wu, A.W., Provonost, P. and Morlock, L. (2002) ICU incident reporting systems. *Journal of Critical Care*, **17**(2), 86–94.

Yong, H. and Kluger, M.T. (2003) Incident reporting in anaesthesia: a survey of practice in New Zealand. *Anaesthesia and Intensive Care*, **31**(5), 555–559.

CHAPTER 6
Measuring safety

In the last decade, considerable efforts have been made to improve the safety of healthcare. Are patients any safer than they were 10 years ago? The answer to this simple question is curiously elusive. While some aspects of safety are difficult to measure for technical reasons (i.e. defining preventability) the more substantive problem is that, for all the energy and activity, measurement and evaluation have not been high on the agenda. This is a curious state of affairs. If you were engaged in trying to reduce heart disease, cancer or road accidents, your first question would be 'how many people have heart disease?' or 'how many road accidents are there each year?' and then you would want to know if numbers were reducing year on year.

Some systems, such as the United States Veterans Affairs, have invested heavily in both financial and quality assessments and as a consequence can monitor and track quality over time. In many healthcare systems, a considerable amount of safety and quality data is collected, but this has relatively little impact on day-to-day practice. The problem in Britain at least is not the paucity of the data but that the available information is widely scattered and not easily accessible to clinical teams and managers. The Bristol Inquiry report for instance, concluded that 'Bristol was awash with data' (Aylin *et al.*, 2004). However, little of this information was available to parents and it did not help in the identification, prior to the Enquiry, of the problems brewing there. A central feature of the recent report by Darzi (2009) is that quality must be the defining principle of the British NHS and that quality needs to be systematically measured.

The measurement of quality is a vast topic, which requires a book in its own right. In this chapter we will principally focus on the specific problems associated with measuring safety, though many of the issues equally apply to measuring effectiveness, efficiency and other quality measures. Examples of measures will be given, but the chapter is mainly designed as a exploration of some of the important issues and as a backdrop and preparation for the discussions of the measurement and evaluation of safety interventions in later chapters.

The critical role of measurement

'You cannot manage what you cannot measure' is a familiar and perhaps rather tired management mantra, but it certainly applies to improving safety and

Patient Safety, 2nd edition. By Charles Vincent. Published 2010 by Blackwell Publishing Ltd.

quality. One of the greatest and rather unexpected challenges of the Safer Patients' Initiative (Chapter 17) was simply getting baseline data on the reliability of clinical processes. Most teams had no idea whether patients were receiving the treatment intended for them and were often surprised to discover the gap between their beliefs and the care actually delivered to patients. There are nevertheless some outstanding examples of major transformations of services grounded in careful, systematic measurement (Chassin, 2002). My colleague, Erik Mayer (2009), provides some examples:

An example of how an evidence-based quality framework can be used to improve healthcare has been seen with improvements in stroke services in the United Kingdom following the implementation of the National Service Framework (NSF) for older people in 2001. . . . The Biannual Sentinel Stroke Audit for 2008 has recently been published, and it demonstrates a continued significant improvement in stroke services. In terms of healthcare structure, 96% of hospitals in the United Kingdom now offer specialist stroke services, with an increasing number of specialist stroke unit beds; 98% of hospitals employ a physician with a specialist interest in stroke. There also have been improvements in process of care measures, including the uptake of thrombolysis services and secondary prevention measures. A similar initiative has been beneficial for coronary heart disease and more recently has been broadly applied to cancer.
(MAYER *ET AL.,* 2009)

Good safety and quality information therefore does exist in certain areas, but is generally neither very reliable nor comprehensive. This has important consequences at every level of healthcare organizations and the wider health economy. Hospital boards for example, are unable to effectively monitor safety and quality or assess the impact of any initiatives or programmes they may launch. They are accountable for something they cannot assess, a most uneasy position. At the level of the clinical directorate and the clinical team, the problem is more acute still. If clinical teams are to ensure or improve safety and quality, they must have data on their performance and an opportunity to reflect on the trends and features of those data over time. Consider also one of the most difficult issues in safety and quality. Why is it so hard to engage clinical staff in safety and quality initiatives? Clinical staff do, of course, care very much about safety and quality; on an individual level, it is at the heart of everything they do. However, they do not necessarily systematically monitor clinical processes and outcomes. There is little hope of real engagement without systematic collected local trend data, relevant to clinical concerns and that can be disseminated and discussed within clinical teams.

Defining measures of safety

Safety in other domains is assessed by the incidence of accidents and injuries; aviation accidents, road accidents, lost time injuries at work and other types of mishap are counted and tabulated by various means. Defining these accidents is

relatively, but not completely, straightforward; while a serious crash is unambiguous, there are many lesser road, rail and air incidents that cause minor
damage or can be considered as near misses. Ideally, we would like to have a
general index of safety, rather like rates of road or rail accidents, so that we
could track progress over time and ask more sophisticated questions about the
safety of different parts of the system and the factors that increased or degraded
safety. However, this reasonable and worthy objective presents a number of
problems, which have been well summarized by Peter Pronovost:

*A prime challenge in measuring safety is clarifying indicators that can be validly
measured as rates. Most safety parameters are difficult or impossible to capture in the
form of valid rates for several reasons: (1) events are uncommon (serious medication
errors) or rare (wrong-site surgical procedure); (2) few have standardized definitions;
(3) surveillance systems generally rely on self-reporting; (4) denominators (the populations at risk) are largely unknown; and (5) the time period for exposure (patient day
or device day) is unspecified. All of these may introduce bias. Creating measurement
systems that are relatively free of such bias would be costly and complex.*
(PRONOVOST, MILLER AND WACHTER, 2006)

Defining harm is a particularly difficult issue in healthcare for a number of
reasons. First, in other arenas, establishing cause and effect between accident
and injury is reasonably straightforward. In contrast, patients are generally,
though not always, sick and separating the harm due to healthcare from that
due to illness is often difficult. Second, some treatments given in healthcare are
necessarily 'harmful' to the patient; radiotherapy and chemotherapy are two
obvious examples. Third, harm from healthcare may not immediately be
detected or may only gradually become apparent. In fact, a cause celebre of
medical error – the chemotherapy overdose of *Boston Globe* reporter Betsy
Lehman – was only discovered on a routine review of research data in the
clinical study in which she was a participant. Finally, even if a patient is harmed,
this does not necessarily point to any deficiencies in care. One patient may get
pneumonia because of a major lapse in basic care; another may receive
exemplary care but still succumb to pneumonia.

The issue of denominators is also critical:

*Deciding on the best denominator is an added dilemma in the error rate equation. In
general, the denominator should quantify exposure to risk for the outcome of interest. For
example, when a patient who is hospitalized experiences a narcotic overdose, is the
appropriate denominator the patient or patient day, the prescribed or dispensed doses, all
administered medication doses, or all administered narcotic doses?*
(PRONOVOST, MILLER AND WACHTER, 2006)

If you consider this for a moment, you will see that the choice of denominator
makes an enormous difference to the error rate and to the interpretation of the
standard of care. Supposing a patient is given 10 different drug doses per day,

stays in hospital for ten days and sustains one adverse drug event from an overdose. You could say, well that's 100 doses over the admission, that's a rate of 1%. Certainly serious, but it doesn't look too bad. However, calculate by the day and the rate is 10%, and by the admission the average becomes 100%. Suddenly what looks like a technical issue for statisticians takes on new life.

Structure, process and outcome: what measures best reflect safety?

We must now consider what to actually measure, which again is not straight-forward. The first question that comes to mind is to ask whether safety is best reflected by examining rates of harm or by examining errors or failures to provide appropriate interventions (Pronovost, Miller and Wachter, 2006). Rather than pose this as a question that must be decided one way or another, it is much more profitable to consider the issue in the broader context of the relationship between various safety critical constructs. Here we are greatly helped by some clear thinking from Richard Lilford and colleagues (Figure 6.1) (Lilford *et al.*, 2004), who set out a conceptual framework to clarify the various factors that might be considered.

Structural measures

The basis of the diagram is the classic distinction between the structure, processes and outcomes of healthcare. Structures represent both physical structures (buildings and equipment), but also basic institutional characteristics such as the number and qualifications of staff (Donabedian, 2003). These characteristics can be changed, but generally only slowly, and the link between these factors and patient outcomes is not yet well understood. Some structural factors, such as staffing levels and the organization of intensive care have been linked to the safety and quality of care (Aiken, Sloane and Sochalski, 1998; Pronovost *et al.*, 1999; Main *et al.*, 2007). Human resource practices, which influence staff morale and working environment, have also been shown to relate to patient outcomes, even including hospital death rates (West *et al.*, 2002). Lilford and colleagues suggest that these influences are mediated by a number of intervening variables (discussed below), such as morale, motivation and safety culture, which affect staff attitudes and behaviour which in turn affect the clinical work carried out.

Outcome measures

Outcomes are changes in the health status of the patient, covering mortality, morbidity and more subtle changes in quality of life, patient satisfaction with care and changes in health related behaviours (such as giving up smoking). Safety outcomes are certainly top priority for patients and families. While you certainly might be concerned by observing errors in your care, your absolute priority is not to come to any harm, to at least leave hospital or emerge from treatment no worse than you were before. Some of the main adverse

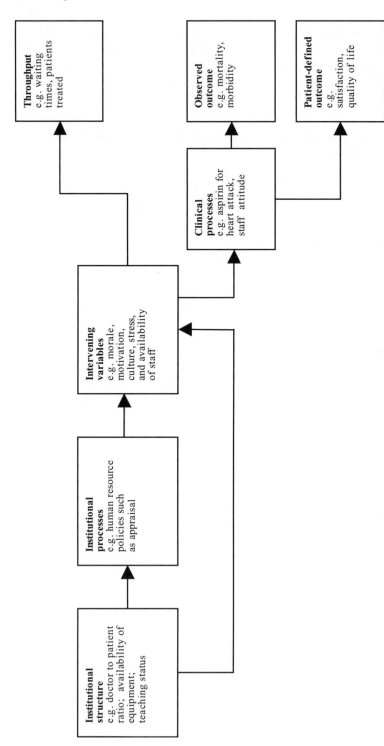

Figure 6.1 Conceptual map linking various structures and process variables to outcome (from Lilford *et al.*, 2004).

outcomes are infections, adverse drug events, pressure ulcers and surgical complications.

Death and surgical complications seem relatively unambiguous outcomes. However, some indicators of morbidity, such as wound infection, anastomotic leak and postpartum haemorrhage are difficult to define with precision (Lilford *et al.*, 2004). Even death can pose difficulties of classification, in the sense that a death in hospital can simply mean the arrival of a terminally ill person who died shortly after admission. A death in those circumstances says nothing at all about the quality or safety of care in that hospital.

Outcomes are determined by a combination of the patient's underlying condition and the care they actually receive. Any kind of outcome indicator, such as wound infection is only a very indirect reflection of the safety and quality of care provided. Comparing units or institutions on such indicators is therefore problematic, as any differences may simply reflect differences in patient populations as well as other factors, such as data quality and random variation. Case mix adjustment, in which rates or mortality or morbidity are statistically adjusted to allow for differences in patient population, is widely used but there will always be some uncertainty about the validity of comparisons based on such data. This is not to suggest that case mix adjustment is not valid or that comparisons should not be made, only to point out that the differences that emerge need thoughtful interpretation (Bottle and Aylin, 2008).

Issues of case mix adjustment matter much less however, if a unit or institution simply wishes to track its own progress over time and use the mortality or morbidity data as a stimulus and measure of improvement. If one makes the reasonable assumption that the patient population is relatively stable over time, then an organization can certainly use mortality or morbidity data as an indicator (Bottle and Aylin, 2008). Any change does reflect, albeit imperfectly, a corresponding change in safety and quality, though it may be difficult to identify which improvements were critical to the overall success.

Process measures

Donabedian describes clinical processes as 'the activities that constitute healthcare – including diagnosis, treatment, rehabilitation, prevention and patient education'. This is basically what healthcare professionals actually do, though it also includes the actions and care provided by patients themselves and their families. It is obviously impossible to capture the quality of fluid, day-to-day clinical work in its entirety. However, it is possible to select and capture specific clinical processes which are clearly indicated, supported by underlying evidence and, ideally, would be agreed as desirable by the clinicians caring for those patients. Examples of such measures would be the use of beta blockers after myocardial infarction and the timing of antibiotics after pneumonia.

When considering safety and quality improvement, process measures have a number of advantages, whether one is comparing organizations or simply monitoring change over time. Richard Lilford and colleagues suggest that monitoring clinical processes have several advantages over outcomes if the primary aim of measurement is to guide efforts to improve performance:

- Process measures focus on violation of agreed evidence or standards, so that deviations are clear cut.
- Measurement can be made close to the point of delivery of care, overcoming the delay between intervention and outcome.
- They can be applied to all institutions, not just the 'worst' 1, 2 or 5%, and therefore offers the hope of improving the average quality of care, yielding far bigger gains to the public health (Lilford et al., 2004).

We should note however that, in practice, it has proved difficult to show that improvements in processes produce improvements in outcomes. For instance, only weak associations have been found between process and outcome for myocardial infarction, a range of acute medical conditions, hip fracture and stroke (Lilford et al., 2004).

Intervening variables

As this book unfolds, you will see that multiple factors potentially affect the safety and quality of care delivered to patients. Teamwork, the performance of individuals, the use of technology, the conditions in which people work, the ethos and culture of the organization may all be relevant. These are the 'intervening variables' in measurement terms. They may only affect care indirectly, but are also potential reflections of the safety of an organization and also of its potential to improve care in the future. We should note however, that assessing safety by what has happened only tells you how safe a system has been in the past and does not tell you how dangerous it is now or will be in the future. Looking further ahead, at the possibility of deriving measures which are more reflective of the likelihood of harm, we might wish to assess the levels of hazard, the ability of systems to recover when errors occur and indices such as safety culture or staffing levels which might reflect overall systems safety. We will examine some of this work at a later stage. For now it is sufficient to note that although many of these factors are almost certainly relevant to safety and quality, the precise form of leadership, for instance, and the way it impacts on safety of care in practice remain to be elucidated.

The integration of safety and quality at the process level

Both measures of harm and assessments of failures in the process of care may reflect overall levels of safety. Failure to give appropriate care may or may not lead to harm, but it certainly seems reasonable to class these failures under the general heading of safety. These process measures however, seem similar if not identical to broader quality measures of effectiveness, reliability and efficiency captured in numerous studies of the quality of care. Does this mean that safety measures are nothing more than quality measures under another name? Not exactly, though when we examine the level of process rather than outcomes, the same measures may reflect both safety (in the sense of potential for harm) and other aspects of quality (efficiency, effectiveness and so on). The reason that this overlap has been slow to emerge is, to my mind, because our concern with safety was initially driven by relatively rare events with serious consequences.

Quality assessments have always been directed at overall standards of care given to populations of patients. In contrast, patient safety initially focused on rarer, often tragic events which had not been captured by traditional assessments of quality. As safety was more systematically studied however, it became clear that the frequency of error and harm were much greater than previously realized and that the safety of all patients needed to be addressed. No longer were we trying to prevent rare events, instead we were facing an epidemic of infection, adverse drug reaction and complications, together with a host of other rarer and less predictable incidents. The gradual *rapprochement* of these concepts, and the need to maintain focus on both, has been eloquently expressed by Vahe Kazandjian and colleagues (2008) in their paper 'Safety is a part of quality: a proposal for a continuum in performance measurement.' This is a long passage but well worth quoting in full:

Indicators of quality assess magnitude (events, frequency of processes, etc.). Through both statistical and clinical decision-making processes, changes in the magnitudes of measurement over time assist organizations in identifying priorities for improvement. For that reason alone, comparative analysis remains essential, be it to an organization's past performance or the performance of peers (while adjusting for confounding variables, if necessary). In the case of safety indicators, however, the philosophy appears entirely different: adverse events, often described with terms ranging from 'never events' to 'near misses', may not require comparative data. Indeed, it could even be proposed that for some safety measures one event is too many. Risk management and risk managers are primarily focused on those singular outcomes. For example, while it was not necessary to establish how many wrong doses of chemotherapy drugs were administered to a patient who developed kidney failure, it was sufficient to know that one patient had developed kidney failure because of wrong chemotherapy dosage. It is the very nature of safety measure events to occur with low frequency, although the associated outcomes can be catastrophic.

As the scientific literature has focused increasingly on the importance of near misses, even the potential for errors, a basic reconsideration of the initial distinction between 'quality' and 'safety' indicators seems in order. Seminal works on errors resulting from the provision of a service in any industry, have well established that errors can occur during any process. Therefore, it appears of much greater importance to understand the environment, structures, processes, as well as the attitudes of the people themselves rather than the outcomes defined as either quantifiable or qualifiable events.

This accounts for the rapprochement *between the concepts on the one hand and the mechanics of defining and designing quality indicators on the other. When analysis of a process is required to understand whether best knowledge at the time (evidence-based practice) was followed or whether the process suffered from inherent predispositions to undesirable outcomes (such as errors), the very distinction between 'quality' on the one hand and 'safety' indicators on the other becomes noticeably blurred.*

(REPRODUCED FROM *JOURNAL OF EVALUATION IN CLINICAL PRACTICE*, KAZANDJIAN ET AL. "SAFETY IS PART OF QUALITY: A PROPOSAL FOR A CONTINUUM IN PERFORMANCE MEASUREMENT". **14**, NO.2, 357–358, 2008.)

Approaches to the measurement of safety

We have already discussed record review and reporting of adverse events as methods of assessing adverse events at a particular point in time. We will now briefly consider whether they can also be used routinely to monitor safety over time.

Systematic record review

Patient safety is of course underpinned by large-scale studies of adverse events. If we want to monitor progress over time, then surely we should repeat these studies, whether on a local or national level. At a national level though, the simple fact is that no country has had the courage to repeat a study of the incidence of adverse events as a formal comparison; The Netherlands, however, has carried out a major study (Zegers *et al.*, 2009) and a follow-up study is planned to assess progress on patient safety.

Case note review is sometimes viewed as time consuming and comparatively expensive. Nevertheless, with experience and refinement and the development of training packages (Olsen *et al.*, 2007), it can be carried out relatively inexpensively, producing systematic, detailed analyses. A few organizations, such as Royal North Shore in Sydney (Harrison, personal communication) carry out formal, annual case note reviews and use these as the basis of their quality assurance and improvement systems. Record reviews could be repeated over time, and trends studied, particularly as we would now be able to define and monitor specific types of adverse events rather than just assess the overall rates. Reliability and validity of judgement of adverse events is not as good as we would wish but could certainly be improved if specific definitions of particular classes of adverse events were developed.

The global trigger tool

There is another class of instrument which is sometimes put forward as a measure of safety, namely 'trigger tools'. Essentially medical records are screened, by a clinician or sometimes electronically, for certain triggers which might indicate that an adverse event has occurred. These might include a return to the operating theatre, a death in hospital or more specifically a low platelet count or the need for renal replacement therapy. Trigger tools have been much used in programmes run by the Institute of Healthcare Improvement, such as the Safer Patients' Initiative, which will be discussed later. This kind of instrument can certainly be useful in providing a 'panoramic view of safety' (Pronovost, Miller and Wachter, 2006) to flag up worrying trends and areas. Whether the trigger tool is a measure of adverse events is not really clear; hospitals might claim 'we achieved a 50% reduction in adverse events', when what they mean is that they had 50% less triggers, which is not quite the same thing. Trigger tools are very similar to the Stage 1 of case record review, a screening tool for potential problems. They are certainly useful as a screen, but the subtle shading into the use of triggers as measures is a little disquieting.

Mandatory reporting of never events

Some safety events are rare. Deaths from injecting intravenous drugs into the spinal cord are, thankfully, very rare. These are the most prominent, most disturbing safety events which most closely correspond to the 'accidents' of other domains. These events are captured in the list of 28 'never events' drawn up by the National Quality Forum in 2004, and since adopted by many organizations as a safety target. We will never be able to systematically measure 'never events' and hopefully will not need to. Identification of these rare but terrible events will always have to rely on reporting, at least until reliable ways of searching electronic medical records emerge.

BOX 6.1 Examples of 'never events'

Surgical events
- Surgery performed on the wrong body part or wrong patient;
- Unintended retention of a foreign object in a patient after surgery;
- Intraoperative or immediately postoperative death in an ASA Class I patient.

Product of device events
- Patient death or serious disability associated with the use of contaminated drugs, devices or biologics provided by the healthcare facility;
- Patient death or serious disability associated with the use or function of a device in patient care in which the device is used or functions other than as intended;
- Patient death or serious disability associated with intravascular air embolism that occurs while being cared for in a healthcare facility.

Patient protection events
- Infant discharged to the wrong person;
- Patient suicide, or attempted suicide, resulting in serious disability while being cared for in a healthcare facility.

Care management events
- Patient death or serious disability associated with a medication error;
- Patient death or serious disability associated with a haemolytic reaction due to the administration of incompatible blood or blood products;

- Maternal death or serious disability associated with labour or delivery in a low-risk pregnancy while being cared for in a healthcare facility;
- Stage 3 or 4 pressure ulcers acquired after admission to a healthcare facility.

Environmental events
- Any incident in which a line designated for oxygen or other gas to be delivered to a patient contains the wrong gas or is contaminated by toxic substances;
- Patient death or serious disability associated with a fall while being cared for in a healthcare facility;
- Patient death or serious disability associated with the use of restraints or bedrails while being cared for in a healthcare facility.

Criminal events
- Abduction of a patient of any age;
- Sexual assault on a patient within or in the grounds of a healthcare facility.

(REPRODUCED WITH PERMISSION FROM THE NATIONAL QUALITY FORUM, COPYRIGHT 2004)

Safety indicators: using routine data

Measurement of clinical information can be time-consuming and staff can be burdened with excessive form-filling and, most irritating, multiple submissions of the same data in slightly different forms to different echelons and outside organization. For instance, there are around 270 national healthcare databases across the United Kingdom (Raftery, Roderick and Stevens, 2005) and about another 105 clinical databases. The prospect of adding further systems geared to collecting safety relevant information has to be considered in the context of the resources it would consume, both in time and money. One potential solution is to make more effective use of the huge and comprehensive administrative databases that healthcare systems have, to monitor basic activity, financial and clinical information. They were not established to monitor safety and quality, but contain much potentially relevant information.

Clinicians tend to distrust this information, as it is often coded by people who, though well intentioned, do not have the clinical understanding to always code medical records correctly. On their side, they may have difficulty contacting clinicians in order to clarify issues. The nature and extent of such problems varies widely between countries. Where items of care are individually billed or where, more broadly, money follows care delivered, much more attention is given to proper and comprehensive coding. No codes, no cash.

A number of important quality indicator programmes have been established around the world, with hospitals signing up on a voluntary basis to share information, benchmark their performance against their peers and learn from each other. In the United States, the Agency for Healthcare Research and Quality has led the way in establishing core sets of indicators, backed by a substantial research programme, that can be used across the United States. There are three sets of indicators: Prevention Quality Indicators, Inpatient Hospital Indicators and most recently, released in 2004, Patient Safety Indicators.

The patient safety indicators were developed with exemplary thoroughness and due attention to a number of key issues affecting the validity and usefulness of the indicators. The full list of indicators is shown in Box 6.2, and some examples of definitions and outstanding issues in Box 6.3. It is critical to appreciate that the indicators do not necessarily indicate unsafe care and still less specific errors; the clinician panels rated only severe transfusion reaction and retained foreign body as very likely to be due to error. While this is important for individual cases however, it is less critical when aggregating data over time. Any organization would like to reduce these events and once they

---

BOX 6.2 AHRQ Patient safety indicators

Complications of Anaesthesia
Death in Low-Mortality diagnostic groups
Decubitus Ulcer
Failure to Rescue
Foreign Body Left During Procedure Iatrogenic Pneumothorax
Selected Infections Due to Medical Care
Postoperative Hip Fracture
Postoperative Haemorrhage or Haematoma
Postoperative Physiologic and Metabolic Derangements
Postoperative Respiratory Failure
Postoperative Pulmonary Embolism or Deep Vein Thrombosis
Postoperative Sepsis
Postoperative Wound Dehiscence
Accidental Puncture or Laceration
Transfusion Reaction
Birth Trauma – Injury to Neonate
Obstetric Trauma – Vaginal with Instrument
Obstetric Trauma – Vaginal without Instrument
Obstetric Trauma – Caesarean Delivery
Foreign Body Left During Procedure
Iatrogenic Pneumothorax
Selected Infections Due to Medical Care
Postoperative Wound Dehiscence
Accidental Puncture or Laceration
Transfusion Reaction
Postoperative Haemorrhage or Haematoma.

(ADAPTED, IN PART, FROM: *PATIENT SAFETY INDICATORS OVERVIEW*. AHRQ QUALITY INDICATORS. FEBRUARY 2006. AGENCY FOR HEALTHCARE RESEARCH AND QUALITY, ROCKVILLE, MD. http://www.qualityindicators.ahrq.gov/psi_overview.htm)

BOX 6.3 Examples of AHRQ patient safety indicators

PSI Name	Definition	Validity Concerns
Complications of Anaesthesia (PSI 1)	Cases of anaesthetic overdose, reaction or endotracheal tube misplacement per 1000 surgery discharges. Excludes codes for drug use and self-inflicted injury	Condition definition varies Under-reporting or screening Denominator unspecific
Death in Low Mortality DRGs (PSI 2)	In-hospital deaths per 1000 patients in DRGs with < 0.5% mortality. Excludes trauma, immunocompromised and cancer patients	Heterogeneous severity
Decubitus Ulcer (PSI 3)	Cases of decubitus ulcer per 1000 discharges with a length of stay of 5 or more days. Excludes patients with paralysis or in MDC 9, MDC 14, and patients admitted from a long-term care facility	Under-reporting or screening Heterogeneous severity Case mix bias
Failure to Rescue (PSI 4)	Deaths per 1000 patients having developed specified complications of care during hospitalization. Excludes patients age 75 and older, neonates in MDC 15, patients admitted from long-term care facility and patients transferred to or from other acute care facility	Adverse consequences Stratification suggested Unclear preventability Heterogeneous severity
Foreign Body Left During Procedure (PSI 5)	Discharges with foreign body accidentally left in during procedure per 1000 discharges	Rare Stratification suggested
Iatrogenic Pneumothorax (PSI 6)	Cases of iatrogenic pneumothorax per 1000 discharges. Excludes trauma, thoracic surgery, lung or pleural biopsy, or cardiac surgery patients, and MDC 14	Denominator unspecific

are monitored, programmes can be put in place to reduce them and the programmes themselves can be evaluated.

Groups around the world have adapted the AHRQ PSIs for use in their own systems. Veena Raleigh and colleagues have recently reported that in both the United States and Britain, indicators are associated with an increased length of stay. For instance, postoperative infections lead to an average additional 10 days in hospital, painful for the patient and expensive for the organization (Raleigh *et al.*, 2008). Paul Aylin and colleagues have translated the indicators for use with English administrative data and tracked the indicators over time for the British National Health Service (Vincent *et al.*, 2008). Deaths in patients expected to have a low mortality ($< 0.5\%$) appear to be decreasing significantly, and fewer foreign bodies were being left in patients after procedures (Figure 6.2). The remaining indicators all appear to be increasing, suggesting that care may be getting steadily less safe. However, at this stage of development, the most likely explanation for the observed trends is improved coding. This means one should, at least for the time being, be cautious about comparing organizations or units.

Targets, standards and the unexpected consequences of measurement

Setting clear targets and standards has undoubtedly brought changes in clinical performance when rigorously applied with standards, but setting measurement in a performance framework is different from considering it in an improvement framework (Bevan and Hood, 2006). The distinction between

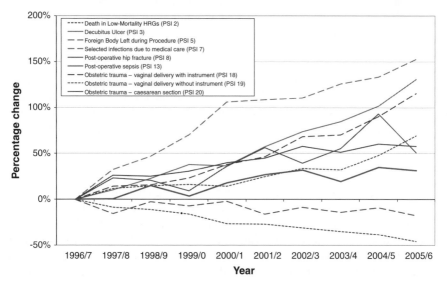

Figure 6.2 Changes in rates of 9 AHRQ derived patient safety indicators (Hospital Episode Statistics 1996/7–2005/6, England).

a measure and a target or standard is a subtle one. The distinction does not really concern the nature of the measure, more the use to which is put, the context in which a target or standard is set and the consequences of meeting or failing to meet a standard. Robert Wachter has explored this thoughtfully in a paper on the unexpected consequences of measurement, giving this example of a target for administration of antibiotics.

In the United States, a target of administration of antibiotics within 8 hours to patients with community acquired pneumonia was introduced in 1998, later reduced to four hours in 2002. Patients with pneumonia obviously need antibiotics as soon as possible, so this seems a reasonable target. However, once introduced, a number of problems began to emerge, such as patients who turned out not to have pneumonia were given antibiotics inappropriately to ensure the target was met. Other patients who received 'poor quality care' were found, on review, to have received entirely appropriate care, with delay occurring for good clinical reasons, such as ruling out more dangerous conditions. Later the rule was relaxed to six hours and further specifications of confirming test results introduced, which resolved some problems but created others (Wachter, 2006).

The standards issue becomes most problematic with patients who have multiple problems. It may be sensible to delay the treatment of pneumonia, for instance, while more urgent investigations and treatments are instituted. An additional problem is that of combining multiple treatments with the risk of adverse drug events and actually producing harm through the application of standard procedures. Wachter (2006) has argued that quality measurement is bewildered by the patient with multiple conditions, which is, of course, most people admitted to hospital and many older people outside hospital. He considers a hypothetical 79-year-old woman with five common diseases: hypertension, osteoporosis, osteoarthritis, type 2 diabetes mellitus and chronic obstructive pulmonary disease:

Had this patient received guideline concordant therapy, she would have been adminis-tered 13 medicines . . . with more than 20 potential drug-disease, drug-drug, and drug-diet interactions. The doctor prescribing this polypharmacy would receive a high ranking on quality measurement metrics, even if adherence to clinical guidelines would have harmed or bankrupted this patient.
(WACHTER, 2006)

Measurement *per se* is arguably a neutral act, though potentially costly in terms of time and resources. However, measurement with real or implied pressure to conform to a standard is not a neutral act but an intervention within a system. This is not to argue against measurement or, necessarily, against performance standards and accountability. However, the potential adverse effects of targets and standards need to be appreciated. Generally speaking, measurement of safety and quality is less problematic when carried out by clinical teams for the benefit of themselves and their patients and used by them to monitor the care they give. Issues of case mix, gaming, organizational pressure and definitions are likely to be less critical and provide less distortion.

Tracking safety over time: are patients any safer?

We will now return to the question posed at the beginning of this chapter. Are patients any safer after all this effort and investment in patient safety? My colleagues and I at Imperial College set out to address this question, taking the case of the British National Health Service as our case study (Vincent *et al.*, 2008). We examined several core areas which reflect the safety of healthcare to determine whether it is possible to assess change and, if so, what changes were apparent. We focused on measures of outcome, in the sense of definable events that happen to patients (infections, morbidity, mortality) and on key measures of process (such as medication errors). The next sections give a flavour of our findings.

Hospital standardized mortality

In-hospital mortality has fallen significantly over the past 11 years, as measured through hospital standardized mortality ratios (HSMR). When measured against mortality in 2000/1 (HSMR = 100), calculations suggest that the ratio has fallen from 114 in 1996/7 to 82 in 2006/7. The HSMR is case mix adjusted for a number of factors, including age, sex, diagnosis, whether the admission is planned/unplanned, socio-economic deprivation, co-morbidity and season, so these changes are not simply due to different types of patients being seen in hospital. Shorter admissions and changing discharge policies may have some bearing on the reduction in hospital mortality, as could more general trends in mortality (both in and out of hospital), and a general increase in longevity. The overall picture, although difficult to interpret, suggests that care is at least as safe and may be improving.

Mortality following surgery

Another approach to examining mortality rates is through professionally led national audits. The Scottish Audit of Surgical Mortality (SASM) for instance, uses case assessment applying proformas that are voluntarily filled by clinicians and then examined by clinical assessors to determine the reasons for the death. SASM has shown that cases in which an adverse event contributed to death have steadily reduced over the years, suggesting that efforts by SASM and others to increase involvement of consultants in decision making and improve interaction between surgical, anaesthetic and ITU teams have borne fruit.

The Society of Cardiothoracic Surgeons has collected data for over 20 years. There is evidence of improved outcomes in cardiac surgery, with a reduction in mortality in the North of England from 2.4% in 1997/8 to 1.8% in 2004/5 (Bridgewater *et al.*, 2007). However, an analysis of HES data indicates that the improvements are seen mainly in low- and medium-volume hospitals (Al Sarira *et al.*, 2007). Whether this improvement is through superior performance of individuals and teams or whether this is due to better case selection is not completely clear.

Healthcare acquired infections

The best measures of harm that we have, and a possible measurement model for patient safety in general (Burke, 2003), are rates of healthcare acquired infections. Most of these infections are preventable and are measured using standardized and well-validated systems and definitions. In the United States, the Centre for Disease Control and Prevention has set out standard definitions, and hospitals have created epidemiology and infection control departments to independently monitor, report and reduce infections.

In Britain, the Health Protection Agency fulfils a similar function. Mandatory reporting for Meticillin resistant *Staphylococcus aureus* (MRSA) bacteraemia has been required since April 2001 and for *Clostridium difficile* since January 2004. Reporting is public, transparent and submissions of MRSA and *C. difficile* data now require monthly Chief Executive sign off, producing strong pressure both for accurate data and the actual reduction of infection. From being a side issue tackled by small harassed infection control teams, it has become a major organizational priority and a matter for statutory regulation.

Voluntary reporting of both MRSA and *C. difficile* saw steadily rising rates in the 1990s, in part because of improved detection, surveillance and reporting. The introduction of mandatory reporting and the accompanying infection control initiatives are now producing a reduction in MRSA nationally, particularly in the acute Teaching trusts. The latest data from the British Health Protection Agency suggest that rates of *C difficile* are now falling, though the agency expresses some caution about whether this can be sustained in the longer term.

Medication errors and adverse drug events

A number of UK studies have been published on the rate of medication error (Table 6.1). Rates of administration error are not decreasing over time, and may even be increasing; no trend is apparent for rates of prescribing error. However, in both cases the possibility of direct comparison is limited as the studies were conducted in different settings and do not share a common methodology. Adverse drug events have many causes and it will never be possible to reduce such events to zero. Nevertheless, many are undoubtedly preventable and the overall level of adverse drug events would be an important indicator of the safety of any healthcare systems. More comprehensive data can be obtained from reviews of medical notes (Barber *et al.*, 2006) but ongoing studies at regular intervals would be needed to identify trends in ADE rates. We have no idea at the moment of national rates or trends for adverse drug events.

Overall, the data we examined present a mixed picture. While there are some difficulties of interpretation, there is reasonable evidence for a reduction in overall hospital mortality and in mortality after certain types of surgery. There is also good evidence for a fall in rates of MRSA, and possibly also

Table 6.1 UK data on medication administration error rates over time

Authors	Year	Error rate	Comments
Ridge *et al.*	1995	3.5% of 3312 doses	
Dean *et al.*	1995	3.0% of 2756 doses	
Gethins	1996	3.2% of 2000 doses	
Ho *et al.*	1997	5.5% of 2170 doses	
Cavell *et al.*	1997	5.5% of 1295 doses	Electronic prescribing
Cavell *et al.*	1997	5.7% of 1206 doses	Manual prescribing
Ogden *et al.*	1997	5.5% of 2973 doses	
Taxis *et al.*	1999	8.0% of 842 doses	
Dean *et al.*	2000	4.3% of 3576 doses	Traditional drug trolley
Dean *et al.*	2000	4.2% of 2491 doses	Bedside lockers
Franklin *et al.*	2006	6.1% of 1796 doses	Pre-educational intervention
Franklin *et al.*	2006	4.2% of 1397 doses	Post-educational intervention
Franklin *et al.*	2007	7.0% of 1473 doses	Paper-based system
Franklin *et al.*	2007	4.3% of 1139 doses	Electronic prescribing, automated ward-based dispensing, barcode administration

All studies are observation-based; all figures exclude intra venous doses (Reproduced from British Medical Journal, Charles Vincent, Paul Aylin, Bryony Dean Franklin et al. "Is health care getting safer?". **337**, no. nov13, [2426], 2008, with permission from BMJ Publishing Group Ltd.)

C. difficile. Of the nine safety indicators (Figure 6.2), seven showed an increase which apparently indicated that care was less safe or, more probably, better coding. For medication errors, adverse drug events and indeed most other safety issues in the NHS, we simply have no idea of long-term trends. The fact that we simply do not know whether patients are safer suggests that much more attention needs to be paid to measurement and evaluation in the next ten years than has been the case in the previous 10 years.

References

Aiken, L.H., Sloane, D.M. and Sochalski, J. (1998) Hospital organisation and outcomes. *Quality in Health Care*, **7**(4), 222–226.

Al Sarira, A.A., David, G., Willmott, S. *et al.* (2007) Oesophagectomy practice and outcomes in England. *The British Journal of Surgery*, **94**(5), 585–591.

Aylin, P., Tanna, S., Bottle, A. and Jarman, J. (2004) Dr Foster's case notes: how often are adverse events reported in English hospital statistics? *British Medical Journal*, **329** (7462), 369.

Barber, N., Franklin, B.D., Comford, T. *et al.* (2006) *Safer, Faster, Better? Evaluating Electronic Prescribing. Report to the Patient Safety Research Programme,* Department of Health, London.

Bevan, G. and Hood, C. (2006) Have targets improved performance in the English NHS? *British Medical Journal,* **332**(7538), 419–422.

Bottle, A. and Aylin, P. (2008) Intelligent information: a national system for monitoring clinical performance. *Health Services Research,* **43**(1 Pt 1), 10–31.

Bridgewater, B., Grayson, A.D., Brooks, N. *et al.* (2007) Has the publication of cardiac surgery outcome data been associated with changes in practice in northwest England: an analysis of 25 730 patients undergoing CABG surgery under 30 surgeons over 8 years. *Heart,* **93**(6), 744–748.

Burke, J.P. (2003) Infection control – A problem for patient safety. *The New England Journal of Medicine,* **348**(7), 651–656.

Chassin, M.R. (2002) Achieving and sustaining improved quality: lessons from New York State and cardiac surgery. *Health Aff. (Millwood.),* **21**(4), 40–51.

Darzi, A. (2009) *High Quality Care for All,* Department of Health.

Donabedian, A. (2003) *An Introduction to Quality Assurance in Health Care,* Oxford University Press, Oxford.

Kazandjian, V.A., Wicker, K.G., Matthes, N. and Ogunbo, S. (2008) Safety is part of quality: a proposal for a continuum in performance measurement. *Journal of Evaluation in Clinical Practice,* **14**(2), 354–359.

Lilford, R., Mohammed, M.A., Spiegelhalter, D. and Thomson, R. (2004) Use and misuse of process and outcome data in managing performance of acute medical care: avoiding institutional stigma. *Lancet,* **363**(9415), 1147–1154.

Main, D.S., Henderson, W.G., Pratte, K. *et al.* (2007) Relationship of processes and structures of care in general surgery to postoperative outcomes: a descriptive analysis. *Journal of the American College of Surgeons,* **204**(6), 1157–1165.

Mayer, E.K., Chow, A., Vale, J.A. and Athanasiou, T. (2009) Appraising the quality of care in surgery. *World Journal of Surgery,* **33**(8), 1584–1593.

Olsen, S., Neale, G., Schwab, K. *et al.* (2007) Hospital staff should use more than one method to detect adverse events and potential adverse events: incident reporting, pharmacist surveillance and local real-time record review may all have a place. *Quality and Safety in Health Care,* **16**(1), 40–44.

Pronovost, P.J., Dang, D., Dorman, T. *et al.* (1999) ICU nurse to patient ratio greater than 1 to 2 associated with an increased risk of complications in abdominal aortic surgery patients. *Critical Care Medicine,* **27**(12), A27.

Pronovost, P.J., Miller, M.R. and Wachter, R.M. (2006) Tracking progress in patient safety – an elusive target. *Journal of the American Medical Association,* **296**(6), 696–699.

Raftery, J., Roderick, P. and Stevens, A. (2005) Potential use of routine databases in health technology assessment. *Health Technology Assessment,* **9**(20), 1–iv.

Raleigh, V.S., Cooper, J., Bremner, S.A. and Scobie, S. (2008) Patient safety indicators for England from hospital administrative data: case-control analysis and comparison with US data. *British Medical Journal,* **337**(oct17_1), a1702.

Vincent, C., Aylin, P., Franklin, B.D. *et al.* (2008) Is healthcare getting safer? *British Medical Journal,* **337**(nov13_1), a2426.

Wachter, R.M. (2006) Expected and unanticipated consequences of the quality and information technology revolutions. *The Journal of the American Medical Association,* **295**(23), 2780–2783.

West, M.A., Borrill, C., Dawson, J. *et al.* (2002) The link between the management of employees and patient mortality in acute hospitals. *International Journal of Human Resource Management*, **13**(8), 1299–1310.

Zegers, M., de Bruijne, M.C., Wagner, C. *et al.* (2009) Adverse events and potentially preventable deaths in Dutch hospitals: results of a retrospective patient record review study. *Quality and Safety in Health Care*, **18**(4), 297–302.

From Accident Analysis to System Design

CHAPTER 7

Human error and systems thinking

Human error is routinely blamed for accidents in the air, on the railways, in complex surgery and in healthcare generally. Immediately after an incident people make quick judgements and, all too often, blame the person most obviously associated with the disaster. The pilot of the plane, the doctor who gives the injection, the train driver who passes a red light, are quickly singled out. However, these quick judgements and routine assignment of blame prevent us uncovering the second story (Cook, Woods and Miller, 1998). This is the story in its full richness and complexity, which only emerges after thoughtful and careful enquiry. While a particular action or omission may be the immediate cause of an incident, closer analysis usually reveals a series of events and departures from safe practice, each influenced by the working environment and the wider organizational context (Vincent, Adams and Stanhope, 1998).

The next two chapters explore the themes of human error, systems thinking and the analysis of accidents and disaster. This chapter addresses the underlying conceptual issues while the next chapter is more practical but, as with medicine itself, until you understand the concepts the practice will elude you. We begin by examining the lessons of major accidents, which will bring out the themes of the two chapters. We then examine the difficult topic of human error, addressing the concept and definitions, the nature of medical error, the psychology of error and the different ways error can be managed.

The lessons of major accidents

Our understanding of how the events preceding a disaster unfold has been greatly expanded in the last 20 years by the careful examination of a number of high profile accidents (Boxes 7.1 and 7.2). The brief summaries of major accidents, and the account of the Columbia Space Shuttle accident, allow us to reflect on the many ways in which failure can occur and the complexity of the story that may unfold during a serious investigation. Human beings have the opportunity to contribute to an accident at many different points in the

Patient Safety, 2nd edition. By Charles Vincent. Published 2010 by Blackwell Publishing Ltd.

process of production and operation. Problems and failures may occur in the design, testing, implementation of a new system, its maintenance and operation. Technical failures, important though they can be, often play a relatively minor part. Looking at other industries, although they are often very different from healthcare, helps us understand the conceptual landscape and some of the practicalities of accident investigation.

BOX 7.1 Major disasters involving human error

Chernobyl (April 1986)

Chernobyl's 1000 MW Reactor No. 4 exploded, releasing radioactivity over much of Europe. Although much debated since the accident, a Soviet investigation team admitted 'deliberate, systematic and numerous violations' of safety procedures.

Piper Alpha (July 1988)

A major explosion on an oil rig resulted in a fire and the deaths of 167 people. The Cullen enquiry (1990) found a host of technical and organizational causes rooted in the culture, structure and procedures of Occidental Petroleum. The maintenance error that led to the initial leak was the result of inexperience, poor maintenance procedures, and deficient learning mechanisms.

Space Shuttle Challenger (January 1986)

An explosion shortly after lift-off killed all the astronauts on board. An 'O ring' seal on one of the solid rocket boosters split after lift-off, releasing a jet of ignited fuel. The causes of the defective O-ring involved a rigid organizational mindset, conflicts between safety and keeping on schedule and the effects of fatigue on decision making.

Herald of Free Enterprise (March 1987)

The roll-on-roll-off ferry sank in shallow water off Zeebruge, Belgium, killing 189 passengers and crew. The enquiry highlighted the commercial pressures in the ferry business and the friction between ship and shore management that led to safety lessons not being heeded. The company was found to be 'infected with the disease of sloppiness'.

Paddington Rail Accident (October 1999)

31 people died when a train went through a red light onto the main up-line from Paddington, where it collided head on with an express approaching the station. The enquiry identified failures in training of drivers, a serious and persistent failure to examine reported poor signal visibility, a safety culture that was slack and less than adequate and significant failures of communication in the various organizations.

(THIS ARTICLE WAS PUBLISHED IN *HUMAN FACTORS IN SAFETY CRITICAL SYSTEMS*, LUCAS D, "CAUSES OF HUMAN ERROR". 38–39, COPYRIGHT ELSEVIER. 1997)

BOX 7.2 The loss of Space Shuttle *Columbia*

The Columbia Accident Investigation Board's independent investigation into the loss on 1 February 2003 of the Space Shuttle *Columbia* and its seven-member crew lasted nearly seven months, involving a staff of more than 120, along with some 400 NASA engineers supporting the Board's 13 members. Investigators examined more than 30 000 documents, conducted more than 200 formal interviews, heard testimony from dozens of expert witnesses, and reviewed more than 3000 inputs from the general public. In addition, more than 25 000 searchers combed vast stretches of the Western United States to retrieve the spacecraft's debris. The Board recognized early on that the accident was probably not an anomalous, random event, but likely to be rooted to some degree in NASA's history and the human space flight programme's culture. The Board's conviction regarding the importance of these factors strengthened as the investigation progressed, with the result that this report placed as much weight on these causal factors as on the more easily understood and corrected physical cause of the accident.

The physical cause of the loss of *Columbia* and its crew was a breach in the Thermal Protection System on the leading edge of the left wing, caused by a piece of insulating foam which separated from the External Tank at 81.7 seconds after launch and struck the wing. During re-entry this breach in the Thermal Protection System allowed superheated air to penetrate through the leading edge insulation and progressively melt the aluminium structure of the left wing, resulting in a weakening of the structure until increasing aerodynamic forces caused loss of control, failure of the wing, and break-up of the Orbiter.

The organizational causes of this accident are rooted in the Space Shuttle Programme's history and culture, including the original compromises that were required to gain approval for the Shuttle, subsequent years of resource constraints, fluctuating priorities, schedule pressures, mischaracterization of the Shuttle as operational rather than developmental, and lack of an agreed national vision for human space flight. Cultural traits and organizational practices detrimental to safety were allowed to develop, including: reliance on past success as a substitute for sound engineering practices; organizational barriers that prevented effective communication of critical safety information and stifled professional differences of opinion; lack of integrated management across programme elements; and the evolution of an informal chain of command and decision-making processes that operated outside the organization's rules.

(ADAPTED FROM US NATIONAL AERONAUTICS AND SPACE ADMINISTRATION, 2003, www.nasa.gov)

The most obvious errors and failures are usually those that are the immediate causes of an accident, such as a train driver going through a red light or a doctor picking up the wrong syringe and injecting a fatal drug. These failures are mostly unintentional, though occasionally they are deliberate, though misguided, attempts to retrieve a dangerous situation. Some of the 'violations of procedure' at Chernobyl were in fact attempts to use unorthodox methods to prevent disaster. Attempts to control an escalating crisis can make matters worse, as when police officers believed they needed to contain rioting football fans who were in fact trying to escape from a fire. Problems may also occur in the management of escape and emergency procedures, as when train passengers were unable to escape from carriages after the Paddington crash.

The immediate causes described above are the result of actions, or omissions, by people at the scene. However, other factors further back in the causal chain can also play a part in the genesis of an accident. These 'latent conditions', as they are often termed, lay the foundations for accidents in the sense that they create the conditions in which errors and failures can occur (Reason, 1997). This places the operators at the sharp end in an invidious position, as James Reason eloquently explains:

Rather than being the instigators of an accident, operators tend to be the inheritors of system defects . . . their part is usually that of adding the final garnish to a lethal brew whose ingredients have already been long in the cooking.
(REASON, 1990)

The accidents described (Box 7.2) allude to poor training, problems with scheduling, conflicts between safety and profit, communication failures, failure to address known safety problems and to general sloppiness of management and procedures. Some of these failures may have been known at the time, in that communication failures between management and supervisors may have been a longstanding and obvious problem. However, latent conditions may also be created by decisions which may have been perfectly reasonable at the time, but in retrospect are seen to have contributed to an accident. For instance, the training budget for maintenance workers may have been cut to avoid staff redundancies. In any organization there are always pressures to reduce training, eliminate waste, act quickly to keep on schedule and so on. Safety margins are eroded bit by bit, sometimes without anyone noticing, eventually leading to an accident.

Another feature of these explanations for accidents, especially the more recent ones, are the references to safety culture and organizational culture. The safety culture of a train company, for instance, is described as 'slack and less than adequate'. The Columbia investigation refers to a number of 'cultural traits and organizational practices detrimental to safety', such as reliance on past success rather than formal testing, barriers to passing on safety information, stifling of dissenting voices and informal decisions that bypassed organizational rules and procedures. These are all broadly speaking cultural, in that they refer to or are embedded in the norms, attitudes and values of the organizations concerned.

Safety culture is hard to define precisely but may become more tangible when one reflects on one's own experience of organizations. In some hospital wards for instance, the atmosphere may be friendly and cheerful, but it is clear that there is little tolerance for poor practice and the staff are uniformly conscientious and careful. In contrast, others develop a kind of sub-culture in which sloppy practices are tolerated, risks are run and potentially dangerous practices allowed to develop. These cultural patterns develop slowly but erode safety and morale. Sometimes these features of the ward or organization are ascribed to the personalities of the people working there, who are viewed as slapdash, careless and unprofessional. The use of the term culture however, points to the powerful influence of social forces in moulding behaviour; we are all more malleable than we like to think and to some extent develop good or bad habits according to the prevailing ethos around us.

We should also note that major accidents in high hazard industries are often the stimulus for wide ranging safety improvements. For instance, the enquiry into the Piper Alpha oil disaster led to a host of recommendations and the implementation of a number of risk reduction strategies, which covered the whole industry and addressed a wide range of issues. These included the setting up of a single regulatory body for offshore safety, relocation of pipeline emergency shutdown valves, and the provision of temporary safe refuges for oil workers, new evacuation procedures and requirements for emergency safety training (Reason, 1990; Vincent, Adams and Stanhope, 1998).

Finally, consider the resources that have been put into understanding these accidents. In the case of Columbia, hundreds of people were involved in intense investigation of all aspects of NASAs functioning. Certainly these accidents were all tragedies; many people died unnecessarily, there was a great deal at stake for the organizations concerned, and enormous political and media pressures to contend with. Unnecessary deaths in healthcare, in comparison, receive relatively little attention and are only occasionally the subject of major enquiries. Large sums of money are spent on the roads and railways on safety measures, again relatively little in health. Patient safety is, thankfully for staff and patients alike, now firmly on the healthcare agenda in many countries. But the resources for keeping patients safe are still pretty minimal.

Is healthcare like other industries?

Aviation, nuclear power, chemical and petroleum industries are, like health-care, hazardous activities carried out in large, complex organizations by, for the most part, dedicated and highly trained people. Commercial, political, social and humanitarian pressures have compelled these industries to raise their game and make sustained efforts to improve and maintain safety. Healthcare, in contrast, has relied on the intrinsic motivation and professionalism of clinical and managerial staff which, while vital, is not sufficient to ensure safety. Hearing other people working in dangerous environments talk about how they treat safety as something to be discussed, analysed, managed and resourced tells us that safety is not just a by-product of people doing their best, but a far more complex and elusive phenomenon.

We should, however, be cautious about drawing parallels between healthcare and other industries. The high technology monitoring and vigilance of anaesthetists and the work of pilots in commercial aviation are similar in some respects, but the work of surgeons and pilots is very different. Emergency medicine may find better models and parallels in the military or in fire fighting than in aviation, and so on. The easy equation of the work of doctors and pilots has certainly been overstated, even though many useful ideas and practices have transferred from aviation to medicine. For instance, simulation and team training in anaesthesia and other specialties was strongly influenced by crew resource management in aviation. However, surgical team training has to be grounded in the particular tasks and challenges faced by surgical teams. We cannot just import aviation team training wholesale. Aviation acts as a motivator and source of ideas, but the actual training has to be developed and tested within the healthcare setting.

Differences between healthcare and other industries
What differences can be identified between healthcare and other industries? First, healthcare encompasses an extraordinarily diverse set of activities. Healthcare encompasses the mostly routine, but sometimes highly unpredictable and hazardous world of surgery; primary care, where patients may have relationships with their doctors over many years; the treatment of acute psychosis, requiring rapid response and considerable tolerance of bizarre behaviour; some highly organized and ultrasafe processes, such as radiotherapy or the management of blood products; and the inherently unpredictable, constantly changing environment of emergency medicine. To this list we can add hospital medicine, care in the community, patients who monitor and treat their own condition and, by far the most important in poorer cultures, care given in people's homes. Even with the most cursory glance at the diversity of healthcare, the easy parallels with the comparatively predictable high-hazard industries, with a relatively limited set of activities, begins to break down.

Work in many hazardous industries, such as nuclear power is, ideally, routine and predictable. Emergencies and departures from usual practice are unusual and to be avoided. Many aspects of healthcare are also largely routine and would, for the most part, be much better organized on a production line basis. Much of the care of chronic conditions, such as asthma and diabetes, is also routine and predictable, which is not to say that the people suffering from these conditions should be treated in a routine standardized manner. However, in some areas, healthcare staff face very high levels of uncertainty. In hospital medicine, for example, the patient's disease may be masked, difficult to diagnose, the results of investigations not clear cut, the treatment complicated by multiple comorbidities and so on. Here, a tolerance for uncertainty on the part of the staff, and indeed the patient, is vital. The nature of the work is very different from most industrial settings.

A related issue is that pilots and nuclear power plant operators spend most of their time performing routine control and monitoring activities, rather than actually doing things. For the most part the plane or the plant runs itself, and the pilot or operator is simply checking and watching. Pilots do, of course, take over manual control and need to be highly skilled, but actual 'hands on' work is a relatively small part of their work (Reason, 1997). In contrast, much of healthcare work is very 'hands on' and, in consequence, much more liable to error. The most routine tasks, putting up drips, putting lines in to deliver drugs, all require skill and carry an element of risk. Finally, and most obviously, passengers in trains and planes are generally in reasonable health. Many patients are very young, very old, very sick or very disturbed, and in different ways vulnerable to even small problems in their care.

The organization of safety in healthcare and other industries

As well as comparing specific work activities, we can also consider more general organizational similarities and differences. David Gaba (2000) has identified a number of ways in which the approach to safety in healthcare differs from other safety-critical industries. First, most high risk industries are very centralized with a clear control structure; healthcare, even national systems such as in England, is fragmented and decentralized in comparison. This makes it very difficult to regulate and standardize equipment and basic procedures; standardizing the design of infusion pumps, for instance, is highly desirable but very difficult to achieve in practice. Second, other industries put much more emphasis on standardizing both the training and the work process. Rene Amalberti (2001) has pointed out that it is a mark of the success and safety of commercial aviation that we do not worry about who the pilot is on a particular flight; we assume they, in his phrase, are 'equivalent actors', who are interchangeable. This is not an insult, but a compliment to their training and professionalism. In healthcare the autonomy of the individual physician, while absolutely necessary at a clinical level, can also be a threat to safety (Gaba, 2000; Amalberti et al., 2005). If nurses, for instance, are constantly responding to different practices of senior physicians in intensive care, unnecessary variability and potential for error is introduced.

Third, safe organizations devote a great deal of attention and resources to ensuring that workers have the necessary preparation and skills for the job; medical school is a long and intensive training, but a young doctor will still arrive on a new ward and be expected to pick up local procedures informally – sometimes with catastrophic consequences, as we will see in the next chapter. Finally, Gaba points out that healthcare is comparatively unregulated compared to other industries. In many countries there is a host of regulatory bodies, each with responsibility for some aspect of education, training or clinical practice. However, regulation still has very little effect day to day on clinical practice. All of these issues are complex and we will return to many of them later in the book. For now however, it is sufficient to note there are many differences, as well as some similarities, between healthcare and other industries in both activity and organization.

What is error?

I kept my tea in the right hand side of a tea caddy for some months and when that was finished kept it in the left, but I always for a week took off the cover of the right hand side, though my hand would sometimes vibrate. Seeing no tea brought back memory.
(CHARLES DARWIN NOTEBOOKS C217 QUOTED IN BROWNE, 2003)

Patient safety is beset by difficulties with terminology and the most intractable problems occur when the term error is used. For instance, you might think that it would be relatively easy to define the term 'prescribing error'. Surely, either a drug is prescribed correctly or not? Yet, achieving a consensus on this term required a full study and several iterations of definitions amongst a group of clinicians, with still room for disagreement (Dean, Barber and Schachter, 2000). Such definitional and classification problems are longstanding and certainly not confined to healthcare. Regrettably, we are not going to resolve the problems here. However, we can at least draw some distinctions and show the different ways that error is defined and discussed. Hopefully this will clear some of the fog that envelops the term and allow us to discern the various uses and misuses in the patient safety literature.

Defining error

In everyday life, recognizing error seems quite straightforward, though admitting it may be harder. My own daily life is accompanied by a plethora of slips, lapses of memory and other 'senior moments', in the charming American phrase, that are often the subject of critical comment from those around me. (How can you have forgotten already?). Immediate slips, such as Darwin's example shown above, are quickly recognized. Other errors may only be recognized long after they occur. You may only realize you took a wrong turning some time later when it becomes clear that you are irretrievably lost. Some errors, such as marrying the wrong person, may only become apparent years later. An important common theme running through all these examples is that an action is only recognized as an error after the event. Human error is a judgement made in hindsight (Woods and Cook, 2002). There is no special class of things we do or don't do that we can designate as errors; it is just that some of the things we do turn out to have undesirable or unwanted consequences. This does not mean that we cannot study error or examine how our otherwise efficient brains lead us astray in some circumstances, but it does suggest that there will not be specific cognitive mechanisms to explain error that are different from those that explain other human thinking and behaviour.

Eric Hollnagel (1998) points out that the term error has historically been used in three different senses: as a cause of something (plane crash due to human error), as the action or event itself (giving the wrong drug) or as the outcome of an action (the death of a patient). The distinctions are not absolute in that many uses of the term involve both cause and consequence to different degrees, but they do have a very different emphasis. For instance, the UK National Patient Safety Agency has found that patients equate 'medical error' with a preventable adverse outcome for the patient. Terms like 'adverse event', although technically much clearer, just seem like an evasion or a way of masking the fact that someone was responsible.

The most precise definition of error, and most in accord with everyday usage, is one that ties it to observable behaviours and actions. As a working definition, Senders and Moray (1991) proposed that an error means that something has been done which:

- was not desired by a set of rules or an external observer;
- led the task or system outside acceptable limits;
- was not intended by the actor.

This definition of error, and other similar ones (Hollnagel, 1998), imply a set of criteria for defining an error. First, there must be a set of rules or standards, either explicitly defined or at least implied and accepted in that environment; second, there must be some kind of failure or 'performance shortfall'; third, the person involved did not intend this and must, at least potentially, have been able to act in a different way. All three of these criteria can be challenged, or at least prove difficult to pin down in practice. Much clinical medicine, for instance, is inherently uncertain and there are frequently no guidelines or protocols to guide treatment. In addition, the failure is not necessarily easy to identify; it is certainly not always clear, at least at the time, when a diagnosis is wrong or when at what point blood levels of a drug become dangerously high. Finally, the notion of intention, and in theory at least being able to act differently, is challenged by the fact that people's behaviour is often influenced by factors, such as fatigue or peer pressure, which they may not be aware of and have little control over. So, while the working definition is reasonable, we should be aware of its limitations and the difficulties of applying it in practice.

Classifying errors

Classifications of error can be approached from several different perspectives. An error can be described in terms of the behaviour involved, the underlying psychological processes, and in terms of the factors that contributed to it. Giving the wrong drug, for instance, can be classified in terms of the behaviour (the act of giving the drug), in psychological terms as a slip (discussed below) and be due, at least in part, to fatigue. To have any hope of a coherent classification systems these distinctions have to be kept firmly in mind, as some schemes developed in healthcare mix these perspectives together indiscriminately.

Human factors experts working in high-risk industries often have to estimate the likelihood of accidents occurring when preparing a 'safety case'

7

ιe regulator that all reasonable safety precautions have been ιaration of a safety case usually involves considering what errors ιw often and in what combinations. To facilitate this, a number ι schemes have been proposed. One of the most detailed, incorporating useful features of many previous schemes, is the one used in the Predictive Human Error Analysis (PHEA) technique (Embrey, 1992; Hollnagel, 1998) (Table 7.1).

PHEA has been developed for industries where the actions of a particular person controlling operations can be fairly closely specified (operations here meaning the operation of the system, not the surgical type). The scheme is deliberately generic, a high level classification scheme which can be applied in many different environments. It covers errors of omission (failure to carry out an operation), errors of commission (doing the wrong thing) and extraneous error (doing something unnecessary). Generally there is quite high agreement when independent judges are asked to classify errors with schemes of this kind,

Table 7.1 PHEA classification of errors

Planning errors	Incorrect plan executed
	Correct, but inappropriate plan executed
	Correct plan, but too soon or too late
	Correct plan, but in the wrong order
Operation errors	Operation too long/too short
	Operation incorrectly timed
	Operation in wrong direction
	Operation too little/too much
	Right operation, wrong object
	Wrong operation, right object
	Operation omitted
	Operation incomplete
Checking errors	Check omitted
	Check incomplete
	Right check on wrong object
	Wrong check on right object
	Check incorrectly timed
Retrieval errors	Information not obtained
	Wrong information obtained
	Information retrieval incomplete
Communication errors	Information not communicated
	Wrong information communicated
	Information communication incomplete
Selection errors	Selection omitted
	Wrong selection made

From Hollnagel, 1998

which at least gives a starting point in describing the phenomena of interest. Looking at such schemes gives one new respect for human beings; the wonder is not how many errors occur but, given the numerous opportunities for messing things up, how often things go well.

Conceptual clarity about error is not just an obsession of academics; it has real practical consequences. Classifications of medical errors often leave a lot to be desired, frequently grouping and muddling very different types of concept. Reporting systems, for instance, may ask the person reporting to define the error made, or select the type of error from a list. In one system I reviewed the causes of an error including 'wrong drug given', 'a mistake' and 'fatigue', and the clinician was meant to choose between them. In reality, any or all of these might be applicable. If the clinician is not presented with a sensible set of choices, there is no hope of learning anything useful from the incident.

Describing and classifying error in medicine

Generic error classification schemes may seem very remote from healthcare, too abstract, too conceptual and only of interest to researchers. However, PHEA maps quite easily onto many standard clinical practices. Consider the checking of anaesthetic equipment before an operation; there are several different types of check to be made, but all the ways of failing to check probably fall into one of the five types listed in PHEA. In operating the anaesthetic equipment, anaesthetic drugs can be given for too long, at the wrong time, the dials can be turned in the wrong direction, the wrong dial can be turned and so on. Communication between the surgeon and anaesthetist about, say, blood loss might not occur, might be incomplete or be misleading. Realizing the importance of clarity and classification, some researchers have sought to clarify the definitions in use and build classification schemes that everyone can agree on. We will briefly examine work on prescribing error and diagnostic error, which present contrasting challenges of both classification and understanding.

Prescribing error

Studies suggest that prescribing errors occur in 0.4–1.9% of all medication orders written and cause harm in about 1% of inpatients. A major problem with interpreting and comparing these studies is that many of the definitions of prescribing error used are either ambiguous or not given at all. To bring some rigour and clarity to the area, Bryony Dean and colleagues (Dean, Barber and Schachter, 2000) carried out a study to determine a practitioner based definition of prescribing error, using successive iterations of definitions until broad agreement was obtained. The final agreed list is shown in Table 7.2 and we can see that this definition of prescribing error covers a wide range of specific failures. A strength of working 'from the ground up' and basing such decisions on the views of pharmacists, doctors and nurses is that the final definition is clinically meaningful and the descriptions of acts and omissions that result are also clearly defined.

Table 7.2 Varieties of prescribing error

Prescriptions inappropriate for patient	Drug that is contraindicated
	Patient has allergy to drug
	Ignoring potentially significant drug
	Inadequate dose
	Drug dose will give serum levels above/below therapeutic range
	Not altering drug in response to serum levels outside therapeutic range
	Continuing drug in presence of adverse reaction
	Prescribing two drugs where one will do
	Prescribing a drug for which there is no indication
Pharmaceutical issues	Intravenous infusion with wrong dilution
	Excessive concentration of drug to be given by peripheral line
Failure to communicate essential information	Prescribing a drug, dose or route that is not that intended
	Writing illegibly
	Writing a drug's name using abbreviations
	Writing an ambiguous medication order
	Prescribing 'one tablet' of a drug that is available in more than one strength
	Omission of route of administration for drug that can be given by more than one route
	Prescribing an intermittent infusion without specifying duration
	Omission of signature
Transcription errors	Not prescribing drug in hospital that patient was taking prior to admission
	Continuing a GPs prescribing error when patient is admitted to hospital
	Transcribing incorrectly when rewriting patient's chart
	Writing 'milligrams' when 'micrograms' was intended
	Writing a prescription for discharge that unintentionally deviates from in hospital prescription
	On admission to hospital writing a prescription that unintentionally deviates from pre-admission prescription

Reprinted from *The Lancet*, **359**, no. 9315, Bryony Dean, Mike Schachter, Charles Vincent and Nick Barber. "Causes of prescribing errors in hospital inpatients: a prospective study." [232–237], © 2002, with permission from Elsevier.

The descriptions are, as the table shows, sensibly couched in terms of behaviour as far as possible, though concepts such as 'intention' also need to be included. Many of the specific types of prescribing error do fall into the general categories in the PHEA scheme. There are, for instance, failures of planning (not prescribing what was intended), failures of operation (writing illegibly, using abbreviations), failures of communication of various kinds (transcription errors) and so on. There may not be a complete mapping of one scheme to another, but comparing the two schemes does show the relationship between generic and specific schemes and that the same errors can, even in behavioural terms, be classified in more than one scheme.

Diagnostic errors

Prescribing errors are a relatively clearly defined type of error in that they do at least refer to a particular act – that is writing or otherwise recording a drug, a dose and route of administration. Diagnosis in contrast is not so much an act as a thought process; whereas prescribing happens at a particular time and place, diagnosis is often more an unfolding story. Diagnostic errors are much harder to specify and the category 'diagnostic error' wider and less defined. The list of examples of diagnostic error in Table 7.3 shows how the label 'diagnostic error' may indicate either a relatively discrete event (missing a fracture when looking at an X-ray) or something that happens over months or even years (missed lung cancer because of failures in the co-ordination of

Table 7.3 Examples of diagnostic errors

Examples	Comment on error
Errors of uncertainty (no-fault errors)	
Missed diagnosis of appendicitis in elderly patient with no abdominal pain	Unusual presentation of disease
Missed diagnosis of Lyme disease in an era when this was unknown	Limitations of medical knowledge
Wrong diagnosis of common cold in patient found to have mononucleosis	Diagnosis reasonable but incorrect
Errors precipitated by system factors (system errors)	
Missed colon cancer because flexible sigmoidoscopy performed instead of colonoscopy	Lack of appropriate equipment or results
Fracture missed by emergency department	Radiologist not available to check initial assessment
Delay in diagnosis due to ward team not informed of patient's admission	Failure to co-ordinate care
Errors of thinking and reasoning (cognitive errors)	
Wrong diagnosis of ventricular tachycardia on ECG with electrical artefact simulating dysrhythymia	Inadequate knowledge
Missed diagnosis of breast cancer because of failure to perform breast examination	Faulty history taking and inadequate assessment
Wrong diagnosis of degenerative arthritis (no further test ordered) in a patient with septic arthritis	Premature decision made before other possibilities considered

Adapted from Graber, Gordon and Franklin, 2002

outpatient care). These examples show that the term error can be an over-simplification of very complex phenomena and sometimes a long story of undiagnosed illness.

Diagnostic errors have not yet received the attention they deserve, considering their probable importance in leading to harm or sub-standard treatment for patients; the emphasis on systems has led us away from examining core clinical skills such as diagnosis and decision making. Diagnostic errors are also very difficult to study, being hard to define, hard to fix at a particular point in time and not directly observable; they have recently been described as the 'next frontier' for patient safety (Newman-Toker and Pronovost, 2009). Graber, Gordon and Franklin (2002), amongst others, have argued for a sustained attack on diagnostic errors, dividing them into three broad types which require different kinds of intervention to reduce them (Table 7.3). They distinguish 'no-fault errors', which arise because of the difficulty of diagnosing the particular condition, 'system errors' primarily due to organizational and technical problems and 'cognitive errors' due to faulty thinking and reasoning.

We should be cautious about accepting a sharp division between no-fault, system and cognitive errors, as this distinction, while broadly useful, is potentially misleading. First, separating out some errors as 'cognitive' is slightly curious; in a sense all error is 'cognitive' in that all our thinking and action involves cognition. The implication of the term cognitive error is really to locate the cause of the diagnostic error in failures of judgement and decision making. Second, the term 'system error', although widely used, is to my mind a rather ghastly and nonsensical use of language. Systems may fail, break down or fail to function, but only people make errors. System error as a term is usually a rather unsatisfactory shorthand for factors that contributed to the failure to make an accurate diagnosis, such as a radiologist not being available or poor co-ordination of care. In reality, diagnosis is always an interaction between the patient and the doctor or other professional, who are both influenced by the system in which they work.

The psychology of error

In the preceding two sections error has mainly been examined in terms of behaviour and outcome. However, errors can also be examined from a psychological perspective. The psychological analyses to be described are mainly concerned with failures at a particular time and probe the underlying mechanisms of error. There is therefore not necessarily a simple correspondence with medical errors which, as discussed, may refer to events happening over a period of time. In his analysis of different types of error, James Reason (1990) divides them into two broad types of error: slips and lapses, which are errors of action, and mistakes which are, broadly speaking, errors of knowledge or planning. Reason also discusses violations which, as distinct from error, are intentional acts which, for one reason or another, deviate from the usual or expected course of action.

Slips and lapses

Slips and lapses occur when a person knows what they want to do, but the action does not turn out as they intended. Slips relate to observable actions and are associated with attentional failures, whereas lapses are internal events and associated with failures of memory. Slips and lapses occur during the largely automatic performance of some routine task, usually in familiar surroundings. They are almost invariably associated with some form of distraction, either from the person's surrounding or their own preoccupation with something in mind. When Charles Darwin went to the wrong tea caddy, he had a lapse of memory. If, on the other hand, he had remembered where the tea was but had been momentarily distracted and knocked the caddy over rather than opening it, he would have made a slip.

Mistakes

Slips and lapses are errors of action; you intend to do something, but it does not go according to plan. With mistakes, the actions may go entirely as planned but the plan itself deviates from some adequate path towards its intended goal. Here the failure lies at a higher level: with the mental processes involved in planning, formulating intentions, judging and problem solving (Reason, 1990). If a doctor treats someone with chest pain as if they have a myocardial infarction, when in fact they do not, then this is a mistake. The intention is clear, the action corresponds with the intention, but the plan was wrong.

Rule based mistakes occur when the person already knows some rule or procedure, acquired as the result of training or experience. Rule based mistakes may occur through applying the wrong rule, such as treating someone for asthma when you should follow the guidelines for pneumonia. Alternatively, the mistake may occur because the procedure itself is faulty; deficient clinical guidelines for instance.

Knowledge based mistakes occur in novel situations, where the solution to a problem has to be worked out on the spot. For instance, a doctor may simply be unfamiliar with the clinical presentation of a particular disease, or there may be multiple diagnostic possibilities and no clear way at the time of choosing between them; a surgeon may have to guess at the source of the bleeding and make an understandable mistake in their assessment in the face of considerable stress and uncertainty. In none of these cases does the clinician have a good 'mental model' of what is happening to base their decisions on, still less a specific rule or procedure to follow.

Violations

Errors are, by definition, unintended in the sense that we do not want to make errors. Violations, in contrast, are deliberate deviations from safe operating practices, procedures, standards or rules. This is not to say that people intend that there should be a bad outcome, as when someone deliberately sabotages a piece of equipment; usually people hope that the violation of procedures won't matter on this occasion or will actually help get the job done. Violations differ from errors in several important ways. Whereas errors are primarily due to our human limitations in thinking and remembering, violations are more closely linked with our attitudes, motivation or the work environment. The social context of violations is very important and understanding them, and if necessary curbing them, requires attention to the culture of the wider organization, as well as the attitudes of the people concerned.

Reason (1990) distinguishes three types of violations:

- A routine violation is basically cutting corners for one reason or another, perhaps to save time or simply to get on to another more urgent task.
- A necessary violation occurs when a person flouts a rule because it seems the only way to get the job done. For example, a nurse may give a drug which should be double checked by another nurse, but there is no one else available. The nurse will probably give the drug, knowingly violating procedure, but in the patient's interest. This can, of course, have disastrous consequences, as we will see in the next chapter.
- Optimizing violations which are for personal gain, sometimes just to get off work early or, more sinister, to alleviate boredom, 'for kicks'. Think of a young surgeon carrying out a difficult operation in the middle of the night, without supervision, when the case could easily wait until morning. The motivation is partly to gain experience, to test oneself out, but there may be a strong element of the excitement of sailing close to the wind in defiance of the senior surgeon's instructions.

The psychological perspective on error has been very influential in medicine, forming a central plank of one of the most important papers in the patient safety literature (Leape, 1994). Errors and violations are also a component of the organizational accident model, discussed in the next chapter. However, attempts to use these concepts in practice in healthcare, in reporting systems for instance, have often foundered. Why is this? One important reason is that in practice the distinction between slips, mistakes and violations is not always clear, either to an observer or the person concerned. The relationship between the observed behaviour, which can be easily described, and the psychological mechanism, are often hard to discern. Giving the wrong drug might be a slip (attention wandered and picked up the wrong syringe), a mistake (misunderstanding about the drug to be given) or even a violation (deliberate oversedation of a difficult patient). The concepts are not easy to put into practice, except in circumstances where the action, context and personal characteristics of those involved can be quite carefully explored.

Perspectives on error and error reduction

As must now be clear, error has many different facets and the subject of error, and how to reduce error, can be approached in different ways. While there are a multitude of different taxonomies and error reduction systems, we can discern some broad general perspectives or 'error paradigms' as they are sometimes called. Following Deborah Lucas (1997) and James Reason (1997) four perspectives can be distinguished: the engineering perspective, psychological, individual and organizational. The psychological perspective has already been discussed and we will not consider it further here. The various perspectives are seldom explicitly discussed in medicine but, once you have read about them, you will certainly have seen them in action in discussions of safety in healthcare. Each perspective leads to different kinds of solutions to the problem of error. Some people just blame doctors for errors and think discipline and retraining is the answer; some want to automate everything; others put everything down to 'the system'. Each perspective has useful features, but unthinking adherence to any particular one is unlikely to be productive.

Engineering perspective

The central characteristic of the engineering perspective is that human beings are viewed as potentially unreliable components of the system. In its extreme form, this perspective implies that humans should be engineered out of a system by increasing automation, so avoiding the problem of human error. In its less extreme form, the engineering approach regards human beings as important parts of complex systems, but places a great deal of emphasis on the ways people and technology interact. For instance, the design of anaesthetic monitors needs to be carefully considered if the wealth of information displayed is not to lead to misinterpretation and errors at times of crisis.

In the manufacture of computers and cars on assembly lines, less human involvement in repetitive tasks has undoubtedly led to higher reliability. However, automation does not always lead to improvements in safety and may actually introduce new problems – the 'ironies of automation' as Lisanne Bainbridge expressed it (Bainbridge, 1987). In particular, the operators of equipment become much less 'hands on' and spend more time monitoring and checking. This is well expressed in the apocryphal story of the pilot of a commercial airliner who turned to his co-pilot and said, of the onboard computer controlling the plane, 'I wonder what it's doing now?' There have, however, been some real life tragedies in which automation led human beings astray with tragic consequences (Box 7.3).

BOX 7.3 The *Vincennes* incident

In 1988, the USS *Vincennes* erroneously shot down a civilian Airbus carrying 290 passengers. The *Vincennes* had been fitted with a very sophisticated Tactical Information Co-ordinator (TIC), which warned of a hostile aircraft close to the ship. The captain also received a warning that the aircraft might be commercial but, under great time pressure, and considering the safety of ship and crew he accepted the TIC warning and shot down the airliner. In another US warship with, paradoxically, less sophisticated warning system, the crew relied less on the automated system and decided the aircraft was civilian.

(THIS ARTICLE WAS PUBLISHED IN *HUMAN FACTORS IN SAFETY CRITICAL SYSTEMS*, LUCAS D, "CAUSES OF HUMAN ERROR". 38–39, COPYRIGHT ELSEVIER. 1997)

Individual perspective: the person model

In daily life, errors are frequently attributed to stupidity, carelessness, forget-fulness, recklessness and other personal defects. The implication is that the person who makes an error has certain characteristics which produce the error and, furthermore, that these characteristics are under their control and they are therefore to blame for the errors they make. This is error seen from the individual perspective; when applied to understanding accidents; James Reason refers to this as the 'person model' (Reason, 2000).

Efforts to reduce error are, from this perspective, targeted at individuals and involve exhortations to 'do better', retraining, or adding new rules and procedures. For errors with more serious consequences, more severe sanctions come into play, such as naming and shaming, disciplinary action, suspension, media condemnation and so on. Legal perspectives on error, and the whole notion of medical negligence, are built on the concepts of personal responsibility, fault, blame and redress. This view is strongly entrenched in healthcare, as seen by the immediate suspension of nurses who make serious errors, with reflection on the incident and investigation coming later, if at all. Blame, when thoughtless and automatic, penalizes individuals sometimes to the point of destroying careers. However, it is also a major barrier to improving safety, hence the importance given to creating an 'open and fair culture', discussed later in the book.

The folly of the crude person model is apparent. However, it is important not to swing to the other extreme and attribute everything to 'the system'. Rather one needs to preserve individual accountability but understand the interplay between the person, the technology and the organization. Individual characteristics may well play a part in the occurrence of an error or in a poor clinical outcome. For instance, motivation and attitude are important determinants of how people behave and whether they work conscientiously. A strong sense of personal responsibility is fundamental to being a good clinician. Patient safety is not a never-never land in which everyone is always motivated and principled. People who deliberately behave recklessly and without regard to their patients' welfare deserve to be blamed, whether or not they make errors.

Organizational perspective: the system model

The quote from James Reason earlier in this chapter perfectly expresses the essence of the organizational view of accidents, often referred to in healthcare as the 'system' model. The essential idea underlying this approach is that errors and human behaviour cannot be understood in isolation, but only in relation to the context in which people are working. Clinical staff are influenced by the nature of the task they are carrying out, the team they work in, their working environment and the wider organizational context; these are the system factors (Vincent, Adams and Stanhope, 1998). From this perspective errors are seen, not so much as the product of personal falliblity, but as consequences of more general problems in the working environment.

In considering how people contribute to accidents therefore we have to distinguish between 'active failures' and 'latent conditions' (Reason, 1997). The active failures are unsafe acts of various kinds (errors and violations) that have already been described. These are committed by people at the 'sharp end' of the system who are actually operating it or working with a patient. The active failures are wrongly opening the bow door of a ferry, shutting down the wrong engine on an airliner, or misreading the anaesthetic monitor. These unsafe acts can, and often do, have immediate consequences.

However, these unsafe acts all occur in a particular context and they can be precipitated by what Reason terms 'latent conditions'. Perhaps the ferry company has become progressively more lax, and the procedures for opening the bow doors are ill defined or ambiguous; the cockpit design and warning signals are misleading; syringe labels do not sufficiently distinguish dangerous drugs; anaesthetists are working excessive hours, becoming tired and less vigilant. These are the latent conditions that stem from decisions made by designers, people who write procedures and guidelines, senior management and others. Note that, while errors can be made by anyone, it is not easy to foresee the long-term effects of design or management decisions, which are themselves made in the face of many competing demands. For instance, there may be pressure on surgical teams to clear the waiting lists of patients waiting for operations. These are, in some respects, well intentioned decisions and yet, pushed too far, make the delivery of healthcare unsafe. Decisions made years before, such as in the design of instruments, can have consequences later when a particular combination of circumstances puts the people and the system under stress. The system model, and its application in healthcare, will be discussed further in the next chapter, when we examine the causes of harm to patients in more detail.

Error, blame and censure

The picture of error and its causes that is emerging is rather different from our everyday understanding of error, accidents and the behaviour of skilled professionals. We have a comforting picture of a world in which we are in safe hands, cared for by infallible professionals trained to perfection who, while of course compassionate, are able to perform with machine-like regularity and precision. Errors, in this scenario, are caused only by recklessness or carelessness and we all too easily blame people who appear to be the cause of accidents.

Without doubt, healthcare has a culture of blame and changing this culture is an essential step in enhancing safety. Yet I have chosen not to discuss the issue of blame until near the end of a chapter on error, which might seem eccentric. The reason is straightforward. The issue of error and blame is often presented without any background understanding of the nature of error and can, at worst, seem to be little more than a plea to be nice to people. More usually it is a very reasonable plea for a fairer and more thoughtful approach to people involved in serious accidents or bad outcomes for patients. However, with more understanding of error and its causes, the arguments for a just and fair culture become much more powerful. Error is frequent, errors are committed by even the best people, error is often precipitated by circumstances beyond our control, indeed is often outside our conscious control; major accidents are seldom due to one person alone and so on. When all these considerations are taken into account, blame becomes not so much morally wrong, as largely irrelevant to the quest for safety. With understanding comes a very different perspective of both the causes of harm to patients and of what an appropriate response might be.

The concept of error: is it useful for the design of safe healthcare systems?

After an entire chapter on error, it may seem still more curious, even perverse, to ask whether the concept of error is useful for patient safety. The heading comes from the title of a chapter written by Jens Rasmussen (Rasmussen, 1997), whose work has influenced every field of safety and who has been a major influence on many of the leading figures in patient safety. We cannot do more than hint at some of his ideas here, but they will set the scene for later chapters on creating safety.

Rasmussen was very influenced in his thinking by his studies of the operators of nuclear power plants (Rasmussen, 2000). Even here, in what one would imagine to be the most highly proceduralized environment, he found enormous flexibility and adaptation to circumstances and departure from guidelines and procedures. This was not because nuclear power workers were especially reckless or wished to endanger others; quite the contrary. The point is that although they were trained in standard procedures and knew about them, they often did not follow them in the practice; rather they tried to get the job done in the way that seemed best at the time. Rasmussen's view of human work is that of our own everyday experience; we are constantly adapting to new circumstances, doing the best we can and coping with a variety of organizational pressures. He further argues, in a wide ranging critique, that error is often an oversimplification, that the accident investigator can never really capture the choices and conflicts facing those involved in the accident, that error often plays a crucial role in learning and that recovery from error is as worthy of study as error. Studying errors and accidents, while certainly illuminating, will never be sufficient. We need to understand how people work and how they adapt to pressures and circumstances.

Furthermore, because of the shifting and changing nature of systems, safety measures themselves affect the system in unanticipated ways. When radar was introduced to improve safety at sea, captains of ships (and their owners) were more able to anticipate bad weather. They were therefore more able to travel in bad weather, could travel more efficiently and thus increase the number of journeys made. A measure to improve safety therefore simultaneously increased danger by exposing ships to worse weather. In a similar vein, Morel, Amalberti and Chauvin (2008) have recently studied deep-sea fishing, an occupation probably with one of the worst recorded accident rates. Captains of deep-sea boats embraced new safety technology to detect other boats more accurately and so avoid collisions. However, they used the technology to knowingly take more risks in the pursuit of larger catches. Paradoxically, each time a system becomes safer, there is more pressure for increased performance, cutting corners and the eventual degrading of safety – until the next accident occurs. Anaesthesia, being generally extremely safe, is vulnerable to pressure from patients and management to achieve more and so put safety at risk (Healzer, Howard and Gaba, 1998).

Reading and reflecting on this view helps one to understand that safety in a system is a much more fluid and dynamic concept than is often thought. Many charged with improving safety regard increasing standardization, more automation, better training and a general tightening up of procedures as the way forward. While we should not underestimate the importance of these approaches, particularly in disorganized healthcare systems, Rasmussen helps us understand that this can never be a complete solution. Safety is, both at the individual and organizational level, very much a question of steering a course in a shifting and changing landscape, rather than setting standards and expecting people to stick to them for all time. The people who work in the system will always be adapting to circumstances, sometimes degrading safety in the process, but more often enhancing safety by their anticipation and improvization in a complex, changing environment.

References

Amalberti, R. (2001) The paradoxes of almost totally safe transportation systems. *Safety Science*, **37**, 109–126.

Amalberti, R., Auroy, Y., Berwick, D. and Barach, P. (2005) Five system barriers to achieving ultrasafe health care. *Annals of Internal Medicine*, **142**(9), 756–764.

Bainbridge, L. (1987) Ironies of automation, in *New Technology and Human Error* (eds J. Rasmussen, K. Duncanand J. Leplat), John Wiley & Sons, Chichester, pp. 271–283.

Browne, J. (2003) *Charles Darwin. Voyaging*, Pimlico Books, London.

Cook, R.I., Woods, D.D. and Miller, C.A. (1998) *A Tale of Two Stories: Contrasting Views of Patient Safety*, US National Patient Safety Foundation.

Dean, B., Barber, N. and Schachter, M. (2000) What is a prescribing error? *Quality in Health Care*, **9**, 232–237.

Embrey, D.E. (1992) *Quantitative and Qualitative Prediction of Human Error in Safety Assessments*, Institute of Chemical Engineering, Rugby.

Gaba, D.M. (2000) Anaesthesiology as a model for patient safety in healthcare. *British Medical Journal*, **320**(7237), 785–788.

Graber, M., Gordon, R. and Franklin, N. (2002) Reducing diagnostic errors in medicine: what's the goal? *Academic Medicine*, **77**(10), 981–992.

Healzer, J.M., Howard, S.K. and Gaba, D.M. (1998) Attitudes toward production pressure and patient safety: a survey of anesthesia residents. *Journal of Clinical Monitoring and Computing*, **14**(2), 145–146.

Hollnagel, E. (1998) *Cognitive Reliability and Error Analysis Method*, Elsevier, Oxford.

Leape, L.L. (1994) Error in medicine. *Journal of the American Medical Association*, **272**(23), 1851–1857.

Lucas, D. (1997) The causes of human error, in *Human Factors in Safety Critical Systems* (eds F. Redmill and J. Rajan), Butterworth Heinemann, Oxford.

Morel, G., Amalberti, R. and Chauvin, C. (2008) Articulating the differences between safety and resilience: the decision-making process of professional sea-fishing skippers. *Human Factors*, **50**(1), 1–16.

Newman-Toker, D.E. and Pronovost, P.J. (2009) Diagnostic errors – the next frontier for patient safety. *JAMA: The Journal of the American Medical Association*, **301**(10), 1060–1062.

Rasmussen, J. (1997) Risk management in a dynamic society: a modelling problem. *Safety Science*, **27**, 183–213.

Rasmussen, J. (2000) The concept of human error. Is it useful for the design of safe systems in healthcare, in *Safety in Medicine* (eds C.A. Vincent and B. de Mol), Elsevier, Oxford.

Reason, J.T. (1990) *Human Error*, Cambridge University Press, New York.

Reason, J.T. (1997) *Managing the Risks of Organisational Accidents*, Ashgate, Aldershot.

Reason, J.T. (2000) Human error: models and management. *British Medical Journal*, **320**, 768–770.

Senders, J.W. and Moray, N. (1991) *Human Error: Course, Prediction and Reduction*, Lawrence Earlbaum Associates, Hillsdale, NJ.

US National Aeronautics and Space Administration (2003) Report of the Columbia Accident Investigation Board.

Vincent, C., Taylor-Adams, S. and Stanhope, N. (1998) Framework for analysing risk and safety in clinical medicine. *British Medical Journal*, **316**(7138), 1154–1157.

Woods, D.D. and Cook, R.I. (2002) Nine steps to move forward from error. *Cognition, Technology & Work*, **4**, 137–144.

CHAPTER 8
Understanding how things go wrong

At approximately 17.00 hrs on Thursday 4th January 2001, Mr David James, a day case patient on Ward E17 at the Queen's Medical Centre Nottingham (QMC), was prepared for an intrathecal (spinal) administration of chemotherapy as part of his medical maintenance programme following successful treatment of leukaemia.

After carrying out a lumbar puncture and administering the correct cytotoxic therapy (Cytosine) under the supervision of the Specialist Registrar Dr Mitchell, Dr North, a Senior House Officer, was passed a second drug by Dr Mitchell to administer to Mr James, which he subsequently did. However, the second drug, Vincristine, should never be administered by the intrathecal route because it is almost always fatal.

Unfortunately, whilst emergency treatment was provided very quickly in an effort to rectify the error, Mr James died at 8.10 a.m. on 2 February 2001.
(TOFT, 2001)

Following an Internal Enquiry at QMC, Professor Brian Toft was commissioned by the Chief Medical Officer of England to conduct an enquiry into the death and to advise on the areas of vulnerability in the process of intrathecal injection of these drugs and ways in which fail-safes might be built in (Toft, 2001). The orientation of the enquiry was therefore, from the outset, one of learning and change. We will use this sad story, and Brian Toft's thoughtful report, to introduce the subject of analysing cases. Although the names of those involved were made public, I have changed them in the narrative, as identifying the people again at this distance serves no useful purpose. This case acts as an excellent, though tragic, illustration of models of organizational accidents and systems thinking.

The systems view of medical error was not, however, the approach taken by the courts. Dr Mitchell was charged with manslaughter, pleaded guilty and was sentenced to eight months imprisonment. David James's parents considered the sentence ridiculous, pointing out that he would have probably served a longer sentence for theft of hospital equipment (Balen, 2004). The anger and

---

Patient Safety, 2nd edition. By Charles Vincent. Published 2010 by Blackwell Publishing Ltd.

desire for justice is more than understandable and some would argue that no one, in whatever profession, should be exempt from charges of manslaughter. Conversely, criminalizing fatal medical mistakes and destroying careers and people may not actually help us improve patient safety. As Dr Mitchell said, when interviewed by police, 'I know it's a lame excuse, but I am a human being' (Holbrook, 2003). The proper role of the law in healthcare is too complex an issue to be discussed properly here, and in any event heavily dependent on culture and wider societal attitudes and values. However, we should note the contrast between, on the one hand, the judicial view of error and the concept of manslaughter and, on the other, the view that emerges from Brian Toft's enquiry. After considering the full circumstances of the case and the way the odds stacked up against the unfortunate patient and doctors involved in this tragedy, the reader can reappraise the verdicts.

Background to the incident

Provided Vincristine is administered intravenously (IV), it is a powerful and useful drug in the fight against leukaemia. The dangers of inadvertent intrathecal administration of Vincristine are well known: there are product warnings to that effect, a literature that stresses the dangers and well publicized previous cases. Medical staff at QMC had put a number of measures in place to prevent inadvertent intrathecal use, and it was clear that these precautions were taken seriously. There was a standard written protocol which, at the request of hospital staff, had been changed so that Cytosine and Vincristine would be administered on different days to avoid any potentially fatal confusion. Drugs for intravenous and for intrathecal use were also supplied separately to the wards, again to reduce the chances of mixing up the different types of drug. Nevertheless, due to a combination of circumstances, all these defences were breached and Mr James died (Box 8.1).

BOX 8.1 The death of David James

Mr James arrived on the ward at about 4.00 p.m.; he was late for his chemotherapy, but staff tried to accommodate him. The pharmacist for the ward had made an earlier request that the Cytosine should be sent up and that the Vincristine should be 'sent separately' the following day. The pharmacy made up the drugs correctly and they were put on separate shelves in the pharmacy refrigerator. During the afternoon the ward day case co-ordinator went to the pharmacy and was given a clear bag containing two smaller bags each containing a syringe – one Vincristine and one Cytosine. She did not know they should not be in the same bag.

Dr Mitchell was informed and approached by Dr North to supervise the procedure, as demanded by the protocol. When it had been established that Mr James's blood count was satisfactory, Dr Mitchell told Dr North that they would go ahead with Mr James's chemotherapy. The staff nurse went to the ward refrigerator and removed the transparent plastic bag, placed there by the day case co-ordinator, within which were two separate transparent packets each one containing a syringe. She noted that the name 'David James' was printed on each of the syringe labels, delivered it and went to carry on her work.

Dr Mitchell looked at the prescription chart noting that the patient's name, drugs and dosages corresponded with the information on the labels attached to the syringes. He did not, however, notice that the administration of Vincristine was planned for the following day or that its route of administration was intravenous. Dr Mitchell, anticipating a cytotoxic drugs system similar to the one at his previous place of work had presumed that, as both drugs had come up to the ward together, both were planned for intrathecal use. He had previously administered two types of chemotherapy intrathecally and it did not therefore seem unusual.

A lumbar puncture was carried out successfully and samples of cerebro spinal fluid taken for analysis. Dr Mitchell then read out aloud the name of the patient, the drug and the dose from the label on the first syringe and then handed it to Dr North. Dr Mitchell did not, however, read out the route of administration. Dr North, having received the syringe, now asked if the drug was 'Cytosine', which Dr Mitchell confirmed. Dr North then removed the cap at the bottom of the syringe and screwed it onto the spinal needle after which he injected the contents of the syringe.

Having put down the first syringe, Dr Mitchell handed the second syringe containing Vincristine to Dr North, again reading out aloud the name of the patient, the drug and dosage. Once again, he did not read out the route of administration. However, Dr Mitchell could not later recall if he:

. . .actually said the word 'Vincristine' but once again I had clearly fixed in my mind that the drug was Methotrexate and not a drug for administration other than intrathecally. If I had consciously appreciated that the drug was Vincristine I would have stopped the procedure immediately and would never have allowed Dr North to administer it.

Dr Mitchell could not explain the fact that he mentally substituted the word 'Methotrexate' for 'Vincristine', except for the fact that his mindset was that drugs for administration by a route other than intrathecal would simply not be available at the same time.

Dr North was surprised when he was passed a second syringe, because on the only other occasion that he had performed a supervised intrathecal injection only one syringe had been used. However, he assumed that on this occasion that '. . .the patient was either at a different stage in his treatment or was on a different treatment regime than the other patient.' Dr North, with the second syringe in his hand, said to Dr Mitchell 'Vincristine?' Dr Mitchell replied in the affirmative. Dr North then said 'intrathecal Vincristine?' Dr Mitchell again replied in the affirmative. After which Dr North removed the cap at the bottom of the syringe and screwed it onto the spinal needle. He then administered the contents of the syringe to Mr James, with ultimately fatal results.

(ADAPTED FROM TOFT, 2001)

Defences, discussed further below, are the means by which systems ensure safety. Sometimes the term is used to encompass almost any safety measure, but it more usually refers to particular administrative, physical or other barriers that protect or warn against deviations from normal practice. Usually these defences and barriers will 'capture' an error and block the trajectory of an accident. In this example, many defences and barriers existed, in the form of procedures and protocols, custom and practice. Administering Cytosine and Vincristine on separate days, for instance, is clearly intended to be a defence against incorrect administration. The separation of the two drugs in pharmacy and the separate delivery to the ward are other examples of defences against error. Having two doctors present checking labels and doses is another check, another barrier against potential disaster. If one or other of these checks fails, the outcome is usually still good. For instance, as long as the correct drug has been delivered, no harm will result if the doctor does not check conscientiously or is distracted while checking. It is nevertheless good practice to always check 'just in case'. Sometimes however, as in this case, a series of defences and barriers are all breached at once. This is brilliantly captured in James Reason's Swiss Cheese (Figure 8.1; Reason, 1990) metaphor of the trajectory of an accident, which gives us the sense of hazard being ever present and occasionally breaking through when all the holes in the Swiss Cheese line up.

Death from spinal injection: a window on the system

From the chronology one can see the classic 'chain of events' leading towards the tragedy. Dr Mitchell was quite new to the ward, unfamiliar with the chemotherapy regime and did not know the patient. The pharmacy somehow, although separating the two drugs, placed them in a single bag. Although the doctors involved can be held responsible for their specific actions and omissions, one can also see that circumstances conspired against them. However, the case also illustrates some much more general themes, issues that pervade healthcare and indeed other organizations, and which are right now, as you read this, putting patients at risk.

Assumption that the system was reliable

The unit where David James died had used these drugs for many years without a major incident. After an event of this kind, and a subsequent analysis, we can

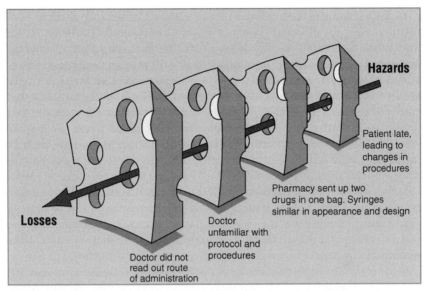

Figure 8.1 Swiss cheese diagram. (Figure adapted from Reason, 1997)

see that the systems, while reasonably robust, were nevertheless far from fault free. Huge reliance was placed on custom and practice and on people simply knowing what they were doing. With experienced staff who know the unit's procedures, this works reasonably well, but when new staff join a unit without clear induction and training, the system inevitably becomes unsafe. In fact, the unit where David James died seems to have been a well run unit, where professionals respected each other's work and things went well on a day-to-day basis. Paradoxically, safety creates its own dangers in that an uneventful routine lulls one into a false sense of security. The safer one becomes, the more necessary it is to remind oneself that the environment is inherently unsafe. This is what James Reason means when he says that the price of safety is chronic unease (Reason, 2001). In fact, the very assumption that all is well can itself be dangerous.

Assumptions about people

Brian Toft introduces his examination of the tacit assumptions of those involved in this case with an apposite quote:

A newcomer assumes that he knows what the organization is about, assumes that others in the setting have the same idea, and practically never bothers to check out these assumptions.

(TOFT, 2001)

Dr Mitchell, the newest member of staff involved, assumed for instance that chemotherapy for different routes of administration could never be on the ward at the same time. He also assumed that he was competent to supervise Dr North, and that Dr North was allowed to give these drugs under supervision. More rashly still, he assumed that Dr North was familiar with Mr James's case and so they did not need to consult his records. Dr North, in his turn, assumed that Dr Mitchell knew what he was doing and was authorized to supervise him. He also assumed that, although he should not have administered the drugs, it was permissible when authorized by Dr Mitchell. This assumptions made by each doctor were unfortunately perfectly matched, each tacitly reassuring the other of their mutual competence and the essential normality of the situation.

Senior doctors on the ward, although not directly involved, made their own assumptions. They assumed that Dr Mitchell knew about the dangers of Vincristine, that there was no need for a formal induction for junior staff, and that Dr Mitchell understood that 'shadowing' meant that he should not administer Cytocine.

None of the assumptions made by anyone was completely unreasonable. We all make such assumptions; in fact we need to just get through the day. People are assumed to be competent who in fact are necessarily 'winging it', doing the best they can in the circumstances. In healthcare this happens all the time as junior staff battle with situations that are unfamiliar to them, or when more senior staff new to a unit feel that they must display more competence than they actually feel. We cannot check everything all the time. However, one can at least realise that many of one's assumptions are likely to be wrong and begin to look, before disaster strikes, for the holes in the Swiss Cheese that permeate one's own organization. We will return to this theme of vigilance and the anticipation of error and hazard later in the book.

The influence of hierarchy on communication

When asked why he did not challenge Dr Mitchell, Dr North said:

First of all, I was not in a position to challenge on the basis of my limited experience of this type of treatment. Second, I was an SHO (junior doctor) and did what I was told to do by the Registrar. He was supervising me and I assumed he had the knowledge to know what was being done. Dr Mitchell was employed as a Registrar by QMC which is a centre for excellence and I did not intend to challenge him.
(TOFT, 2001)

Dr North was in a very difficult position. He assumed Dr Mitchell, as a registrar, knew what he was doing and reasonably points out that he himself had limited experience of the treatment. However, he did know that Vincristine should not be given intrathecally, but he failed to speak up and challenge a senior colleague. Criticism might be made here of both Dr North, for not having the courage to request further checks, and of the Dr Mitchell for not taking the junior doctor's query more seriously and at least halting the procedure while checks were made.

The interaction can also be seen as reflecting the more general problem of authority gradients in clinical teams. In a survey asking whether junior members of a team should be able to question decisions made by senior team members, pilots were almost unanimous in saying that they should (Helmreich, 2000). The willingness of junior pilots to question decisions is not seen as a threat to authority but as an additional defence against possible error. In contrast, in the same survey, almost a quarter of consultant surgeons stated that junior members of staff should not question seniors.

Physical appearance of syringes containing cytotoxic drugs

Syringes containing Vincristine were labelled 'for intravenous injection' and syringes containing Cytosine 'for intrathecal use'. You might think this is fairly clear cut, but on a busy ward with numerous injections being given every day, the design and packaging of drugs is an important determinant of the likelihood of error. In the final few minutes leading up to the fatal injection, the doctors involved were not helped by the similarity in appearance and packaging of the drugs. First, the labels were similar and, while the bold type of the drug and dose stood out there were no other strong visual cues to draw a reader's eye to the significance of the route of administration. Second, the syringes used to administer the two drugs were of similar size; the size of the syringe did not give any clues as to the route of administration to be used. Third, both drugs were clear liquids administered in similar volumes; neither colour nor volume gave any indication of the proper route of administration. Finally, the most dangerous physical aspect of all, in Toft's opinion, is 'that a syringe containing Vincristine can also be connected to the spinal needle that delivers intrathecal drugs to patients. Clearly, once such a connection has been made, the patient's life is in danger as there are no other safeguards in place to prevent the Vincristine from being administered.' (Toft, 2001: p. 14)

We can see therefore, first that the syringes and labelling are unnecessarily similar and second that there are potential design solutions which would reduce, or even eliminate, this type of incident. Most obviously syringes of drugs for intrathecal use could have their own specific, unique fitting, colour and design. While this might not eliminate the possibility of injecting the correct drug, it does add a powerful check to wrong administration. In the same way, fatalities in anaesthesia that resulted from switching oxygen and nitrous oxide supplies were eliminated by the simple expedient of making it impossible to connect the nitrous oxide line to the oxygen input. In daily life, there are thousands of such checks and guides to behaviour. When you fill your car with unleaded petrol you use a small nozzle; larger nozzles for leaded or diesel will simply not fit into the filling pipe. In many areas of healthcare, we still have to learn these lessons and make these obvious improvements.

Unnecessary differences in practice between hospitals

The Joint Council for Clinical Oncology had published guidelines for the administration of cytotoxic chemotherapy. However, these were only advisory, and indeed the Council probably did not have the power to make them mandatory. Thus, what any particular doctor knew about the practice of administering cytotoxic drugs depended, to some extent at least, on local custom and practice. When moving from post to post therefore, new practices are encountered and there is every possibility of confusion, particularly in the first few weeks.

The administration of cytotoxic drugs cries out for the adoption of national standards, aided by good design and training. Simply having the same procedures in place throughout the country would, if they were well designed, in itself be a safety measure. As an example of a much overdue standardization, the British National Patient Safety Agency has done the NHS a great service by the simple expedient of standardizing the hospital crash call number across the country; previously several different numbers were in use.

Much more could, and has, been said about the death of David James. Our purpose here, however, is not to resurrect this particular tragedy or to criticize the people involved, but to use the story to show the complexity of events that lead to harm and illuminate the many facets of patient safety. We can see that a combination of individual errors, assumptions about the workplace, poor design, communication problems, problems in team working and other contributory factors brought about this death. In fact, as we saw in the last chapter, this same blend of personal, design and organizational factors underlies many accidents and disasters. We will now look at this more formally by examining James Reason's model of organizational accidents and its application in healthcare (Reason, 2001).

Aetiology of 'organizational' accidents

Many of the accidents in both healthcare and other industries need to be viewed from a broad systems perspective if they are to be fully understood. The actions and failures of individual people usually play a central role, but their thinking and behaviour is strongly influenced and constrained by their immediate working environment and by wider organizational processes. James Reason has captured the essentials of this understanding in his model of an organizational accident (Reason, 1997). We should emphasise though, before describing the model, that not every slip, lapse or fall needs to be understood in terms of the full organizational framework; some errors are confined to the local context and can be largely explained by individual factors and the characteristics of the particular task at hand. However, major incidents almost always evolve over time, involve a number of people and a considerable number of contributory factors; in these circumstances the organizational model (Figure 8.2) proves very illuminating.

The accident sequence begins (from the left) with the negative consequences of organizational processes, such as planning, scheduling, forecasting, design, maintenance, strategy and policy. The latent conditions so created are transmitted along various organizational and departmental pathways to the

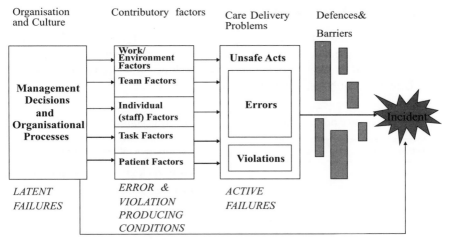

Figure 8.2 Organizational accident model (adapted from Reason, 1997).

workplace (the operating theatre, the ward, etc.), where they create the local conditions that promote the commission of errors and violations (e.g. high workload or poor human equipment interfaces). Many unsafe acts are likely to be committed, but very few of them will penetrate the defences to produce damaging outcomes. The fact that engineered safety features, such as alarms or standard procedures, can be deficient due to latent failures as well as active failures, is shown in the figure by the arrow connecting organizational processes directly to defences.

The model presents the people at the sharp end as the inheritors rather than as the instigators of an accident sequence. Reason points out that this may simply seem as if the 'blame' for accidents has been shifted from the sharp end to the system managers. However, managers too are operating in a complex environment and the effects of their actions are not always apparent; they are no more, and no less, to blame than those at the sharp end of the clinical environment (Reason, 2001). Also, any high level decision, whether within a healthcare organization or made outside it by government or regulatory bodies, is a balance of risks and benefits. Sometimes, such decisions may be obviously flawed, but even prima facie reasonable decisions may later have unfortunate consequences.

As well as highlighting the difficulty of assessing the wisdom of strategic decisions, this analysis also extends the analysis of accidents beyond the boundaries of the organization itself to include the regulatory environment. In healthcare many external organizations, such as manufacturers, government agencies, professional and patient organizations, also impact on the safety of the patient. The model shown in Figure 6.2 relates primarily to a given institution, but the reality is considerably more complex, with the behaviour of other organizations impinging on the accident sequence at many different points.

Seven levels of safety

We have extended Reason's model and adapted it for use in a healthcare setting, classifying the error producing conditions and organizational factors in a single broad framework of factors affecting clinical practice (Vincent, Taylor-Adams and Stanhope, 1998) (Table 8.1).

Table 8.1 Framework of contributory factors influencing clinical practice

Factor Types	Contributory Influencing Factor
Patient Factors	Condition (complexity and seriousness)
	Language and communication
	Personality and social factors
Task and Technology Factors	Task design and clarity of structure
	Availability and use of protocols
	Availability and accuracy of test results
	Decision-making aids
Individual (staff) Factors	Knowledge and skills
	Competence
	Physical and mental health
Team Factors	Verbal communication
	Written communication
	Supervision and seeking help
	Team leadership
Work Environmental Factors	Staffing levels and skills mix
	Workload and shift patterns
	Design, availability and maintenance of equipment
	Administrative and managerial support
	Physical environment
Organizational and Management Factors	Financial resources and constraints
	Organizational structure
	Policy, standards and goals
	Safety culture and priorities
Institutional Context Factors	Economic and regulatory context
	National health service executive
	Links with external organizations

(Reproduced from British Medical Journal, Charles Vincent, Sally Taylor-Adams, Nicola Stanhope. "Framework for analysing risk and safety in clinical medicine". **316**, no. 7138, [1154–1157], 1998, with permission from BMJ Publishing Group Ltd.)

At the top of the framework are patient factors. In any clinical situation the patient's condition will have the most direct influence on practice and outcome. Other patient factors such as personality, language and psychological problems may also be important as they can influence communication with staff. The design of the task, the availability and utility of protocols and test results may influence the care process and affect the quality of care. Individual factors include the knowledge, skills and experience of each member of staff, which will obviously affect their clinical practice. Each staff member is part of a team within the inpatient or community unit, and part of the wider organization of the hospital, primary care or mental health service. The way an individual practises, and their impact on the patient, is constrained and influenced by other members of the team and the way they communicate, support and supervise each other. The team is influenced in turn by management actions and by decisions made at a higher level in the organization. These include policies for the use of locum or agency staff, continuing education, training and supervision and the availability of equipment and supplies. The organization itself is affected by the institutional context, including financial constraints, external regulatory bodies and the broader economic and political climate.

The framework provides the conceptual basis for analysing clinical incidents, in that it includes both the clinical factors and the higher-level, organizational factors that may contribute to the final outcome. In doing so, it allows the whole range of possible influences to be considered and can therefore be used to guide the investigation and analysis of an incident. However, it has also been used to frame and guide broader inquiries and in the design of reporting systems such as the ICU-SRS described in Chapter 5. For instance, Bryony Dean and colleagues used this framework in an analysis of a series of 88 potentially serious prescribing errors (Dean *et al.*, 2002). Interviews with prescribers who made 44 of these errors provided a rich account of the factors contributing to these errors, which were analysed and classified using the seven levels framework, although in practice the influence of higher level factors could not be identified directly (Box 8.2). Staff identified staffing and workload issues as fundamental, followed by lack of skills and knowledge and physical health as being the most important contributory factors.

The investigation and analysis of clinical incidents

A clinical scenario can be examined from a number of different perspectives, each of which may illuminate facets of the case. Cases have, from time immemorial, been used to educate and reflect on the nature of disease. They can also be used to illustrate the process of clinical decision making, the weighing of treatment options and sometimes, particularly when errors are discussed, the personal impact of incidents and mishaps. Incident analysis, for the purposes of improving the safety of healthcare, may encompass all of these perspectives but critically also includes reflection on the broader healthcare system.

BOX 8.2 Classification of factors contributing to 88 potentially serious prescribing errors

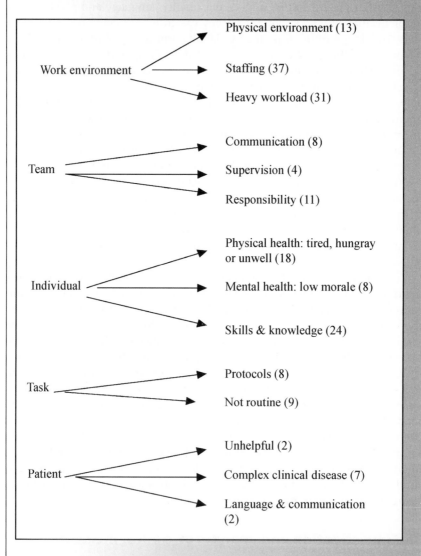

Methods of investigation

There are a number of methods of investigation and analysis available in healthcare, though these tend to be comparatively underdeveloped in comparison with methods available in industry. In the United States, the most familiar is the root cause analysis approach of the Joint Commission, an intensive process with its origins in Total Quality Management approaches to healthcare improvement (Spath, 1999). The Veterans Hospital Administration has developed a highly structured system of triage questions, which is being disseminated throughout their system. In our unit we have developed a method based on Reason's model and our framework of contributory factors. The British National Patient Safety Agency has developed a method of root cause analysis, which is an amalgam of elements of all these approaches. We do not have space to examine all potential methods, which vary in their orientation, theoretical basis and basic approach. All, however, to a greater or lesser extent, uncover factors contributing to the final incident. We will summarize the approach developed by the Clinical Safety Research Unit over the years with many London based colleagues, known, imaginatively, as the *London Protocol* (www.cpssq.org).

Systems analysis or root cause analysis?

For reasons that are now lost in history, most other approaches to analysing incidents in healthcare are termed 'root cause analysis'; in contrast we have described our own approach to the analysis of incidents as a systems analysis as we believe that it is a more accurate and more fruitful description. The term root cause analysis, while widespread, is misleading in a number of respects. To begin with, it implies that there is a single root cause, or at least a small number. Typically, however, the picture that emerges is much more fluid and the notion of a root cause is a gross oversimplification. Usually there is a chain of events and a wide variety of contributory factors leading up to the eventual incident. However, a more important and fundamental objection to the term root cause analysis relates to the very purpose of the investigation. Surely the purpose is obvious? To find out what happened and what caused it. Certainly it is necessary to find out what happened and why, in order to explain to the patient, their family and others involved. However, if the purpose is to achieve a safer healthcare system, then it is necessary to go further and reflect on what the incident reveals about the gaps and inadequacies in the healthcare system in which it occurred. The incident acts as a 'window' on the system – hence systems analysis. Incident analysis, properly understood, is not a retrospective search for root causes but an attempt to look to the future. In a sense the particular causes of the incident in question do not matter, as they are now in the past. However, the system weaknesses revealed are still present and could lead to the next incident (Vincent, 2004); the *London Protocol* aims to guide reflection on incidents in order to reveal these weaknesses.

Systems analysis of clinical incidents: the London Protocol

During an investigation, information is gleaned from a variety of sources. Case records, statements and any other relevant documentation are reviewed.

Structured interviews with key members of staff are then undertaken to establish the chronology of events, the main care delivery problems and their respective contributory factors, as perceived by each member of staff. The key questions are: What happened? (the outcome and chronology); How did it happen? (the care delivery problems); and Why did it happen? (the contributory factors). Examples of care delivery problems and a summary of the process are shown in Boxes 8.3 and 8.4.

BOX 8.3 Examples of care delivery problems

- Failure to monitor, observe or act
- Delay in diagnosis
- Inadequate risk assessment (i.e. of suicide risk)
- Inadequate handover
- Failure to note faulty equipment
- Failure to carry out pre-operative checks
- Not following an agreed protocol (without clinical justification)
- Not seeking help when necessary
- Incorrect protocol applied
- Treatment given to incorrect body site
- Wrong treatment given.

(FROM THE *LONDON PROTOCOL* www.cpssq.org)

BOX 8.4 A summary of the process of investigation and analysis

Care Delivery Problems (CDPs)
The first step in any analysis is to identify the care delivery problems. These are actions or omissions, or other deviations in the process of care which had a direct or indirect effect on the eventual outcome for the patient.

Clinical Context and Patient Factors
For each care delivery problem identified, the investigator records the salient clinical events or condition of the patient at that time (e.g. bleeding heavily, blood pressure falling) and other patient factors affecting the process of care (e.g. patient very distressed, patient unable to understand instructions).

Contributory Factors
Having identified the CDP, the investigator then considers the conditions in which errors occur and the wider organizational context. These are the contributory factors. For each CDP, the investigator uses the framework

both during interview and afterwards, to identify the factors that led to that particular care management problem. For example:

- Individual factors may include lack of knowledge or experience of particular staff.
- Task factors might include the non-availability of test results or protocols.
- Team factors might include inadequate supervision or poor communication between staff.
- Work environment might include high workload, inadequate staffing or limited access to vital equipment.

(FROM THE *LONDON PROTOCOL* www.cpssq.org)

Once the chronology of events is clear, there are three main considerations: the care delivery problems identified within the chronology; the clinical context for each of them; and the factors contributing to the occurrence of the care delivery problems. Any combination of contributory factors might contribute to the occurrence of a single care delivery problem. The investigator needs to differentiate between those contributory factors that are only relevant on that particular occasion and those which are longstanding or permanent features of the unit. For instance, there may be a failure of communication between two midwives which might be an isolated occurrence or might reflect a more general pattern of poor communication on the unit. Ideally the patient, or a member of their family, should also be interviewed, though as yet this does not often happen.

While a considerable amount of information can be gleaned from written records, interviews with those involved are the most important method of identifying the contributory factors. This is especially so if the interview systematically explores these factors and so allows the member of staff to collaborate in the investigation. In the interview, the story and 'the facts' are just the first stage. The staff member is also encouraged to identify both the care delivery problems and the contributory factors, which greatly enriches both the interview and investigation.

Analyses using this method have been conducted in hospitals, primary care settings and mental health units. The protocol may be used in a variety of formats, by individual clinicians, researchers, risk managers and by clinical teams. A clinical team may use the method to guide and structure reflection on an incident, to ensure that the analysis is full and comprehensive. For serious incidents, a team of individuals with different skills and backgrounds would be assembled, though often only a risk manager or an individual clinician will be needed. The protocol may also be used for teaching as a vehicle for introducing systems thinking. While reading about systems thinking is helpful, actually analysing an incident brings systems thinking alive.

The contributory factors that reflect more general problems in a unit are the targets for change and systems improvement. When obvious problems are identified, action may be taken after a single incident, but when more substantial changes are being considered, other incident analyses and sources of data (routine audits and outcome data) should also be taken into account. Recommendations may be made in a formal report but it is essential to follow these up with monitoring of action and outcome and to specify who is responsible for implementation.

An illustrative case example

Stephen Rogers (2002) adapted this method for use in primary care and family medicine settings, also producing a very clear format for presenting the findings of both the analysis and recommendations for action. He describes a case in which a 70-year-old widow who was living alone in a ground floor Housing Association flat had a fall at home. Her first language was Portuguese and her English was poor. The patient had suffered from osteoarthritis of the knees for years; she had been referred for an orthopaedic opinion and was waiting for an appointment. After her fall she was taken by ambulance to her local hospital and admitted for assessment. During her hospital stay she was seen by an orthopaedic surgeon who included her in his operating list for a knee replacement the following week. The patient developed pyrexia after the operation, but no cause was found and she was sent home, with instructions to complete a course of antibiotics. A week later, a neighbour called the district nurses' office because no one had visited the patient. After two visits by nurses her primary care doctor assessed her and was concerned to find that the patient's knee was hot and painful. He admitted her to hospital with a provisional diagnosis of septic arthritis. A methicillin-resistant *Staphylococcus aureus* infection of the knee joint was confirmed and the patient required arthroscopic washout and long-term antibiotics. The primary care doctor reviewed the case, as he felt that the patient's diagnosis had been unnecessarily delayed. (Adapted from Rogers, 2002)

The analysis is summarized in Table 8.2. In this case, the analysis centres round the delay in diagnosis and summarizes the contributory factors from several points in the process of care. Rogers focuses on one particular problem in the process care, the delay in diagnosis of infection following discharge from hospital; in this instance, this spans a period of several days and involves quite a number of clinical staff. The initial problem in fact stemmed from her being discharged from hospital without the cause of the infection being ascertained, which could have been separately examined as a care delivery problem. However, once discharged, a combination of misunderstanding of the purpose of the antibiotics, inadequate communication from the hospital, slow communication between members of the primary care team and other factors led to a week in which the infection went unrecognized. This delay certainly had consequences for the patient, but the eventual outcome was good. The importance of the example lies in the fact that even a relatively ordinary incident can be used to examine weaknesses in the process of care and to suggest points where improvements might be made.

Table 8.2 Care delivery problem: there was delay in recognizing the seriousness of the patient's complaint

Patient Factors	The patient was not able to make her worries and concerns clear to her doctor
Individual Factors	The visiting nurse assumed that the antibiotics prescribed by the hospital were for the patients 'wound infection'
Task Factors	The patient's discharge letter arrived nine days after the patient was sent home
Team Factors	There was no call from the orthopaedic ward to indicate a need for district nurse visit
	The visiting nurse did not discuss the case in detail with nursing colleagues, nor with the doctors
	District nurses had no reliable means of communicating with doctors typically passing messages via reception
Work environment Factors	The visiting nurse was temporarily seconded to the team and not familiar with the local doctors
Organizational Management and Institutional Factors	Measures designed to optimise bed management can compromise other aspects of the hospital admission and discharge process
	Recruitment problems in district nursing lead to teams being understaffed

(Adapted from Rogers, 2002)

An action plan based on the framework of contributory factors was set out to address a number of the issues identified. These included appraising the skills of one member of staff, reviewing arrangements for cover during times of staff shortages, reviewing the practice policy on home visits and the means by which visiting nurses communicated with the family doctors. Note that even such a detailed analysis as this does not necessarily lead immediately to recommendations for change. The widespread practice of insisting that all formal analyses include a list of recommendations has some dangers. While it is understandable and commendable that people want to see change, it is not always either possible or desirable to see what those changes ought to be from the analysis of a single case. Case analysis sometimes identifies glaring problems that just need to be fixed. More often though, the analyses tell you where problems might lie but not how extensive they are or how best to make the system more reliable. In addition, recommendations accumulate which are never followed through; if a hospital analyses 20 cases a year in depth, each of which produces five recommendations, there could be as many as 100 action plans floating around, which is clearly unworkable. Better to use the cases to identify a small number of core vulnerabilities which can then be systematically and sensibly addressed in long-term improvement and evaluation projects.

Human reliability analysis

Analyses of specific incidents, especially when systematic and thorough, can illuminate systemic weaknesses and help us understand how things go wrong. We have seen how there is frequently a chain of events leading to an incident and a variety of contributing factors. Having understood these principles, we are now able to approach the examination of system weaknesses from a different perspective. Rather than take a case, analyse it and see where it leads us, an alternative approach is to begin with a process of care and systematically examine it for possible failure points. This is the province of human reliability analysis.

Human Reliability Analysis or Assessment (HRA) has been defined as the application of relevant information about human characteristics and behaviour to the design of objects, facilities and environments that people use (Kirwan, 1994). HRA techniques may be used in the analysis of incidents, but are more commonly used to examine a process or system. Human reliability analytic techniques of various kinds have been in use in high-risk industries and military settings for over 50 years. Failure Modes and Effects Analysis (FMEA) for instance, was developed in 1949 by the US military to determine the effects of system and equipment failures and was used by NASA in the 1960s to predict failures, plan preventative measures and back-up systems in the Apollo Space Program (Kirwan, 1994). Since then, HRA has been applied in many safety critical industries, including aviation and aerospace, rail, shipping, air traffic control, automobile, offshore oil and gas, chemical, and all parts of the military. HRA has been applied at all stages of the 'life-cycle' of a process from design of a system, normal functioning of the process, maintenance and decommissioning (Lyons *et al.*, 2004).

Techniques which purport to assess reliability of systems in advance of their operations have been particularly closely associated with the development of the nuclear industry; in order to gain public acceptance and an operating licence designers and builders of nuclear power plants have to demonstrate *in advance* that the designs and proposed methods of operation are safe. This requires a minutely detailed specification of the actual processes, a quantitative assessment of the likelihood of different kinds of failure, a quantitative assessment of the likelihood of different kinds of human error and, finally, modelling the combined effects of all possible combinations of error and breakdown to give an overall assessment of safety.

Techniques of human reliability analysis

There are a vast number of these analytic techniques, derived by different people in different industries for different purposes. Most are commercial in origin, often not published in the academic literature and not subject to formal evaluation or validation (Lyons *et al.*, 2004). Some techniques are primarily aimed at providing a close description of a task or to map out the work sequence. For instance, in hierarchical task analysis, the task description is broken down into sub-tasks or operations; this approach has been applied with much success to error analysis in endoscopic surgery (Joice, Hanna and Cuschieri, 1998). Human error identification and analysis techniques build on a basic task analysis to provide a detailed description of the kinds of errors that can occur, the points in the sequence where they are likely to occur and the contextual or environmental factors that make errors more or less likely to occur.

The goal of human error quantification is to produce error probabilities, building on task analysis and error identification techniques to provide a probabilistic risk assessment (PRA). This provides numerical estimates of error likelihood and of the probability of overall likelihood of system breakdown. Quantification of error is the most difficult aspect of HRA, often heavily reliant on expert judgement, rather than the more rigorous approach of actual observation and recording of error frequencies. Such techniques are little used in healthcare but have been successfully applied to anaesthesia (Pate-Cornell and Bea, 1992). Nevertheless, some hospital tasks, such as blood transfusion, are highly structured and the quantification of errors probabilities would seem to be eminently feasible (Lyons *et al.*, 2004).

Box 8.5 summarizes some of the best known approaches to give a general sense of the range of methods. Some of the approaches focus on mapping a

---

BOX 8.5 Techniques of human reliability analysis

Fault Tree Analysis starts with a potential, or actual, undesirable event and works backwards seeking the immediate cause, preceding causes and combinations of causes.

Event Tree Analysis works forward from events (such as equipment failure) and assesses their possible consequences in different unfolding scenarios.

Failure Modes and Effects Analysis analyses potential failures of systems, components or functions and their effects. Each component is considered in turn, its possible modes of failure defined and the potential effects delineated.

Hazard Analysis and Critical Control Points (HACCP) is a systematic methodology for the identification, assessment and control of hazards, mostly used in food production.

Hazard and Operability Study (HAZOP) is a team-based, systematic, qualitative method to identify hazards (or deviations in design intent) in process industries.

Probabilistic Risk Assessment (PRA) builds on such techniques as FMEA and HAZOP, by adding modelling of fault and event trees and assignment of probabilities to events and outcomes.

Tripod Delta An integrated system of safety management which assesses general failure types, such as maintenance and design problems, and their potential impact on safety.

Human Error Assessment and Reduction Technique (HEART) examines particular task types and their associated error probabilities using tables of task types and factors which impact on the performance of the task.

(FROM REDMILL AND RAJAN, 1997; REASON, 1997)

process and identifying points of weakness or hazard. These include Event Tree Analysis, Fault Tree Analysis, and Failure Modes and Effects Analysis. These are all general approaches used in a variety of ways. The Hazard and Operability Study (HAZOP), used particularly in the chemical industry, offers a specific methodology and approach to this basic question. Probabilistic Reliability Analysis (PRA) goes one step further, taking a basic fault tree, and adding specific probabilities to the various branches so that an overall assessment of risk can be derived. Finally there are approaches which address the conditions in which people work, rather than the process itself emphasizing, as Reason's accident model does, the importance of assessing latent factors and organizational processes. These include Tripod Delta, developed by Reason and colleagues for use in the oil industry, and Human Error Assessment and Reduction Technique (HEART), developed by Jeremy Williams, an ergonomist, to assess the influence of error producing conditions in various contexts (Williams, 1985; Reason, 1997). These techniques are just beginning to be systematically explored in healthcare and are mainly being applied to existing systems. Examples of successful application are few and far between as yet but are very likely to increase in both number and importance in the next few years. We will examine the most common technique used in healthcare so far and provide examples of its application.

Failure modes and effects analysis (FMEA)

The Joint Commission in the United States, the National Patient Safety Agency in the United Kingdom and the US Veterans Administration (VA) are all encouraging the use of FMEA. Guidelines are provided on the respective Web sites and the VA in particular has taken steps to review available methods and customize them for use in healthcare, using elements of classical FMEA, their own root cause analysis framework and the HACPP approach (Box 8.6). The main steps of the VA process are summarized in Box 8.6 (DeRosier *et al.*, 2002). Immediately, we can see that this is a substantial undertaking, but clearly necessary when dealing with a complex, sophisticated and hazardous process. A great strength of the VA approach is their insistence on the involvement and backing of senior management.

To give a sense of how FMEA works in practice, we will review an analysis carried out in the Good Samaritan Hospital, Ohio (Burgmeier, 2002). The

BOX 8.6 Healthcare failure modes and effects analysis: a summary of the Veterans Administration process

Step 1 Define the HFMEA Topic
This will usually be a high-risk area that warrants a sustained safety programme.

Step 2 Assemble a Multidisciplinary Team
All relevant disciplines should be represented. Including people who are not familiar with the process under review encourages critical thinking.

Step 3 Map out the Process Using Flowcharts and Diagrams:
- Create a high level flow diagram.
- If the process is complex, identify the area to focus on.
- Identify all sub processes.
- Create a flow diagram for sub-processes.

Step 4 Conduct a Hazard Analysis
- List all potential failures modes for each process and sub-process:
- Assess the severity of failure at any particular point.
- Decide whether the failure mode warrants further action.

Step 5 Actions and Outcome Measures:
- Determine whether you want to eliminate, control or accept each potential cause of failure.
- Identify possible courses of action to eliminate or control failure modes.
- Identify outcome measures that will be used to test the redesigned process.
- Identify a single responsible individual to act and monitor the outcomes.
- Test to make sure that new vulnerabilities have not been introduced in the system as a result of the changes.

(ADAPTED FROM DEROSIER *ET AL.*, 2002)

hospital's Safety Board, aware of healthcare's vulnerability to error, decided to proactively assess high-risk processes. Blood transfusion was the first process to be studied as it affected a large number of patients, haemolytic reactions to blood could be fatal and because the procedure had become very complicated; numerous steps and double checks had been added to safeguard patients and meet regulatory requirements. Well-intentioned efforts to increase safety, by adding checks, had introduced a new hazard, that of complexity.

The team assembled was quite large and appropriately senior and multidis-ciplinary. There were representatives from risk management, blood transfusion services, and administration, surgery, intensive care and high use patient areas. Roles were defined and a total of four days set aside for the initial mapping and analysis. The difficulties in simply producing the flowchart were extremely illuminating. There were two organizational policies, five nursing procedures, and a multitude of special considerations; for example, certain kinds of filtered tubing are inappropriate for some blood products. It is probable that no one person in this organization fully understood this process until they sat down and mapped it out. Looking at such hospital processes one marvels not so much at the level of error as at people's ability to navigate these bewildering imperfect systems.

For each step in the process, the team considered what could go wrong (the failure mode), why the failure might occur (cause) and what could happen if it did occur (effects). An example of the analysis of a failure mode is shown in Box 8.7. A total of 40 failure modes were identified, each of which was then rated on a 10-point scale for Occurrence (how easily it could happen), Severity and Detectability (if it did occur, how likely it is that the failure would go undetected). These three scores are then multiplied together to give a rough

---

BOX 8.7 A failure mode in the blood transfusion process

Failure Mode
Two people do not always check order entry for blood products.

Causes:
- Immediate patient care elsewhere is often more important.
- Nurses do not fully understand the consequences of a decision not to enter an order when they give priority to a patient elsewhere.
- Nurse entering order prefers to 'get things done' rather than follow process carefully and correctly.
- Current policy is not explicit that two people must check the order

Potential Effects of Failure:
- Waste of personnel and resources;
- Delay in treatment to appropriate patient;
- Ties up scarce blood resources;
- Increases patient's level of risk;
- Increases length of stay.

Design Action (Solutions):
- Blood specific order form used by all departments that is completed by physician;
- Order form faxed through to Blood Transfusion Service and double-checked against computer entry;
- Training given to everyone participating in blood transfusion process;
- In the longer term, physician will enter order directly into computer.

(REPRODUCED FROM *JOINT COMMISSION JOURNAL ON QUALITY IMPROVEMENT*, BURGMEIER, J. "FAILURE MODE AND EFFECT ANALYSIS: AN APPLICATION IN REDUCING RISK IN BLOOD TRANSFUSION" **28**, NO.6. 331–339, 2002)

index of hazard. The most highly rated potential failure modes are shown in Box 8.8.

BOX 8.8 Most serious failure modes in blood transfusion process

- Failure to accurately match the right blood to the right patient;
- Nurse may not remain with patient for full 15 minutes after start of transfusion;
- The patient's stated name and ID band may not be compared when the type and cross-match specimen is drawn;
- The person applying the label to the type and cross-match specimen may not verify the patient's ID band;
- The person applying the label to the type and cross-match specimen may accept verbal instructions instead of requiring a printed requisition;
- Two people may not check the order entry;
- The order may be interpreted differently from the physician's intent.

(ADAPTED FROM BURGMEIER, 2002)

The FMEA process produced a series of recommendations for immediate change, and for longer-term moves to computerized physician order entry and bar coding. The immediate changes included the introduction of a standardized form for blood products, allowing physicians to check boxes for ordering, while documenting the reasons for the transfusion; a blood barrier system which restricted access to the blood until a patient code was dialled in; and a video to provide the required training. Most importantly, the multitude of policies and procedures relating to blood transfusion were combined into a single comprehensive policy that incorporated a flowchart of the new process.

Looking at these changes in a more generic way, we can see a strong element of simplification and standardization at the core. Simplify the policies and procedures, make the flowchart explicit, develop a standard form used by everyone and provide training to get the new systems started. In addition, an additional 'defence' was put in place in the form of the blood barrier system. Monitoring of the changes showed a steady reduction in variances and problems as the system bedded down and no instances of serious error or harm to patients in the initial months. The final judgement of the team was that although FMEA had many advantages, as an approach it was not to be employed lightly. Tackling FMEA had involved substantial investment of time, money and energy and they planned to reserve its use for high priority processes only (Burgmeier, 2002).

Integration and evaluation of analytic techniques

Incident analysis is usually seen as retrospective, while techniques such as FMEA, which examine a process of care, are seen as prospective and, therefore, potentially superior. The idea is that by using prospective analysis we can prevent the next incident, rather than using case analysis to look back at something that has already gone wrong. We might think that as healthcare becomes safer, these prospective analyses will eventually supplant incident analysis. Leaving aside the fact that healthcare has rather a long way to go before the supply of incidents dries up, there are a number of reasons for continuing to explore individual incidents as well as examining systems prospectively.

To begin with, there is no sharp division between retrospective and prospective techniques; as argued above, the true purpose of incident analysis is to use the incident as a window onto the system, in essence looking at current weakness and future potential problems. Conversely, so-called prospective analysis relies extensively on the past experience of those involved. Probabilities and hazards assessed in failure modes and effects analysis are derived almost exclusively from groups of clinicians on the basis of their past experience. Techniques such as FMEA are, in addition, very expensive in terms of time and resources. The analysis of single incidents, whether or not they have a bad outcome, can be scaled to the time and resource available, be it ten minutes or ten days. A single incident, a story, almost always engages a clinical group and can be analysed by an individual risk manager or a whole clinical team. The future lies in a judicious application of both forms of techniques, using systems analyses of incidents to generate both enthusiasm and hypotheses as a basis for more resource intensive analyses of whole processes and systems.

A major concern with all the techniques discussed is the lack of formal testing and evaluation. In one of the few reviews of these techniques, Jeremy Williams began by saying 'It must seem quite extraordinary to most scientists engaged in research into other areas of the physical and technological world that there has been little attempt by human reliability experts to validate the human reliability assessment techniques which they so freely propagate, modify and disseminate', a view echoed by later authors (Williams, 1985; Redmill and Rajan, 1997). Healthcare, although coming late to these approaches, may in fact have much to offer because of the much stronger tradition of use of evidence, comparative clinical trials, evaluation and quantitative research. However, while some rigorous evaluation of the value of the various techniques described in this chapter would be welcome, we should be cautious about the status of the knowledge derived from these methods. Incident analyses provide a wonderful window on the wider system but essentially produce hypotheses about where problems may lie, which need to be followed up with further, more systematic investigation. Human reliability techniques can produce more systematic empirical data but are often reliant on expert opinion, which may also need to be further validated by observation. Accident and incident analysis and other methods do however reveal a great deal about the vulnerabilities in our systems and show us the range of factors which need to be addressed if we are to design a safer, high quality healthcare system.

From accident analysis to system design

We are now at a transitional point in the book between the understanding and analysis of incidents and the coming chapters, which discuss methods of prevention and quality improvement. The seven-levels framework has outlined the patient, task and technology, staff, team, working environment, organizational and institutional environmental factors that are revealed in analyses of incidents. These same factors also point to the means of intervention and different levels on which safety and quality must be addressed, which we will explore systematically as the book unfolds.

Pascale Carayon and colleagues have rightly pointed out however, that the frameworks set out by James Reason, myself and others were primarily aimed at understanding and analysing incidents and accidents. Such analyses have clear implications for change and system design, but this is not explicitly set out in the models. Carayon and colleagues have taken the understanding gained from accident analyses and other sources to set out a model of work system design for patient safety: (System Engineering Initiative for Patient Safety (SEIPS).

Their systems engineering approach to patient safety is anchored within the industrial engineering subspecialty of human factors. The discipline of human factors emphasizes interactions between people and their environment that contribute to performance, safety and health, and quality of working life, and the goods or services produced (Carayon *et al.*, 2006). The model builds on Donabedian's structure–process–outcome model and incorporates the main themes discussed in the frameworks earlier in the chapter. There are some differences of perspective: task and technologies are separated, patient and staff

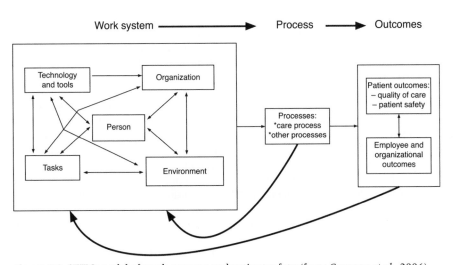

Figure 8.3 SEIPS model of work systems and patient safety (from Carayon *et al.*, 2006).

are together represented by the person component and team working is integrated within the organizational component. Whereas Donabedian's model places most emphasis on the performance of individual healthcare providers, Carayon's model puts the focus on the wider systems and the interactions between the components. Importantly, outcomes in the SEIPS model includes staff outcomes as well as patient outcomes, in the sense that they imply that a healthy work organization will provide safety and excellent care for patients, while simultaneously providing a safe and productive environment for the workforce. As they point out, healthcare workers experience many negative consequences of poor system design, such as job dissatisfaction, burnout, mental health problems and injuries.

The SEIPS model has been used in a study of outpatient surgery centres and is also being tested in other studies. In the surgical context, it had two broad purposes: first, to guide the assessment of systems, processes and outcomes in each outpatient surgery centre for the development of system redesign interventions; and second, to guide the evaluation of the system redesign interventions. While we will not explicitly link the remaining sections of the book to the SEIPS model, it provides a valuable conceptual bridge for us to the later sections of the book, by explicitly articulating the requirements for improving healthcare systems. In later chapters we will address the roles of design and technology, of the patient and staff, of teamwork and organizations and the difficult question of the integration of these various components in long-term programmes of sustained improvement. Before that however, we must deal with a subject still given far too little attention in healthcare, namely the aftermath of error and harm for patients, families and clinical staff.

References

Balen, P. (2004) Gross negligence manslaughter. *Clinical Risk*, **10**, 25–27.

Burgmeier, J. (2002) Failure mode and effect analysis: an application in reducing risk in blood transfusion. *Joint Commission Journal on Quality Improvement*, **28**(6), 331–339.

Carayon, P., Schoofs Hundt, A., Karsh, B.T. *et al.* (2006) Work system design for patient safety: the SEIPS model. *Quality and Safety in Health Care*, **15**(suppl_1), i50–i58.

Dean, B., Schachter, M., Vincent, C.A. and Barber, N. (2002) Causes of prescribing errors in hospital inpatients: a prospective study. *The Lancet*, **359**(9315), 1373–1378.

DeRosier, J., Stalhandske, E., Bagian, J.P. and Nudell, M.S. (2002) Using health care failure mode and effect analysis: the VA National Center for Patient Safety's prospective risk analysis system. *Joint Commission Journal on Quality & Safety*, **28**, 248–267.

Holbrook, J. (2003) The criminalisation of fatal medical mistakes. *British Medical Journal*, **327**(7424), 1118–1119.

Helmreich, R.L. (2000) On error management: lessons from aviation. *British Medical Journal*, **320**, 781–785.

Joice, P., Hanna, G.B. and Cuschieri, A. (1998) Errors enacted during endoscopic surgery – a human realiability analysis. *Applied Ergonomics*, **29**(6), 409–414.

Kirwan, B. (1994) *A Guide to Practical Human Reliability Assessment*, Taylor and Francis, London.

Lyons, M., Adams, S., Woloshynowych, M. and Vincent, C.A. (2004) Human reliability analysis in healthcare: a review of techniques. *International Journal of Risk and Safety in Medicine*, **16**(4), 223–237.

Pate-Cornell, M.E. and Bea, R.G. (1992) Management errors and system reliability: a probabilistic approach and application to offshore platforms. *Risk Analysis*, **12**(1), 1–18.

Reason, J.T. (1990) *Human Error*, Cambridge University Press, New York.

Reason, J.T. (1997) *Managing the Risks of Organisational Accidents*, Ashgate, Aldershot.

Reason, J.T. (2001) Understanding adverse events: the human factor, *Clinical Risk Management: Enhancing Patient Safety*, 2nd edn (ed. C. Vincent), BMJ Books, London.

Redmill, R. and Rajan, J. (1997) *Human Factors in Safety Critical Systems*, Butterworth Heinemann, Oxford.

Rogers, S. (2002) A structured approach for the investigation of clinical incidents in healthcare: application in a general practice setting. *British Journal of General Practice*, **52**(supp), S30–S32.

Spath, P. (1999) *Error Reduction in Health Care: A Systems Approach to Improving Patient Safety*, AHA Press, Washington.

Toft, B. (2001) *External Inquiry into the Adverse Incident that Occurred at Queen's Medical Centre, Nottingham*, Department of Health, London.

Vincent, C., Taylor-Adams, S. and Stanhope, N. (1998) Framework for analysing risk and safety in clinical medicine. *British Medical Journal*, **316**(7138), 1154–1157.

Vincent, C.A. (2004) Analysis of clinical incidents: a window on the system not a search for root causes. *Quality & Safety in Health Care*, **13**(4), 242–243.

Williams, J.C. (1985) Validation of human reliability assessment technique. *Reliability Engineering*, **11**, 149–162.

SECTION FOUR
The Aftermath

CHAPTER 9

Caring for patients harmed by treatment

Previous chapters have shown that many patients experience errors during their treatment, whether they realize it or not, and some are inadvertently harmed by healthcare. The harm may be minor, involving only inconvenience or discomfort, but can involve serious disability or death. Almost all bad outcomes will have some psychological consequences, ranging from worry and distress through to depression and even despair. Most of this book is devoted to understanding how adverse events occur and how they can be prevented. What happens after such events, however, may be just as important as what happens before; injured patients are sometimes treated by hospitals and their legal representatives in ways that are quite abhorrent and make a mockery of healthcare ethics. Arnold Simanowitz, a pioneering campaigner in this area, used to tell medical audiences 'You would be appalled if you knew what was being done in your name.'

Thankfully there is now strong advocacy for open disclosure in several countries, sometimes backed by legislation; this is an important first step to a more humane and thoughtful treatment of patients and families. As yet however, much less attention has been paid to the long-term consequences for injured patients and very few healthcare organizations have shouldered the full responsibility of looking after people they have harmed. The experiences of these people tend not to be fully appreciated, and yet understanding the impact of such injuries is a prerequisite of providing useful and effective help. The aim of this chapter is to convey something of the experience of injured patients and their families and to give some guidance on how they can be helped.

Injury from medical treatment is different from other injures

Patients and relatives may suffer in two distinct ways from a medically induced injury. First from the injury itself and second from the way the incident is handled afterwards. Many people harmed by their treatment suffer further

---

Patient Safety, 2nd edition. By Charles Vincent. Published 2010 by Blackwell Publishing Ltd.

trauma through the incident being insensitively and incompetently handled. Conversely, when staff come forward, acknowledge the damage and take positive action, the support offered can ameliorate the impact both in the short and long term. Injured patients need an explanation, an apology, to know that changes have been made to prevent future incidents, and often also need practical and financial help (Vincent, Young and Phillips, 1994). The problems arise when ordinary impulses to help are blunted by anxiety, shame or just not knowing what to say.

The emotional impact is particularly complex because a medical injury differs from most other accidents in some important respects. First, patients have been harmed, unintentionally, by people in whom they placed considerable trust, and so their reaction may be especially powerful and hard to cope with. Imagine the complex of emotions you might experience if you were injured by a member of your own family. Second, they are often cared for by the same professions, and perhaps the same people, as those involved in the original injury. As they may have been very frightened by what has happened to them, and have a range of conflicting feelings about those involved, this too can be very difficult, even when staff are sympathetic and supportive.

The impact of medical injury

A medical injury will have both physical and psychological consequences, and may affect many other aspects of a person's life.

Physical injury

All patients who suffer adverse events by definition experience harm of some kind. Sometimes the physical effects are fairly minor, amounting simply to some discomfort and extra time in hospital. For a proportion however, the injuries are major. Consider for instance the injuries sustained by some of the patients I have personally interviewed in the past. Injuries sustained by patients themselves included: young women having their womb removed unnecessarily; untreated cancers; unnecessary mastectomy; many cases of chronic pain; scarring and all the associated problems of adjustment and revulsion; incontinence and loss of bowel function; and many other cases with a long legacy of disability.

Psychological injury

Patients are often in a vulnerable psychological state, even when diagnosis is clear and treatment goes according to plan. Even routine procedures and normal childbirth may produce post-traumatic symptoms (Clarke *et al.*, 1997; Czarnocka and Slade, 2000). When they experience harm or misadventure therefore, their reaction is likely to be particularly severe.

Traumatic and life-threatening events produce a variety of symptoms, over and above any physical injury. Sudden, intense, dangerous or uncontrollable events are particularly likely to lead to psychological problems, especially if accompanied by illness, fatigue or mood disturbances (Brewin, Dalgleish and Joseph, 1996). Awareness under anaesthesia is an example of such an event. When people experience such a terrifying, if short-lived, event, they often later suffer from anxiety, intrusive and disturbing memories, emotional numbing and flashbacks. Almost everyone experiences such memories after stressful events, such as a divorce or bereavement and, while distressing, they gradually die down. However, they can be intense, prolonged and cause considerable suffering. In severe cases, the person may suffer from the full syndrome of post-traumatic stress disorder.

Post-traumatic stress disorder is a term that is bandied about fairly indiscriminately, and a word of caution is needed about its use. Properly conceived, it is a formal psychiatric diagnosis with strict, specific criteria. We have no idea how many people suffer from the full syndrome after medical treatment but the number is probably small. However, the incidence of some of the symptoms is probably very much greater. Many injured patients suffer from nightmares about their treatment and time in hospital, from persistent and intrusive recollections of their care and other problems, but nevertheless not from the full constellation of symptoms that makes up post-traumatic stress disorder. Depression appears to be a more common long-term response to the chronic problems of medical injury (Vincent and Coulter, 2002), although there is little research in this area. Whether people actually become depressed and to what degree will depend on the severity of their injury, the support they have from family, friends and health professionals and a variety of other factors (Kessler, 1997).

When a patient dies, the trauma is obviously more severe still, and may be particularly severe after a potentially avoidable death (Lundin, 1984). For instance, many people who have lost a spouse or child in a road accident continue to ruminate about the accident and what could have been done to prevent it for years afterwards. They are often unable to accept, resolve or find any meaning in the loss (Lehman, Wortman and Williams, 1987). Relatives of patients whose death was sudden or unexpected may therefore find the loss particularly difficult to bear. If the loss was avoidable in the sense that poor treatment played a part in the death, their relatives may face an unusually traumatic and prolonged bereavement. They may ruminate endlessly on the death and find it hard to deal with the loss.

Wider impact on family, life and work

The full impact of some incidents only becomes apparent in the longer term. A perforated bowel for example, may require a series of further operations and time in hospital. As with all injuries, the effects and associated problems can multiply over time, especially if recovery is only partial. Chronic pain for instance will affect a person's mood, ability to care for their children, ability to work, their family and social relationships and their sexual relationship. As relationships deteriorate, the person may become more isolated, less engaged and consequently more prone to depression; this in turn makes work and child care more difficult and so on (Vincent, Pincus and Scurr, 1993). The whole scenario may be compounded by the financial problems induced by not being able to work, and the anxiety about the future that this causes. Much of this is unseen by the healthcare organization who caused the injury in the first place (Duclos *et al.*, 2005).

The experiences of injured patients and their relatives

Adverse event is a useful but deliberately neutral technical term. It does not, and is not intended to, capture the often awful human stories that lie behind this innocuous term and it can be difficult to grasp the full extent of the trauma that people sometimes face. The stories in this section, and there are many more available, give an indication of what happens to people when things go wrong. This is the heart of patient safety and its justification.

Appreciating and understanding the experiences of injured patients is essential if one is going to provide individually appropriate and practical help. The two true stories retold here illustrate some of the principal forms of psychological trauma that result from serious adverse events: chronic pain and depression, anxiety and other post-traumatic reactions. The focus of each case description is on the experiences and effects on the people involved, rather than the clinical events that preceded them. The quotations are the patient's or relative's own words taken from interviews. Names and other details have been changed to protect the identity of those involved.

BOX 9.1 Perforation of the colon leading to chronic pain and depression

Mrs. Long underwent a ventrosuspension – the fixation of a displaced uterus to the abdominal wall. After the operation she awoke with a terrible pain in her lower abdomen which became steadily worse over the next four days. She was very frightened and repeatedly told both doctors and nurses but they dismissed it as 'wind'.

On the fifth day the pain reached a crescendo and she felt a 'ripping sensation' inside her abdomen. That evening the wound opened and the contents of her bowel began to seep through the dressings. Even then, no one seemed concerned. Finally, the surgeon realized that the bowel had been perforated and a temporary colostomy was carried out.

The next operation, to reverse the colostomy, was 'another fiasco'. After a few days there was a discharge of faecal matter from the scar, the wound became infected, and the pain was excruciating, especially after eating. She persistently asked if she could be fed with a drip but the nursing staff insisted she should keep eating. For two weeks she was 'crying with the pain, really panicking – I just couldn't take it any more.' She was finally transferred to another hospital where she was immediately put on a liquid diet.

A final operation to repair the bowel was successful but left her exhausted and depressed. She only began to recover her strength after a year of convalescence. Three years later she was still constantly tired, irritable, low in spirits and 'I don't enjoy anything any more.' She no longer welcomes affection or comfort and feels that she is going downhill, becoming more gloomy and preoccupied.

Her scars are still uncomfortable and painful at the time of her periods. Her stomach is 'deformed' and she feels much less confident and attractive as a result. As her depression has deepened, she has become less interested in sex and more self-conscious about the scar. Three years later, the trauma of her time in hospital is still very much alive. She still has nightmares about her time in hospital and is unable to talk about it without breaking into tears. She feels very angry and bitter that no one has ever apologized to her or admitted that a mistake has been made.

(ADAPTED FROM VINCENT, 2001)

Mrs Long suffered a series of avoidable surgical complications over a period of several months which left her in considerable pain. Traumatic experiences, chronic pain and physical weakness combined to produce a serious depression which lasted several years. The depression was marked by classical symptoms of low mood, tiredness, fatigue, low self esteem and sleep disturbance – but nevertheless unnoticed by any of the health professionals involved in her care. There were many problems with her surgical treatment and care on the wards. However, her problems were compounded by the lack of explanation or apology, a lack of interest or response from the hospital where all the problems occurred and a complete failure of anyone involved in her care to realize how deeply she had been affected (Vincent, 2001). This is the 'second trauma' following the original injury.

BOX 9.2 Neonatal death: bereavement and post-traumatic stress disorder

Mr Carter's son, Jamie, sustained injuries at birth, due to inadequate obstetric care, causing irreparable spinal cord injury. He died when he was two months old, without regaining consciousness.

Three days after the birth a paediatrician confirmed that their son was, as they suspected, severely handicapped. He suffered from fits and was partially sighted. He never cried or made any sounds because his vocal cords had been damaged. In spite of these injuries he continued to grow and put on weight. Two weeks after Jamie's birth they were told that he would not live. They then spent a terrible two months, mostly at the hospital, waiting for him to die.

Mr and Mrs Carter had a number of meetings with hospital staff but Mr Carter never felt he had received a full explanation. He remembers being told that 'it was just one of those things – that really sent me sky-rocketing. No one said it was a mistake, that's what wound me up. Till this day I've got many questions. No-one acted quickly enough. No doctor came at all until the paediatrician arrived.'

Mr Carter's reaction to Jamie's death was intense, violent and prolonged. For a year he suffered from disturbing memories and horrific dreams. He became quiet, withdrawn and remote even from his wife, feeling 'empty and hopeless'. He was tormented by disturbing images and memories of Jamie, of the birth, his slow death and particularly of his small, shrunken skull towards the end. Images of Jamie's birth still 'popped into my head at the most unexpected times. Very vivid, just like looking in on it. It just grabs you round the throat . . . ' He suffered from a persistent stress-related stomach disorder. His sleep was interrupted by violent nightmares of a kind he had never previously experienced. 'There was all this blood and gore, fantasy-like stuff.' During the day violent images, sometimes of killing people, would come into his head, which absolutely horrified him.

Before Jamie's death, Mr Carter had always been a relaxed and easy-going person. Now he was easily irritated and there were many arguments between him and his wife. At work, his irritability would often turn to anger, leading to confrontations and sometimes to fights. 'I was really angry all the time, so aggressive – I wanted to hurt people, and I'm not like that at all. I felt I had to blame someone all the time for everything.'

About a year later, Mrs Carter became pregnant again. Mr Carter was very anxious during the pregnancy but his symptoms began to subside after their daughter was born. Two years on he still breaks down and cries occasionally, and is generally a sadder and quieter person. When he passes the cemetery where his son is buried he still becomes angry, but now the feelings subside.

(ADAPTED FROM VINCENT, 2001)

Many of the symptoms and experiences reported by Mr Carter are common in any bereavement. Depression, distressing memories, feelings of anger and dreams of the person who has died are not unusual. However, the intensity, character and duration of Mr Carter's reaction indicate that this was far from an ordinary bereavement. Anger of that intensity and violent day-dreams are not usual and suggested, together with his other symptoms, that he was suffering from post-traumatic stress disorder. The staff of the paediatric unit clearly tried to help Mr and Mrs Carter, although they did not seem to understand the extent of his suffering and did not ask about traumatic reactions. Given the strength of Mr Carter's emotional reaction, it would probably still have been very difficult for him to accept an explanation early on, even if the death had been unavoidable. The necessary explanation would have to have been given gradually, over several meetings, and combined with some attempts to support him and ease the intensity of his reaction (Vincent, 2001).

What do injured patients need?

Imagine that you or your husband, mother or child has, inexplicably, suffered a medical injury. What would you want? Well, I imagine you would want to know what happened, you would want an apology, you would want to be looked after and, later on, you might want steps to be taken to prevent such things happening again to anyone else. If the injury led to you being off work or unable to care for your children, you would certainly appreciate some financial support to help you during the recovery period. If the person concerned was not going to recover, then long-term support would be needed. In an early study of the reasons for litigation, my colleagues and I found exactly this; people wanted an explanation, an apology, preventative action and, in some but not all cases, compensation. Most wanted the clinicians concerned to realize what they were experiencing; feeling ignored or not heard was a particularly painful and intensely frustrating experience, which potentially delayed recovery and adjustment (Vincent, Young and Phillips, 1994). As one patient said to me, 'If only I had been told honestly I could have faced it so much better.'

All this seems pretty obvious when one reflects for a moment on what one might want oneself. Yet most healthcare organizations have proved, in the past at least, extraordinarily bad at dealing with injured patients, resorting at times, particularly during litigation, to deeply unpleasant tactics of delay and manipulation which seriously compounded the initial problems. My phrase 'second trauma' is not just a linguistic device, but an accurate description of what some patients experience.

Every injured patient has their own particular problems and needs. Some will require a great deal of professional help, while others will prefer to rely on family and friends. Some will primarily require remedial medical treatment, while in others the psychological effects will be to the fore. In the short term, the two most important principles are to believe the patient and to be as honest and open as possible, which means that the error or harm must be disclosed to the patient and their family.

Being open: patients' and physicians' attitudes to disclosing error

Acknowledging that an adverse event has occurred can be hard and facing up to an injured patient or bereaved family can be even harder. But the alternative scenario of silence and abandonment is worse: for patients, their families and their health professionals. (BISMARK AND PATERSON, 2005)

A patient harmed by treatment poses acute and painful dilemmas for the staff involved, as Bismark and Paterson describe (2005). It is natural to avoid that pain by avoiding the patient, yet the staff's response is crucial to the patient's recovery. When patients think that information is being concealed from them, or that they are being dismissed as troublemakers, it is much more difficult for them to cope with the injury. A poor explanation fuels their anger, may affect the course of their recovery and may lead patients to distrust the staff caring for them. They may then avoid having further treatment – which in most cases they very much need. In contrast, an honest explanation and a promise to continue treatment may enhance the patient's trust and strengthen the relationship.

The ethics of open disclosure of errors are crystal clear and expressed in many clinical codes of ethics. Here is an example from the American Medical Association:

Patients have a right to know their past and present medical status and to be free of any mistaken beliefs concerning their conditions. Situations occasionally occur in which a patient suffers significant medical complications that may have resulted from the physician's mistake or judgement. In these situations the physician is ethically required to inform the patient of all the facts necessary to ensure understanding of what has occurred.

(REPRINTED WITH PERMISSION FROM AMERICAN MEDICAL ASSOCIATION)

While the principle of being honest and open is hard to disagree with, in practice a host of questions immediately arise. Should everything be disclosed, even minor errors with no consequences? Should all serious injuries be disclosed, even when knowing about the damage will make no material difference to the patient or family? Will patients become unduly anxious once they know how frequently errors occur? These are all reasonable questions which are beginning to be systematically explored.

Both focus groups and surveys of patients, whether or not they have experienced errors, have found that the great majority would like to be informed of any error; most would like to know immediately, though about a quarter preferred to wait until the full picture is known (Hobgood *et al.*, 2002). Most patients are strongly of the view that they wanted to be told about all harmful errors, and to know what happened, how it happened, how it would be mitigated and what will be done to prevent recurrence (Gallagher *et al.*, 2003). A number of studies have presented patients with hypothetical scenarios, depicting errors with different degrees of associated harm and with varying reactions from the clinicians concerned. The manner and speed of disclosure of the error is a powerful determinant of patients' response, with slow or inadequate disclosure leading to more negative ratings of the care provided, their attitudes to the clinicians concerned and the reputation of the hospital (Cleopas *et al.*, 2006). Failing to disclose also makes it more likely that the patient would seek to change doctors and, in some cases, increases the likelihood of complaint or litigation. Studies of obstetricians with high levels of litigation, compared with colleagues, suggests that those with litigation histories are distinguished not by the quality of their care, but by different attitudes, insensitivity and poorer communication skills (Entman *et al.*, 1994; Hickson *et al.*, 1994). Conversely, a positive, empathic response, in which responsibility is accepted, maintains trust and respect and reduces the wish for disciplinary action (Schwappach and Koeck, 2004; Mazor *et al.*, 2006).

Doctors as a group tend to underestimate the information that patients would like about errors and adverse outcomes. This might be a genuine difference of view, but is possibly also due to the clinicians' appreciation of the nuances and practical aspects of disclosure. In one focus group study, the physicians who took part agreed that harmful errors should be disclosed, but were generally more circumspect in the language they used. Often this simply meant speaking truthfully and very factually about what had occurred, without using the word error. 'You were given too much insulin. Your blood sugar was lowered and that's how you arrived in the intensive care unit . . . ' (Gallagher *et al.*, 2003 p. 1004). If the patient wanted to know more, they would go on to explain how the problem had arisen. Opinions in both groups were more varied when near misses were considered, some patients and many physicians thinking it would make patients unduly fearful and lead to unnecessary loss of trust.

Open disclosure: policy and practice

Hospitals and other healthcare organizations are beginning to take their disclosure responsibilities seriously and risk managers and clinicians are beginning to follow up injured patients and consider their longer-term needs. Although the task of dealing with adverse outcomes falls mainly on individual clinicians, they need to be backed by those senior to them and by the organization as a whole. Successful handling of adverse outcomes relies on the sensitivity and courage of individual clinicians and risk managers, but also requires a commitment to certain basic principles at the highest level of the organization. All healthcare organizations need a strong proactive policy of active intervention and monitoring of those patients whose treatment has caused harm. It is quite unrealistic, indeed unfair, to expect openness and honesty from individuals without the backing of a policy of honesty and openness approved by the governing body of the organization concerned.

Open disclosure policies have been increasingly adopted in a number of countries. In the United States, JCAHO mandated open disclosure as part of its accreditation policies in 2001 but, one year later, only a third of its hospitals had a policy in place and there was still considerable reluctance to disclose preventable, as opposed to unpreventable, harm (Lamb *et al.*, 2003); however, by 2005 this figure had increased to 69% (Gallagher, Studdert and Levinson, 2007). The British National Patient Safety Agency has a comprehensive 'Being Open' policy which, while not mandatory, is a strong stimulus for healthcare organizations to proactively promote such policies. The Canadian Patient Safety Institute has produced guidelines and several Canadian states have enacted apology legislation (Silversides, 2009). Open disclosure is moving slowly from a rarely practiced ideal towards being standard organizational policy.

One of the most impressive approaches has been that of the Australian Safety and Quality Council, which has produced a standard information sheet for patients (Box 9.3) and now educational and training materials for staff. The open disclosure standard set out by the Safety and Quality council is thoughtful and wide ranging. Many key themes have been built in: a commitment to openness, support over time, letting patients know the results of investigations, telling them what will be done to prevent future incidents and so on. Notice especially that open disclosure is spoken of as a process, not a one-off event. From the case histories at the beginning of the chapter, we can see that serious incidents may have a long time course to resolution. Even less serious incidents may require more than one meeting and some ongoing contact; in the first meeting, patients may be too shocked to take much in, coming back later, having thought things over, to ask more questions.

BOX 9.3 Patient information sheet on open disclosure

When we need to visit a healthcare professional we can expect to receive the safest healthcare available. But sometimes things may not work out as expected. For example, a patient may be given the wrong dose of medicine. Or there may be complications after surgery that mean the result is not as good as expected. Most adverse events are minor and do not result in harm. When a patient is harmed they have a right to know what has happened and why.

If an adverse event occurs, the hospital needs to follow a process of open disclosure. This means that the patients and their family or carers are told, as soon as possible after the event, what has happened and what will be done about it. An important part of the process is finding out exactly what went wrong, why it went wrong and actively looking for ways to stop it happening again.

What can I expect if something goes wrong?

If something goes wrong during your hospital visit, a member of the hospital staff will talk to you and your family and carers about what happened. You can also discuss any changes to your ongoing care plan because of the adverse event.

In this situation you have the right:
- to have a support person of your choice present at the discussion;
- to ask for a second opinion from another healthcare professional;
- to pursue a complaints process; and
- to nominate specific people (family or carers) who you'd like to be involved.

To make the process easier, we'll ask you to nominate someone (a member of your family, close friend or hospital patient advocate) to support you during your stay in hospital.

Who at the hospital will speak to me?

The person who talks to you about what happened is likely to be one of the healthcare team that is looking after you. However, if you have difficulty talking to this person you can nominate someone else. Ideally this will be someone who:

- you are comfortable with and can talk to easily;
- has been involved in your care and knows the facts; and
- has enough authority to begin action to stop the problem happening again.

Who else will be present?

The person who will be discussing what happened is also able to have someone there to assist and support them. When something goes wrong it is distressing for the patient and their carers, but is also traumatic for the healthcare team involved. Sometimes discussion after the event can become quite emotional or heated. Having someone there who is not as closely involved can help you to make the discussion more constructive. This is likely to assist you as well as the health team member.

What will happen afterwards?

As part of the open disclosure process, if something does go wrong, steps are taken to prevent it from happening again. The hospital will investigate what went wrong. You will be informed of the results and the changes that will be made to prevent the same thing from happening to someone else. If the investigation takes a long time, you will be kept up to date with its progress. If you wish, a meeting will be arranged for you to discuss the results of the investigation when it is finished.

(THE AUTHOR, CHARLES VINCENT, ACKNOWLEDGES THE VALUABLE WORK OF THE OFFICE OF SAFETY AND QUALITY IN HEALTHCARE (OSQH) AT THE WESTERN AUSTRALIAN DEPARTMENT OF HEALTH IN DEVELOPING THE *WA OPEN DISCLOSURE POLICY: COMMUNICATION AND DISCLOSURE REQUIREMENTS FOR HEALTH PROFESSIONALS WORKING IN WESTERN AUSTRALIA (2009)* ON WHICH THIS *OPEN DISCLOSURE PATIENT INFORMATION PAMPHLET* IS BASED. CHARLES VINCENT THANKS THE OSQH FOR PERMISSION TO USE THIS DOCUMENT)

Notice too that the policy specifically says that the patient has a right to complain and, presumably, to seek compensation. Open disclosure is, occasionally, seen as a way of reducing complaints and litigation. Say sorry, and they won't sue. It is certainly true that a failure to receive explanations and apologies is a powerful motivator to legal action (Vincent, Young and Phillips, 1994). However, finding out what happened is simply the patient's right. While open disclosure may indeed reduce claims and complaints, that is not its purpose or rationale. People may still wish to seek compensation, and that is also their right in most legal systems. More importantly, they may need compensation, to care for an injured child for instance. At the moment the legal process generally needs to be invoked before a patient receives compensation, except in jurisdictions such as Sweden and New Zealand, who have introduced systems of no fault compensation. However, even without no fault compensation there is absolutely no need for a protracted legal process in less serious cases. Healthcare organizations could easily be much more proactive in stepping in with offers of help and, if necessary, financial assistance.

Finally, the patient information leaflet rightly draws attention to the impact on staff, discussed in the next chapter. Injured patients may not, quite understandably, be thinking much about the staff but everyone involved in a serious incident will be affected to some degree. However, it is perhaps unfortunate that according to the policy statement, the patient and their carers are described as distressed, but the incident is said to be traumatic for the healthcare team. Much as we want to acknowledge the impact on staff, the outcome is more usually distress for the staff and trauma for the patient. Some patients feel that the phrase 'second victim' to describe the experience of staff obscures and denigrates the much more profound suffering of the patient.

The Australian Open Disclosure policy has recently been evaluated by Rick Iedema and colleagues in a series of interviews with 23 patients and family members and 131 staff involved in an early series of open disclosure meetings. Some of the errors had no long-term consequences, but most were serious; there were, for instance, a number of drug overdoses and several of the patients had died, though not necessarily because of the error. Families appreciated the open process, were very appreciative of supportive staff but some described conflicting accounts, and partial or grudging apologies. Patients and families generally wanted to meet clinical staff involved in the incident, and were disappointed if this did not happen.

Staff were consistent in regarding the meetings as valuable if difficult experiences and patients, while not always satisfied with the outcomes, did not regret taking part. Many of the difficulties derived from the fact that the process was new to all concerned and still evolving; staff particularly felt that they were in a 'grey zone' in which open disclosure was being advised, but the support, knowledge and training to underpin it were still being developed. The experiences of all involved allowed the researchers to flesh out the process and begin to outline the essential features of a successful open disclosure meeting (Box 9.4). When successful, the experience could be very powerful as this staff member recollects:

I'll never forget it, there must've been about 15 people and a couple of relatives because the patient was unconscious at that time. And it was just the most powerful thing I've ever seen, this [clinician] saying 'I really don't know what happened. I really can't explain what happened, but it shouldn't have happened, and I have to take the responsibility for that. I was the one that had the responsibility for it.' You could see he was gutted and the family responded to that. This was a human, and their loved one was in there not well and really nobody knew how things were going to progress. [But the patient] did wake up, and the relationship that was formed between the patient and her partner and the clinician was really quite phenomenal and they both learnt such a lot from that whole episode.
(IEDEMA *ET AL.*, 2008)

BOX 9.4 Characteristics of a good open disclosure process as identified by patients and their families

The process must:
- allow staff to show respect to the patient (and/or family members) by offering an immediate and sincere apology;
- be conducted as much as possible by those originally involved in the patient's care;
- allow patients to appoint a support person;
- allow patients to indicate the matters they want to see clarified and action taken on;
- allow staff to give carefully structured feedback as matters come to light, rather than delaying feedback until the end of a closed-door investigation;
- prevent different staff expressing conflicting perspectives on the causes of the unexpected outcome;
- minimise different staff engaging consumers in repeated questioning about the case;
- be deployed as a formal process for all high-severity adverse events.

(IEDEMA RAM ET AL. **THE NATIONAL OPEN DISCLOSURE PILOT: EVALUATION OF A POLICY IMPLEMENTATION INITIATIVE**. MJA 2008; 188 (7): 397-400. © COPYRIGHT 2008. *THE MEDICAL JOURNAL OF AUSTRALIA* – REPRODUCED WITH PERMISSION)

Barriers to open disclosure

Advocates of openness and proactive approaches to distressed or injured patients are frequently questioned by more cautious colleagues about the problems that may arise. Generally clinicians want to be more open, but are anxious about the disapproval of colleagues, complaints and litigation, the mindless assaults of the media or the anger and bitterness of patients and relatives. Clearly there is an ethical imperative to inform patients of adverse outcomes, but the fear of legal action and media attention can act as a major disincentive (Box 9.5).

BOX 9.5 Barriers to open disclosure

Environmental factors:
- Resource and time pressures of busy clinical environments;
- Inadequacy of existing adverse incident reporting and learning systems;
- Lack of organizational protocols;
- Lack of demonstrated good stories on how to practice 'open disclosure' well.

Professional factors
- Lack of personal and peer support for healthcare professionals involved;
- Feelings of guilt, shame and disappointment;

- Lack of experience and training in disclosure;
- Debate about when open disclosure is needed;
- Culture of secrecy around professional failings;
- Fear of medico-legal risk consequences;
- Fear of damage to professional reputation;
- Perceptions that open disclosure is another 'bureaucratic imposition';
- Perceptions that patient may be over-reacting to relatively minor events;
- Questioning of patients' motive in seeking open disclosure.

Patient factors
- Patients finding it hard to 'speak up,' ask questions and have their needs for information met;
- Lack of knowledge about medical issues of relevance to their case;
- Persistence of a 'doctor as god' attitude;
- Patients feeling physically unwell and vulnerable;
- Anxiety about staff distancing themselves because of a perceived lack of gratitude for care received.

(JAMES PICHERT & GERALD HICKSON. COMMUNICATING RISKS TO PATIENTS AND FAMILIES. IN "CLINICAL RISK MANAGEMENT: ENHANCING PATIENT SAFETY. 2ND EDITION: CHARLES VINCENT, EDITOR. (PP 573; £47.50). LONDON: BMJ BOOKS, 2001. ISBN 0 7279 1392 1 263–282, 2001, WITH PERMISSION FROM BMJ PUBLISHING GROUP LTD.)

There are also a number of practical issues which remain to be worked out. One major issue is simply the time it would take to disclose all errors fully. Given the scale of error and harm to patients, the potential time involved could be huge. We have yet to work out styles of disclosure appropriate to what has occurred. At one end of the scale, openness and honesty might only require a 10-second acknowledgement of a minor problem and a simple apology. At the other, it could involve a series of meetings over several months; in serious cases, disclosure and ongoing support may literally have life-long implications for some patients. Another issue to resolve is who should disclose the error; at the moment disclosure is often thought of as a doctor-patient encounter, but there is evidence that many nurses feel excluded from the process and believe disclosure should be seen as coming from the team (Shannon *et al.*, 2009). The test must be, of course, what is right for the patient and family. The initial disclosure of a serious incident may best be handled quietly and sensitively by one or two people; later a meeting with a larger team might be necessary.

From the little information available, it does seem clear that those organizations that have followed the path of open disclosure have not been overwhelmed by lawsuits. To the contrary, the experience has been positive and they have argued strongly for others to follow. One hospital in the United States initiated a policy of open disclosure in 1987, deciding to both take a more proactive approach to managing defensible claims and also to come forward and acknowledge when a serious error had been made. This commendable ethical position has led to five major settlements over the years of cases where the patient was unaware that an error had been made. Overall, however, the financial cost of claims since the policy was initiated has been moderate and comparable to other similar institutions (Kraman and Hamm, 2002). After implementing an open disclosure initiative, The University of Michigan Health system reported that frequency of litigation decreased substantially in the five years after its implementation, with annual litigation expense reduced from $3 million to $1 million and the number of claims reduced by 50% (Clinton and Obama, 2006).

Breaking the news about error and harm

A young doctor or nurse will not (or should not) be expected to shoulder the burden of breaking the news of a serious adverse outcome or to deal with the longer-term consequences. A senior doctor would usually discuss the incident with the family, although often accompanied by more junior staff. Nevertheless, it is important for clinicians to understand the principles at any stage in their career for two reasons. The first is that they will need to put these principles into practice at some point, and this could be sooner than they think. More importantly, even very junior staff will already be dealing with adverse outcomes, even though they may not see them as such. A painful injection, a prolonged infection or a frightening procedure are all, in a sense, adverse outcomes for the patient, especially if unexpected. The principles of accepting the patient's response, explaining patiently and being open about what has occurred still apply and are a useful basis for coping later with more serious incidents.

When something has gone wrong, healthcare staff should take the initiative to seek out the patient and/or family and face the situation openly and honestly. Avoiding or delaying such a meeting unnecessarily will only suggest there is something to hide. A senior member of staff needs to give a thorough and clear account of what exactly happened. At the first interview, junior staff involved with the patient may also be present. The patient and their relatives need to have time to reflect on what was said and to be able to return and ask further questions. Remember that people may be numb with shock after an incident and be unable to cope with very much information. Several meetings may be needed over the course of weeks or months. Similar considerations, of course, apply when doctors are breaking bad news of any kind (Finlay and Dallimore, 1991).

Telling patients or their families about disappointing results and dealing with their reactions is not easy. Nevertheless, if done with care and compassion, such communication maintains trust between the people involved and can greatly help the patient's adjustment to what has happened. To help clinical staff faced with these difficult meetings, James Pichert and Gerald Hickson have developed some guidelines (Box 9.6) (Pichert and Hickson, 2001). While they are aimed at fairly serious adverse outcomes, the general principles apply to explaining any unforeseen problem that has arisen in a patient's care and which has caused distress.

> **BOX 9.6** Communication after an error or adverse outcome
>
> - Give bad news in a private place, where the patient and/or family may react and you can respond appropriately.
> - Clearly deliver the message. The adverse outcome must be understood. 'I'm sorry to report that the procedure resulted in ...'
> - Wait silently for a reaction. Give the patient/family time to consider what has happened and formulate their questions.
> - Acknowledge and accept the initial reaction. The usual reaction to bad news is a mixture of denial, anger, resignation, shock and so on. Listen.
> - Resist the urge to blame or appear to blame other health professionals for the outcome.
> - Discuss transition support. Tell the patient/family what steps will be taken to provide medical, social or other forms of support.
> - Finish by reassuring them about your continued willingness to answer any questions they might have. Discuss next steps.
> - Consider scheduling a follow-up meeting. Some patients will want to talk only after the crisis has subsided
> - Afterwards, document a summary of the discussion. Ideally share this with the patient and family.
>
> (ADAPTED FROM PICHERT AND HICKSON, 2001)

In the longer term

When serious harm has been done, acknowledging and discussing the incident is just the first stage. The longer-term needs of patients, families and staff need to be considered. We cannot possibly cover all the eventualities here; however, there are a few basic and useful things to bear in mind.

Ask specific questions about emotional trauma

A common theme in interviews with injured patients is that none of the professionals involved in their care appreciated the depth of their distress. I can recall several patients left in severe pain who were deeply depressed and at times suicidal; although great efforts were being made to deal with their physical problems, no one had thought to ask about their mental state. Risk managers, clinicians and others involved with these patients can ask basic questions without fear of 'making things worse'. The case histories illustrate some of the most common reactions and experiences of people suffering from depression and post-traumatic stress disorder. Other crucial areas of enquiry are feelings of anger, humiliation, betrayal and loss of trust – all frequently experienced by injured patients.

When something truly awful has happened, staff are naturally also affected. In most clinical situations the need to think clearly and act decisively means that emotions must be kept under control. Similarly, it is of no help whatever to patients, and may be quite damaging, if staff are obviously unable to cope with the tragedy that has occurred. However, this does not mean that staff need to be remote or uninvolved. Many patients have derived comfort from the empathy and sadness of staff involved in tragic incidents, describing, for instance, the warmth and support they found in the staff's own sadness at the event.

A proportion of patients are likely to be sufficiently anxious or depressed to warrant formal psychological or psychiatric treatment. It is unrealistic to expect the staff of say, a surgical unit, to shoulder the burden of formal counselling. They have neither the time nor the necessary training to deal with the more serious reactions. When a referral to a psychologist or psychiatrist is indicated, it must be carefully handled. Injured patients are understandably very wary of their problems being seen as 'psychological' or 'all in the mind'. When symptoms of anxiety, for instance, are approached sensitively and practically, the resultant trauma can be considerably reduced (Box 9.7).

BOX 9.7 Anaesthetic awareness: reducing the fear of future operations

A woman was admitted for an elbow replacement. During the operation she awoke, paralysed and able to hear the discussions amongst the surgical team. She was terrified, in great pain and absolutely helpless. The lack of anaesthetic was fortunately noticed, and she was next aware of waking in recovery screaming.

The risk manager visited the patient at home as soon as practicable, maintained contact, offered psychological treatment for trauma, and advised her on procedures for compensation, including an offer to pay for an independent legal assessment of the eventual offer of compensation. As in the above example, emotional trauma was the principal long-term concern, particularly anxiety about future operations. As this woman suffered chronic conditions requiring further surgery, this problem required some additional, imaginative measures.

Some months later, when the patient felt ready, she was given a tour of the operating theatre and the anaesthetic failure was explained in great detail, as were the procedural changes that had been made subsequent to the incident. This was immensely important in reducing her understandable fear of future operations and minimizing the long-term impact of the incident.

(ADAPTED FROM VINCENT, 2001)

Continuing care and support

Injured patients may receive support, comfort and practical help from many sources. It may come from their spouse, family, friends, colleagues, doctors or community organizations. An especially important source of support will be the doctors, nurses and other health professionals who are involved in their treatment. It is vital that staff continue to provide the same care and do not withdraw from the patient through guilt or embarrassment. After an initial mistake, it is extremely reassuring for a patient to be overseen by a single senior doctor who undertakes to monitor all aspects of their treatment, even if it involves a number of different specialties. Where care has been sub-standard, the patient must be offered a referral elsewhere if that is what they wish but if the incident is dealt with openly and honestly, then trust may even be strengthened.

Financial assistance and practical help

Injured patients often need immediately practical help. They need medical treatment, counselling and explanations, but they may need money too. They may need to support their family while they are recovering, pay for specialist treatment, facilities to cope with disability and so on. In less serious cases, relatively small sums of money to provide therapy, alterations to the home, or additional nursing may make an enormous difference to the patient both practically and in their attitude to the hospital. Protracted and adversarial medico-legal negotiations can be very damaging, frustrating and above all incomprehensible to the patient and their family. One only has to imagine oneself in a similar position to appreciate this. If you were injured in a rail or aviation accident, you would hope and expect the organization concerned to help you. What would your reaction be if, as is still the case for many patients, the message you received was that 'you will be hearing from our lawyers in due course?' (Box 9.8)

BOX 9.8 Explanations and apology after iatrogenic cardiac arrhythmia

Mrs A was admitted for minor day case surgery, expecting to return home later that day. A surgeon requested a weak solution of adrenaline to induce a blood free field, but was given a stronger solution than requested. As soon as the liquid was applied the patient developed a serious cardiac arrhythmia, the operation was terminated and she was transferred to the Intensive Therapy Unit, where she gradually recovered.

The clinical risk manager was alerted immediately and assessed the likely consequences for the patient and her family. The first task was clearly to apologize and provide a full explanation. However, with both the patient and family in a state of shock, this had to be carried out in stages. The consultant and risk manager had a series of short meetings over a few days, to explain what had happened and keep the family informed about ongoing remedial treatment. Each time the family was given the opportunity to reflect on what they had been told and come back with further questions. A small package of compensation was also arranged, primarily aimed at providing the necessary clinical and psychological support. The whole incident was resolved within six months and the patient expressed her thanks to the hospital for the way in which the incident had been handled, particularly the openness about the causes of the incident.

(ADAPTED FROM VINCENT, 2001)

Inform patients of changes

Patients' and relatives' wish to prevent future incidents can be seen both as a genuine desire to safeguard others and as an attempt to find some way of coping with their own pain or loss. The pain may be ameliorated if they feel that, because changes were made, then at least some good came of their experiences. Relatives of patients who have died may express their motives for litigation in terms of an obligation to the dead person to make sure that a similar accident never happens again, so that some good comes of their death. The implication of this is that if changes have been made as a result of the adverse outcome, it is very important to inform the patients concerned. While some may regret that the changes were made too late for them, most will appreciate the fact that their experience was understood and acted upon.

BOX 9.9 Support organizations founded by patients

MRSA Action UK – founded by a group of people who all had life changing experiences or lost a loved one through contracting MRSA – all volunteers who share a common purpose – to relieve the distress and suffering experienced by patients who contract healthcare infections.

Consumers Advancing Patient Safety (CAPS) – a consumer-led, non-profit organization formed to be a collective voice for individuals, families and healers who wish to prevent harm in healthcare encounters through partnership and collaboration. Susan Sheridan, Co-founder and President, became involved in patient safety after her family experienced two serious medical system failures.

Person United Limited Substandard and Errors (PULSE) – a non-profit organization working to improve patient safety and reduce the rate of medical errors using real life stories and experiences. Survivors of medical errors are encouraged to use their experience to educate the community and advocate for a safer healthcare system.

Medically Induced Trauma Support Services (MITSS), Inc – a non-profit organization whose mission is 'To Support Healing and Restore Hope' to patients, families and clinicians who have been affected by an adverse medical event. Set up by Linda Kenney, who experienced an error and nearly died, and Rick van Pelt, an anaesthetist. The organization is aimed at promoting honesty, error disclosure and support for traumatized patients.

Compassion in action

Injured or bereaved patients may go much further than seeking reassurance from the hospital that changes will be made. A number of patient safety champions have emerged in many countries, supported by the World Alliance for Patient Safety, who have brought the patient voice to patient safety and who campaign for safer healthcare on behalf of the patient. Often this takes the form, initially, of recounting the story of their particular tragedy to healthcare audiences so that they may fully appreciate what is at stake when patient safety is discussed. Increasingly however, such people are finding a wider role in actively working on the design of healthcare services, in policy and in wider safety initiatives, a subject we will return to in a later chapter. Some injured patients have gone further still in establishing organizations which are specifically aimed at supporting patients and families who are the victims of error and harm. As I once heard it expressed, such actions are, amongst other things, 'a way of bringing meaning to the loss.'

References

Bismark, M. and Paterson, R. (2005) 'Doing the right thing' after an adverse event. *The New Zealand Medical Journal*, **118**(1219), U1593.

Brewin, C.R., Dalgleish, T. and Joseph, S. (1996) A dual representation theory of post-traumatic stress disorder. *Psychological Review*, **103**, 670–686.

Clarke, D.M., Russell, P.A., Polglase, A.L. and McKenzie, D.P. (1997) Psychiatric disturbance and acute stress response in surgical patients. *Australia and New Zealand Journal of Surgery*, **67**, 115–118.

Cleopas, A., Villaveces, A., Charvet, A. *et al.* (2006) Patient assessments of a hypothetical medical error: effects of health outcome, disclosure, and staff responsiveness. *Quality and Safety in Health Care*, **15**(2), 136–141.

Clinton, H.R. and Obama, B. (2006) Making patient safety the centerpiece of medical liability reform. *The New England Journal of Medicine*, **354**(21), 2205–2208.

Czarnocka, J. and Slade, P. (2000) Prevalence and predictors of post-traumatic stress symptoms following childbirth. *British Journal of Clinical Psychology*, **39**, 35–52.

Davis, R.E. (2009) *Patient Involvement in Patient Safety*, Imperial College, London.

Duclos, C.W., Eichler, M., Taylor, L. *et al.* (2005) Patient perspectives of patient-provider communication after adverse events. *International Journal for Quality in Health Care*, **17**(6), 479–486.

Entman, S.S., Glass, C.A., Hickson, G.B. *et al.* (1994) The relationship between malpractice claims history and subsequent obstetric care. *Journal of the American Medical Association*, **272**(20), 1588–1591.

Finlay, I. and Dallimore, D. (1991) Your child is dead. *British Medical Journal*, **302**, 1524–1525.

Gallagher, T.H., Waterman, A.D., Ebers, A.G. *et al.* (2003) Patients' and physicians' attitudes regarding the disclosure of medical errors. *Journal of the American Medical Association*, **289**(8), 1001–1007.

Gallagher, T.H., Studdert, D. and Levinson, W. (2007) Disclosing harmful medical errors to patients. *The New England Journal of Medicine*, **356**(26), 2713–2719.

Hickson, G.B., Clayton, E.W., Entman, S.S. *et al.* (1994) Obstetricians' prior malpractice experience and patients' satisfaction with care. *Journal of the American Medical Association*, **272**(20), 1583–1587.

Hobgood, C., Peck, C.R., Gilbert, B. *et al.* (2002) Medical errors – what and when: what do patients want to know? *Academic Emergency Medicine*, **9**(11), 1156–1161.

Iedema, R., Sorensen, R., Manias, E. *et al.* (2008) Patients' and family members' experiences of open disclosure following adverse events. *International Journal for Quality in Health Care*, **20**(6), 421–432.

Kessler, R.C. (1997) The effect of stressful life events on depression. *Annual Review of Psychology*, **48**, 191–214.

Kraman, S.S. and Hamm, G. (2002) Risk management: extreme honesty may be the best policy. *Annals of Internal Medicine*, **131**(12), 963–967.

Lamb, R.M., Studdert, D.M., Bohmer, R.M. *et al.* (2003) Hospital disclosure practices: results of a national survey. *Health Affairs*, **22**(2), 73–83.

Lehman, D.R., Wortman, C.B. and Williams, A.F. (1987) Long-term effects of losing a spouse or child in a motor vehicle crash. *Journal of Personality and Social Psychology*, **52** (1), 218–231.

Lundin, T. (1984) Morbidity following sudden and unexpected bereavement. *British Journal of Psychiatry*, **144**, 84–88.

Mazor, K.M., Reed, G.W., Yood, R.A. *et al.* (2006) Disclosure of medical errors: what factors influence how patients respond? *Journal of General Internal Medicine*, **21**(7), 704–710.

Pichert, J. and Hickson, G. (2001) Communicating risk to patients and families, *Clinical Risk Management*, 2nd edn (ed. C.A. Vincent), BMJ Publications, London, pp. 263–282.

Schwappach, D.L. and Koeck, C.M. (2004) What makes an error unacceptable? A factorial survey on the disclosure of medical errors. *International Journal for Quality in Health Care*, **16**(4), 317–326.

Shannon, S.E., Foglia, M.B., Hardy, M. and Gallagher, T.H. (2009) Disclosing errors to patients: perspectives of registered nurses. *Joint Commission Journal on Quality and Patient Safety*, **35**(1), 5–12.

Silversides, A. (2009) Empathy and understanding down under. *Canadian Medical Association Journal*, **181**(8), E180.

Vincent, C., Young, M. and Phillips, A. (1994) Why do people sue doctors? A study of patients and relatives taking legal action. *Lancet*, **343**, 1609–1613.

Vincent, C.A., Pincus, T. and Scurr, J.H. (1993) Patients' experience of surgical accidents. *Quality in Health Care*, **2**, 77–82.

Vincent, C.A. (2001) Caring for patients harmed by treatment, *Clinical Risk Management. Enhancing Patient Safety*, 2nd edn (ed. C.A. Vincent), BMJ Publications, London, pp. 461–479.

Vincent, C.A. and Coulter, A. (2002) Patient safety. What about the patient? *Quality and Safety in Healthcare*, **11**(1), 76–80.

CHAPTER 10
Supporting staff after serious incidents

Human beings make frequent errors and misjudgements in every sphere of activity, but some environments are less forgiving of error than others. Errors in academia, law or architecture, for instance, can mostly be remedied with an apology or a cheque. Those in medicine, in the air, or on an oil rig may have severe or even catastrophic consequences. This is not to say that the errors of doctors, nurses or pilots are more reprehensible, only that they bear a greater burden because their errors have greater consequences. Making an error, particularly if a patient is harmed because of it, may therefore have profound consequences for the staff involved, particularly if they are seen, rightly or wrongly, as primarily responsible for the outcome. The typical reaction has been well expressed by Albert Wu in the quotation below, which is taken from his aptly titled paper 'the second victim'. All these observations apply to some degree to other health professionals, though the little research in this area is almost entirely restricted to doctors.

Social, legal and personal imperatives drive us to condemn people who make serious mistakes and harm others. Our gut feeling, however much systems thinking we have absorbed, is that this is just appalling and the person concerned must be brought to book. Atul Gawande, an American surgeon, explores this theme, after a description or his own involvement in a near disaster:

Consider some other surgical mishaps. In one, a general surgeon left a large metal instrument in a patient's abdomen, where it tore through the bowel and the wall of the bladder. In another a cancer surgeon biopsied the wrong part of a woman's breast and thereby delayed her diagnosis of cancer for months. A cardiac surgeon skipped a small but key step during a heart valve operation, thereby killing the patient . . .

How could anyone who makes a mistake of that magnitude be allowed to practice medicine? We call such doctors 'incompetent', 'unethical' and 'negligent'. We want to see them punished. And so we've wound up with the public system we have for dealing with error: malpractice lawsuits, media scandal, suspensions, firings.

Patient Safety, 2nd edition. By Charles Vincent. Published 2010 by Blackwell Publishing Ltd.

There is however a central truth in medicine that complicates this tidy vision of misdeeds and misdoers: all doctors make terrible mistakes. Consider the cases I've just described. I gathered them simply by asking respected surgeons I know – surgeons at top medical schools - to tell me about mistakes they had made in the last year.
(GAWANDE, 2002)

BOX 10.1 Death of a child

When I was an inexperienced registrar some eight years ago, a child died under my care. Her death was largely preventable, but caused by a series of errors. I had been a registrar for 24 months, and I had on duty with me a senior house officer who was new to paediatrics. It was an exceptionally busy day covering the wards and accident and emergency department, with cases including a child with tubercular meningitis and another with acute subdural haemorrhage from non-accidental injury. After 5 p.m. I was also responsible for the neonatal intensive care unit, which had 15 intensive care cots.

The child who died was admitted in the morning with a seizure. I had seen her before in the outpatient clinic and during a previous admission with an 'atypical febrile convulsion', when she had been noted to be hypoglycaemic and had had further tests. We initially checked her electrolytes, gave her rectal then intravenous diazepam, and did an infection screen in view of a low grade fever. She was hypoglycaemic on admission, which we corrected.

After admission she appeared to stabilize but later started having another seizure. I ordered a clonazepam infusion, and saw her several times during the day. The professor rang mid-afternoon and asked how things were. I expressed concern about the child, but he suggested no new management. Later that evening, while I was busy on the neonatal unit, the nursing staff notified me that the child was having yet another seizure. I rang the subspecialist. We discussed the case but he sounded uninterested. He suggested I perform a lumbar puncture. I thought this was too risky and my decision was fortunate in the end. She died four hours later from coning secondary to status epilepticus and might have died during the lumbar puncture if I had done what was suggested. In retrospect I had confused the masking effect of clonazepam (half life 72 hours) with cessation of her seizure. At her arrest call, resuscitation went reasonably smooth but the child did not respond. I asked for flumazenil (an antidote drug to diazepam). It was not in the emergency drug cupboard. We called an anaesthetist who went to another ward by mistake. It took several hours for an intensive care bed to be found and she subsequently died.

Things could have gone better if there had been protocols for the management of status epilepticus (there were none on the ward). Double cover of busy neonatal and general paediatric units still goes on and should cease entirely. Intensive care availability has improved but needs to continue to do so. In retrospect, there were various things I should have done, such as recognizing that the child was still having a seizure, arranging transfer to intensive care earlier, and getting a neurological opinion.

I was never given an opportunity to discuss this case in a non-critical forum. If a more junior colleague rings a senior colleague at home, the onus is on that colleague to offer to come in and review the case. I didn't feel able to ask. Rather than look ourselves in the mirror we tend to blame others when things go wrong. In a spirit of openness this needs to change'.

REPRINTED FROM *THE LANCET*, **359**, NO. 9323, ALASTAIR G SUTCLIFFE. "DEATH OF A CHILD." [2104], © 2002, WITH PERMISSION FROM ELSEVIER.

Reactions to error and adverse outcomes in medicine are greatly magnified because so much can be at stake. Few other professions face the possibility of causing the death of another person with such regularity, although the likelihood of this obviously varies in different areas of healthcare. The preventable death of a child under one's care is one of the worst clinical experiences for a doctor or nurse. The brave and thoughtful account reproduced here (Box 10.1) foreshadows many of the themes of this chapter. The doctor concerned acknowledges his personal contribution and responsibility in not appreciating the increasing frequency and severity of the seizures. Yet it is clear that he was failed by others and that organizational problems contributed to the delays and possibly to the final outcome. Although the personal impact on the doctor is not directly discussed it was probably profound, as the case is still vivid eight years later. Although a child died, and he was the clinician with immediate responsibility, he was never able to discuss the case in way that would have helped him personally or foster any clinical learning. The phrase 'a spirit of openness' exemplifies the cultural shift that he believes is needed.

The experience of error

Virtually every clinician knows the sickening feeling of making a bad mistake. You feel singled out and exposed – seized by the instinct to see if anyone has noticed. You agonize about what to do, whether to tell anyone, what to say. Later, the event replays itself in your mind. You question your competence but fear being discovered. You know you should confess, but dread the prospect of potential punishment and of the patient's anger.

REPRODUCED FROM *BRITISH MEDICAL JOURNAL*, ALBERT W WU. "MEDICAL ERROR: THE SECOND VICTIM". **320**, NO. 7237, [726–727], 2000, WITH PERMISSION FROM BMJ PUBLISHING GROUP LTD.

For decades there was very little public debate or discussion of the impact of errors on clinicians. Those that tried to bring the subject into the open did not always fare well at the hands of their colleagues. For instance Hilfiker, (1984) argued that 'We see the horror of our own mistakes, yet we are given no permission to deal with their enormous emotional impact... The medical profession simply has no place for its mistakes' (Hilfiker, 1984: p. 118). This paper drew some supportive correspondence, but also some summary and dismissive comment such as 'This neurotic piece has no place in the New England Journal of Medicine' (Anderson, 1984: p. 1676). Hilfiker hoped that others would follow his example and write about their own errors, but was apparently disappointed that progress was slow thereafter (Ely, 1996).

For some young doctors mistakes are the most memorable events of their training. In interviews Mizrahi (1984) found that half of the young doctors he interviewed had made serious and even fatal mistakes in the first two months of their jobs. Jenny Firth Cozens found that British junior doctors singled out making mistakes, together with dealing with death and dying, relationships with senior doctors and overwork, as the most stressful events they had to deal with (Firth-Cozens, 1987); a missed diagnosis by one young doctor made him reject a career in subspecialties that involved 'a lot of data collection and uncertainty'. This echoes the experience of Carlo Fonsecka (1996), who recounted the personal impact of mistakes in a remarkable personal paper that began 'Error free patient care is the ideal standard but in reality unattainable. I am conscious of having made five fatal mistakes during the past 36 years' (Fonsecka, 1996: p. 1640). Fonsecka wrote that, with hindsight, he believes that the impact of the first case was so great, that he no longer felt able to carry on with clinical work and turned eventually to a laboratory based career.

Medical students anticipate the mistakes they will make as doctors, even before entering medical school (Fischer *et al.*, 2006):

I think one of the scariest things about becoming a doctor is realising how much responsibility you have and that human error happens all the time. I thought about it even before I decided that I definitely wanted to go to medical school.
(FISCHER *ET AL.*, 2006)

Students and young trainees regarded errors as inevitable and part of the practice of medicine, though their responses to errors were influenced by a number of different factors. The nature of the error made, the attitude of their supervisor and the consequences of the error all played a part in their response. However, they were also influenced by what Fischer describes as the 'hidden curriculum', the subtle education in the mores, attitudes and values of one's chosen profession which are powerful and pervasive, though seldom explicitly stated. The culture of medicine as exemplified and inculcated in the hidden curriculum could override personal ethics and beliefs (Box 10.2).

BOX 10.2 The hidden curriculum

'In my mind I know what I think is the right thing to do, but sometimes it's a little different than culture dictates'

'Part of the medical community does not want you to speak up about what you've done that was wrong. If I [apologized for making a serious error] there would be a number of people who would be upset at me for being too much like a bleeding heart and not enough of a tough professional and not being aware enough of the current litigious medical situation.'

'In the past I've automatically thought of myself as somebody who's going to go and own up directly to the person, and maybe now I'm not as sure I would do that.'

'The more I get into the medical profession the more I kind of want to defend doctors in making mistakes.'

FROM FISCHER *ET AL.*, 2006

In a series of 11 in-depth interviews with senior doctors, Christensen *et al.* (1992) discussed a variety of serious mistakes, including four deaths. All the doctors were affected to some degree, but four clinicians described intense agony or anguish as the reality of the mistake had sunk in. The interviews identified a number of general themes: the ubiquity of mistakes in clinical practice; the infrequency of self-disclosure about mistakes to colleagues, friends and family; the emotional impact on the physician, such that some mistakes were remembered in great detail, even after several years; and the influence of beliefs about personal responsibility and medical practice. After the initial shock the clinicians had a variety of reactions that had lasted from several days to several months. Some of the feelings of fear, guilt, anger, embarrassment and humiliation were unresolved at the time of the interview, even a year after the mistake. A few reported symptoms of depression, including disturbances in appetite, sleep and concentration. Fears related to concerns for the patient's welfare, litigation and colleagues discovery of their 'incompetence'.

BOX 10.3 Reactions to mistakes

'I missed the diagnosis of pulmonary embolism and treated the patient as a case of severe pneumonia until the day after. The patient's condition deteriorated and only then was the diagnosis put right. I felt guilty and lost confidence.'

'Missing a diagnosis of perforated peptic ulcer in a patient – at least she is now well and survived. It made me feel useless at my job though.'

'I was really shaken. My whole feelings of self-worth and abilities were basically profoundly shaken.'

'I was appalled and devastated that I had done this to somebody.'

'This case has made me very nervous about clinical medicine. I worry now about all febrile patients since they may be on the verge of sepsis.'

'It was hard to concentrate on anything else I was doing because I was so worried about what was happening, so I guess that would be anxiety. I felt guilty, sad, had trouble sleeping, wondering what was going on.'

'I've made quite a few mistakes in my time. They come back to haunt me late at night. Missing a diagnosis, prescribing a wrong drug, botching a procedure. Sometimes, patients have died as a result of my mistakes. Other times, my mistakes have increased their suffering. When they come back to me, late at night, I hold court in my mind, replaying events, wondering whether they were honest mistakes, forgivable mistakes, or if not, how I can go on.'

(FROM FIRTH-COZENS, (1987); CHRISTENSEN *ET AL.* (1992))

Although relatively few studies have focused on nurses or other professions, studies that do exist suggest that nurses also suffer similarly in the aftermath of errors. Not surprisingly they experience the same basic human responses of shame, guilt and anxiety about the consequences. In one study on medication error, nurses were more likely than doctors or pharmacists to report strong emotional responses to making an error and fear of disciplinary action or punishment (Wolf *et al.*, 2000; White *et al.*, 2008), which perhaps reflects the different disciplinary culture of nursing.

The wider impact on clinical staff

Surveys of clinical staff show that the reactions described above are common responses to making a serious error (Aasland and Forde, 2005; Schwappach and Boluarte, 2009). In an early study, Wu *et al.* (1991) sent questionnaires to 254 doctors in training in the United States asking the respondents to describe the most significant mistake in patient care they had made in the last year. Almost all the errors had serious outcomes and almost a third involved a death; feelings of remorse, anger, guilt and inadequacy were common and over a quarter of the doctors feared negative repercussions from the mistake. Accepting responsibility for the error was most likely to result in constructive changes in practice but was also associated with higher levels of distress. Studies have also begun to examine longer-term effects on physicians. Waterman and colleagues examined the effects of medical error experience on five work and life domains in a large survey of 3171 physicians in the United States and Canada (Waterman *et al.*, 2007). Over 90% remembered a specific error or adverse event. Increased anxiety about future errors was reported most frequently (61%) as response to being involved in error, followed by loss of confidence (44%), sleeping difficulties (42%), reduced job satisfaction (42%), and harm to reputation (13%). Experience of one of these reactions was significantly more likely if responders were involved in a serious rather a minor medical error.

Once mood and well-being are affected, the likelihood of making an error can become greater in a cycle of poor clinical performance and deteriorating psychological state. West *et al.* (2006) carried out a remarkable study in which doctors completed self assessments of burn out, depression and capacity for empathy every three months. Doctors who reported a major error were more likely to feel emotionally exhausted and depressed, but also likely to become more depressed and emotionally exhausted in the subsequent three months. In other studies, doctors with high burn out scores were also more likely to report providing sub-optimal care such as 'making treatment errors that were not due to lack of experience' or discharging patient simply to make the service more manageable. These results suggest that personal distress and self-reported error involvement are related in a reciprocal cycle. Feeling responsible for a serious medical error can induce depression and exhaustion, which in turn increases the likelihood of sub-optimal patient care and future errors (Schwappach and Boluarte, 2009).

The suicide of a patient under one's care is a particularly disturbing event. Alexander *et al.* (2000) studied the impact on psychiatrists who were asked to describe their most distressing suicide; 159 consultant psychiatrists provided information on suicides that had happened between 1 month and 20 years ago. While the study does not specifically concern mistakes, any suicide by a patient in one's care raises the spectre of blame and personal responsibility, coupled with anxiety about the critical reactions of both the patient's family and colleagues. The most common reactions were irritability at home, being less able to deal with routine family problems, poor sleep, low mood, preoccupation with the suicide and decreased self confidence. Although none of the psychiatrists took time off work, the effects of the suicide were very persistent, with a number seriously considering early retirement. These salutary experiences, not surprisingly, also affected their clinical management of suicidal patients, generally moving them towards more structured management, more use of suicide observations, more detailed communication about records, a greater willingness to intervene and a more cautious approach to suicide risk.

What makes an error traumatic?

When a patient is harmed, the errors made are often only part of a chain of events inseparable from a web of organizational background causes. Seldom, after close analysis, is it possible to lay the blame for an adverse outcome solely at the door of one individual, however tempting this may be. Junior doctors for instance, may find themselves forced to deal with events that are well beyond their competence, inheriting problems that originate elsewhere in the organization. For them to then take responsibility and shoulder all the blame may be both unwarranted and personally damaging.

What then singles out a mistake as being particularly traumatic for a clinician? Errors, as we have seen, are frequent. Yet only a small proportion bring anguish, regret and shame in their wake. There is almost no research on this issue to my knowledge, but the nature of the error, personal characteristics and medical culture probably all play a part in determining the personal impact.

The error and the reactions of those involved

First, and most obviously, the outcome will be severe. Hindsight bias applies in this area, in that a bad outcome makes one more critical, and indeed more self critical, of the care given. If you 'get away with it', the feeling is likely to be more relief than guilt. Second, it will be a clear departure from the clinician's usual practice, rather than a close call in a genuinely uncertain situation. The reaction of colleagues, whether supportive or defensive and critical, may be equally powerful. The reaction of the patient and their family may be especially hard to bear, especially when the outcome is severe and if there has been a close involvement over a long period. For instance, psychologists or psychiatrists may find the suicide of a patient very hard to face if there has previously been a long therapeutic relationship.

Personal standards and self criticism

Clinicians, like everyone else, vary in temperament, resilience and attitude to their own errors. Jenny Firth-Cozens (1997) has found that a tendency to self criticism is predictive of stress; this tendency may be rooted in earlier relationships, which in turn may find an echo in relationships with senior colleagues. For a highly self critical person, errors and mistakes will be particularly disturbing; in serious cases the clinician may enter a vicious downward spiral of anxiety, shame and deteriorating performance. There is a fine balance to be struck between personal high standards and undue self criticism. The high personal standards of excellent clinicians may in fact make them particularly vulnerable to the impact of mistakes.

Attitudes to error and the culture of medicine

In his landmark paper on error in medicine, Lucian Leape (1994) argued that one of the most important reasons that clinicians have difficulty dealing with error is because of the culture of medical practice. He argued that physicians are socialized from the very first days of medical school to believe that errors are simply not acceptable. While error-free practice is a worthy ambition it is, of course, completely unattainable, so an internal conflict is inevitable:

Physicians, not unlike test pilots, come to view an error as a failure of character – you weren't careful, you didn't try hard enough. This kind of thinking lies behind a common reaction by clinicians: 'How can there be an error without negligence.'
(LEAPE, 1994: P 1852)

All clinicians recognize the inevitability (though perhaps not the frequency) of error. However this seldom carries over into open recognition and discussion. There is therefore a curious, and in some ways paradoxical, clash of beliefs. On the one hand we have an enterprise fraught with uncertainty, where knowledge is inadequate and errors are bound to occur. On the other hand those working in this environment foster a culture of perfection, in which errors are not tolerated, in which a strong sense of personal responsibility both for errors and outcome is expected. With this background it is not surprising that mistakes are hard to deal with, particularly when so much else is at stake in terms of human suffering.

Beliefs about control and the power of medicine

Beliefs about the degree of control the clinician has, will strongly affect their sense of personal responsibility for adverse outcomes and attitudes to mistakes. A certain degree of realism about the likelihood of mistakes, especially with increasing constraints on practice, pressure of work and the need to take short cuts at times, tempers reactions to individual mistakes and makes it less likely that someone will generalize from a single, regrettable mistake to a more general belief that they are incompetent. For instance, in the study of the impact of suicide, discussed above, Alexander *et al.* (2000) comment that psychiatrists have to strike a balance in their attitude to the suicide of their patients. If they regard suicide as unavoidable, they protect themselves and their profession, but consequently end up in a position of therapeutic nihilism. If, on the other hand, they view every suicide as preventable, they lay themselves open to blame and guilt and would probably eventually be unable to continue their work.

The impact of litigation

The impact of errors and mistakes is compounded and deepened when followed by a complaint or litigation. Even the investigation of a serious incident, if badly handled by senior staff, may be very disturbing for a young nurse or doctor. Patients now demand much more of the doctor or nurse, and may be less forgiving when their own expectations of outcome are not fulfilled, though are rightly angry when no apology or explanation is given. The considerable media attention given to medical catastrophes has also made the public much more aware of the potential for harm as well as benefit from medical treatment.

The experience of being sued in a prolonged and difficult case was dramatically documented in Charles and Kennedy's (1985) book, Defendant: A Psychiatrist on Trial for Medical Malpractice. The psychiatrist in question described feeling utterly alone and isolated from colleagues, later finding that this was quite a common experience for those accused of malpractice. The case lasted five years, seemed to swallow up her life completely, demanded constant attention and made her anxious and insomniac. She felt she had lost her integrity as a person and as a doctor (Charles and Kennedy, 1985).

Charles and Kennedy's book broke new ground in bringing the experience of litigation into the open. Later studies of the wider impact of litigation suggested that these experiences were by no means unique (Shapiro *et al.*, 1989; Martin *et al.*, 1991; Bark *et al.*, 1997). Depression, anger and other nervous symptoms were common responses to litigation. Some doctors find their work less rewarding, at least for a time. In Martin *et al.*'s (1991) study of physicians who had been sued, anxiety, depression and traumatic responses were highest in the two years following litigation, but gradually reduced thereafter, though not to the level of physicians who had not been sued. In contrast, feelings of shame and doubt, though prominent at an early stage, did return to ordinary levels, particularly in those who had won their case. Older physicians however, seemed less affected and more able to put litigation into perspective, as a job hazard rather than an indictment of their ability.

Litigation can clearly be very unpleasant, and sometimes traumatic, but the impact of litigation should not be overstated. We should remember though that in the last 20 years our understanding of the extent and causes of patient harm been transformed; a claim for compensation need not be seen as a shameful personal attack on the responsible doctor. Often, when the case is clear cut and the harm not severe, or at least not permanent, it may be little more than tedious. In most countries very few cases ever reach trial, almost all being settled by lawyers and risk managers, sometimes with little involvement of the clinical staff (which is sometimes welcome and sometimes not). Although some people will always complain, and a few unpleasant or deluded characters delight in litigation, very few injured patients sue; this is partly because, whatever the rights and wrongs of the case, it is a deeply wearing experience in which they constantly have to recall experiences they would much prefer to forget.

We should also just step back for a moment and reflect, from the perspective of both clinician and patient, why litigation has to happen at all? When patients do sue it is for explanations, apologies, to bring about change in the system and, to a widely varying extent, for money (Vincent, Young and Phillips, 1994). For most of the deserving cases, all of these things could be provided by proactive healthcare organizations without litigation and in fact without the need for legislation or no fault compensation. This in turn would make life a great deal easier for the staff involved; when care had been sub-standard, they would know the patients and family were being looked after. When care had been satisfactory, and a case had to be defended, they would have the organization firmly on their side.

Strategies for coping with error, harm and their aftermath

Many of the doctors interviewed in these various studies had not discussed the mistakes or their emotional impact with colleagues. Shame, fears of humiliation, fear of punishment and all acted to deter open discussion and isolate people from their colleagues. When the case was discussed, it would be with close friends or colleagues whom they had come to trust over a long period. The doctors involved wanted the emotional support and professional reaffirmation, but their culture did not often permit such open discussions (Christensen, Levinson and Dunn, 1992; Newman, 1996).

> **BOX 10.4** Strategies for coping with error and harm
>
> Be open about error and its frequency. Senior staff talking openly about past mistakes and problems is particularly effective.
>
> Accept that a need for support is not a sign of weakness. Clinicians have to be resilient but almost all are grateful for the support of colleagues when disaster strikes.
>
> Provide clear guidelines for discussion of error with patients backed up by board level policy on open disclosure.
>
> Offer training in the difficult task of communicating with patient and families in the aftermath of an adverse event is undoubtedly important.
>
> Provide basic education in the law and the legal process, which should reduce some of the anxiety about legal action.
>
> Offer support to staff after major incidents. This may simply be informal support from a colleague.
>
> For a particularly profound reaction, perhaps to the death of a child, formal psychological intervention may be valuable.

People, organizations and culture vary enormously in their approaches and response to error and attitudes to error are changing. Hopefully, as patient safety evolves, healthcare staff will be able to be more open about error and more open about their need for support when errors do occur. While there is little formal guidance, and almost no research on this topic, the following suggestions may be useful.

Potential for error must be acknowledged

First, the potential for error in medicine, as in other activities, needs to be recognized and openly acknowledged. Education about the ubiquity of error, its causes and likely consequences, would promote a more realistic attitude and constructive approach. In clinical medicine, open discussion of error, particularly by respected senior figures, is very powerful because it provides a mandate for such discussions to occur at other times. In effect, the junior nurse or doctor learns that it is acceptable to discuss errors openly because their seniors do it. Modelling of behaviour, as the psychologists call it, is one of the most powerful influences on who we are and what we do. Over time, such changes in attitude and behaviour become embedded as the culture of a unit or organization as 'how we do things round here'.

During the student years, it may also be possible to identify those students who may be vulnerable to excessive reactions to errors – for example, those in whom tutors see signs of self-blame in clinical discussions. High self criticism is a way of thinking, a cognitive style in which self blame occurs whenever things go wrong; it could potentially be changed by teaching students how to allocate responsibility less destructively (Firth-Cozens, 1997).

Agreed policy on openness with injured patients

Many initiatives which are aimed to help patients, such as a policy of open disclosure, can also be a considerable help to staff. Supporting patients and supporting staff are not separate activities, but inextricably intertwined. Many staff are still torn between their own desire for a more open stance and the more cautious approach that they perceive to be demanded, rightly or wrongly, by managers, colleagues and medico legal organizations. This can turn an already very difficult situation into a real conflict that is traumatic for staff and patient alike. This brings home the extent to which a different approach to error and adverse events on the part of clinicians needs to be mirrored by a similar shift in attitudes on the part of managers, lawyers, and indeed patients and relatives.

Support from colleagues

Being understanding of others when they are in the unenviable position of having made a serious error is a vital step towards a more open, indeed a safer, culture. Individual clinicians can do a great deal here, whatever their profession or seniority, to promote a more constructive and supportive approach to errors by simply empathizing with the experience. Albert Wu suggests a personal assignment of structured reflection:

Think back to your last mistake that harmed a patient. Talk to a colleague about it. Notice your colleague's reactions and your own. What helps? What makes it harder? Physicians will always make mistakes. The decisive factor will be how we handle them. Patient safety and physician welfare will be served if we can be more honest about our mistakes to our patients, our colleagues, and ourselves.
(WU, 2000)

In Alexander *et al.*'s (2000) study of the impact of a suicide, the most common and effective sources of help were team members, other psychiatrists, and the psychiatrists' own families and friends. Team meetings and critical incident reviews after a suicide were generally experienced as helpful; one can imagine that exploring the full range of causes of such an event might put individual contributions, or omissions, in perspective. Legal and disciplinary proceedings, and fatal accident enquiries, with their judicial or quasi judicial status were, although uncommon, viewed as stressful and critical.

Professional colleagues were particularly important because they shared an understanding of the professional responsibilities and also prevented those dealing with the aftermath of a suicide from slipping into a dangerous professional isolation. Family members, who themselves were indirectly affected, provided a different kind of help. Talking it through with a colleague brought perspective, whereas talking it over with a husband or wife brought comfort. Patients' families could be very supportive but, understandably, sometimes critical, depending presumably on their own assessment of the care the patient had received and their own relationship with the person before the suicide.

Education and training

Part of the horror of a complaint or threat of litigation lies, for a young clinician at least, simply in ignorance of what is involved. Hospital policies for the investigation of serious incidents for instance, are often expressed in threatening and quasi legal terms that are more likely to provoke fear and paranoia than reflection and learning. Legal procedures vary from country to country but, in Britain for instance, there is no trial by jury for medical negligence and the great majority of cases are settled without a trial of any kind. Education in legal matters for all staff, together with specific information about the likely course of any complaint or claim, can reduce a great deal of unnecessary distress (Genn, 1995). Many doctors act as experts and have considerable experience of the litigation process and therefore represent an important educative resource for their peers and for the junior staff (Hirst, 1996).

Training in disclosing and explaining error is also critical. Facing a patient harmed by treatment, or their naturally distressed and angry relatives, is a particularly difficult clinical situation for which little guidance or training is available. Both patients and staff will benefit if clinical staff have some training in helping dissatisfied, distressed, or injured patients and their relatives.

Formal support and access to confidential counselling

Clinicians are resilient people, but anyone may be vulnerable, because of personality, position or circumstance, to distressingly severe reactions to error. While younger clinicians may be more vulnerable, anyone can be affected at any stage in their career, unless they have become so arrogant or damaged as to be insensitive to the impact of mistakes on their patients.

Understanding and acceptance from colleagues is always important but sometimes people need more than general support and expressions of confidence. The range of potential support extends from a quiet word in a corridor to the offer of extended psychotherapy. Sometimes a private discussion with a colleague or a senior figure will be sufficient; some hospitals employ recently retired senior doctors as mentors. In Bark et al.'s (1997) study, over a quarter of doctors suggested the formal provision of a counselling service and nominated mentors to whom they could refer. A link with a psychiatrist or psychologist from another organization can be useful when the strain is severe or prolonged, as occurs when a member of staff feels responsible for a serious injury or death (Hirst, 1996).

The decision to accept support must, however be left to the individual concerned, who should feel free to ask for a greater or lesser degree of involvement as time goes on. Managers tempted to provide 'stress counselling', especially from paid sources outside the organization, should remember that support from immediate colleagues is usually much more welcome and appropriate (Hirst, 1996). Psychiatrists involved in a suicide felt that it was important that there was access to support and more formal methods of treatment, such as counselling or debriefing; however, they were adamant that these should simply be offered and no attempt should be made to push people into treatment (Alexander et al., 2000).

Peer support after adverse medical events

Few organizations have put staff support service into practice in an organized and effective way or fully understood the need for such a service. In Waterman's study in the United States, 90% of clinicians stated that their organization did not provide adequate support for stress due to medical errors. Brigham and Women's Hospital in Boston is an exception, the home of a remarkable experiment in both patient and staff support that has its origins in a near disaster in 1999 in which Linda Kenney, the founder of Medically Induced Trauma Support Services, experienced a grand mal seizure during an operation for which the anaesthetist, Frederick van Pelt felt responsible. His initial experience sets the scene:

As is typical during medical emergencies, we were focused on the resuscitation with our emotions on hold. Only after the patient had been stabilised on bypass did the impact of what I had just done begin to sink in. I felt personally responsible for what had happened and compelled to communicate with the family. I thought I would be able to provide a factual account of the event to the husband but to my shock, the husband came at me with full emotional and physical force; fortunately the orthopaedic surgeon intercepted him. I was now forced to confront my own emotional distress and I realised my complete lack of training in how to manage this situation. In an instant, the years of clinical training, my board certification and the respect of my colleagues as a competent anaesthesiologist had become irrelevant and meaningless. I felt lost and alone.

REPRODUCED FROM QUALITY & SAFETY IN HEALTH CARE, F VAN PELT. "PEER SUPPORT: HEALTHCARE PROFESSIONALS SUPPORTING EACH OTHER AFTER ADVERSE MEDICAL EVENTS". **17**, NO. 4, [249–252], 2008, WITH PERMISSION FROM BMJ PUBLISHING GROUP LTD.

Linda Kenney was successfully treated and, although severely traumatized, eventually recovered. The hospital passed the incident to the risk management department who sent her impersonal legalistic letters that distressed and angered her. Dr van Pelt was told not to communicate further with the family. Eventually however:

My profound sense of responsibility broke through my fear and compelled me to do the right thing. I chose to write the patient a letter of apology without informing the hospital and invited the patient to open communication if and when she was ready.

REPRODUCED FROM QUALITY & SAFETY IN HEALTH CARE, F VAN PELT. "PEER SUPPORT: HEALTHCARE PROFESSIONALS SUPPORTING EACH OTHER AFTER ADVERSE MEDICAL EVENTS". **17**, NO. 4, [249–252], 2008, WITH PERMISSION FROM BMJ PUBLISHING GROUP LTD.

Doctor and patient spoke on the telephone and eventually, two years after the incident, met and shared their experiences. They began in parallel to establish support services for patients (MITSS, see previous chapter) and a peer support programme for clinical staff. Support services did exist but surveys showed that few people used them because of the stigma attached to using services aimed primarily at mental health problems. The Peer Support Programme focused instead on using colleagues as the primary support, following an approach that has been successfully used in the police, fire and emergency medical services. The programme is now used for a broad range of incidents including personal crisis, medical error and support during litigation. The programme aims to recruit credible, experienced clinical staff with personal understanding of the impact of error, whom are immediately available to provide confidential reflection and support. An education and training programme runs in parallel that aims to challenge the culture of denial of emotional response to serious errors and events. In addition to an active commitment to disclosure and apology, Brigham and Women's Hospital has started to develop an Early Support Activation (ESA) with MITSS for patients and families in conjunction with the hospital's departments of social services and patient relations. The long-term strategy is to have a comprehensive emotional support response for patients, families and care providers (van Pelt, 2008).

References

Aasland, O.G. and Forde, R. (2005) Impact of feeling responsible for adverse events on doctors' personal and professional lives: the importance of being open to criticism from colleagues. *Quality and Safety in Health Care*, **14**(1), 13–17.

Alexander, D.A., Klein, S., Gray, N.M. *et al.* (2000) Suicide by patients: questionnaire study of its effect on consultant psychiatrists. *British Medical Journal*, **320**(7249), 1571–1574.

Anderson, M. (1984) Facing our mistakes. *New England Journal of Medicine*, **310**, 1676.

Bark, P., Vincent, C., Olivieri, L. and Jones, A. (1997) Impact of litigation on senior clinicians: implications for risk management. *Quality in Health Care*, **6**, 7–13.

Charles, S.C. and Kennedy, E. (1985) *Defendant: A Psychiatrist on Trial for Medical Malpractice*, Free Press, New York.

Christensen, J.F., Levinson, W. and Dunn, P.M. (1992) The heart of darkness: the impact of perceived mistakes on physicians. *Journal of General Internal Medicine*, **7**, 424–431.

Ely, J.W. (1996) Physicians' mistakes. Will your colleagues offer support? *Archives of Family Medicine*, **5**, 76–77.

Firth-Cozens, J. (1987) Emotional distress in junior house officers. *British Medical Journal*, **295**, 533–536.

Firth-Cozens, J. (1997) Predicting stress in general practitioners: 10-year follow-up postal survey. *British Medical Journal*, **315**, 34–35.

Fischer, M.A., Mazor, K.M., Baril, J. *et al.* (2006) Learning from mistakes. Factors that influence how students and residents learn from medical errors. *Journal of General Internal Medicine*, **21**(5), 419–423.

Fonsecka, C. (1996) To err was fatal. *British Medical Journal*, **313**, 1640–1642.

Gawande, A. (2002) *Complications: A Surgeons Notes on An Imperfect Science*, Picador, New York.

Genn, H. (1995) Supporting staff involved in litigation, in *Clinical Risk Management* (ed. C.A. Vincent), BMJ Publications, London, pp. 453–472.

Hilfiker, D. (1984) Facing our mistakes. *New England Journal of Medicine*, **310**(2), 118–122.

Hirst, D. (1996) Supporting staff during litigation – managerial aspects. *Clinical Risk*, **2**, 189–194.

Leape, L.L. (1994) Error in medicine. *Journal of the American Medical Association*, **272**(23), 1851–1857.

Martin, C.A., Wilson, J.F., Fiebelman, N.D. III *et al.* (1991) Physicians' psychological reactions to malpractice litigation. *Southern Medical Journal*, **84**(11), 1300–1304.

Mizrahi, T. (1984) Managing medical mistakes: ideology, insularity and accountability among internists-in-training. *Social Science & Medicine*, **19**(2), 135–146.

Newman, M.C. (1996) The emotional impact of mistakes on family physicians. *Archives of Family Medicine*, **5**(2), 71–75.

Schwappach, D.L. and Boluarte, T.A. (2009) The emotional impact of medical error involvement on physicians: a call for leadership and organisational accountability. *Swiss Medical Weekly*, **139**(1–2), 9–15.

Shapiro, R.S., Simpson, D.E., Lawrence, S.L. *et al.* (1989) A survey of sued and non-sued physicians and suing patients. *Archives of Internal Medicine*, **149**, 2190–2196.

Sutcliffe, A.G. (2002) Death of a child. *The Lancet*, **359**(9323), 2104.

van Pelt, F. (2008) Peer support: healthcare professionals supporting each other after adverse medical events. *Quality and Safety in Health Care*, **17**(4), 249–252.

Vincent, C., Young, M. and Phillips, A. (1994) Why do people sue doctors? A study of patients and relatives taking legal action. *The Lancet*, **343**(June 25), 1609–1613.

Waterman, A.D., Garbutt, J., Hazel, E. *et al.* (2007) The emotional impact of medical errors on practicing physicians in the United States and Canada. *Joint Commission Journal on Quality and Patient Safety*, **33**(8), 467–476.

West, C.P., Huschka, M.M., Novotny, P.J. *et al.* (2006) Association of perceived medical errors with resident distress and empathy: a prospective longitudinal study. *Journal of the American Medical Association*, **296**(9), 1071–1078.

White, A.A., Gallagher, T.H., Krauss, M.J. *et al.* (2008) The attitudes and experiences of trainees regarding disclosing medical errors to patients. *Academic Medicine*, **83**(3), 250–256.

Wolf, Z.R., Serembus, J.F., Smetzer, J. *et al.* (2000) Responses and concerns of healthcare providers to medication errors. *Clinical Nurse Specialist*, **14**(6), 278–287.

Wu, A. (2000) Medical error: the second victim. *British Medical Journal*, **320**, 726–727.

Wu, A.W., Folkman, S., McPhee, S.J. and Lo, B. (1991) Do house officers learn from their mistakes? *Journal of the American Medical Association*, **265**(16), 2089–2094.

Design, Technology and Standardization

CHAPTER 11

Clinical interventions and process improvement

Guy Cohen was Director of Quality, Safety and Reliability at NASA until the mid-1990s. Don Berwick, then working on improving the quality of healthcare in the Harvard Community system, had asked how to improve healthcare faster and more effectively; in their first five-hour meeting Cohen had barely started telling him what he had learned about quality and safety (Berwick, 1998). Berwick recalls the response to his initial question:

'How do you get good enough to go to the moon'? Guy Cohen had no one-liners to offer me. He didn't say 'report cards' or 'market forces' or 'incentive pay' or even 'accountability'. In fact, as I recall, not one of those words came up in the time we spent together. His view of human nature, organisations, systems, and change would not permit one-line answers.

(BERWICK DM. "TAKING ACTION TO IMPROVE SAFETY: HOW TO IMPROVE THE CHANCES OF SUCCESS." PRESENTATION AT THE ANNENBERG CENTER FOR HEALTH SCIENCES CONFERENCE, *ENHANCING PATIENT SAFETY AND REDUCING ERRORS IN HEALTH CARE*, IN RANCHO MIRAGE, CALIFORNIA. NOVEMBER 8-10, 1998. REPRODUCED WITH PERMISSION FROM INSTITUTE FOR HEALTHCARE IMPROVEMENT)

In healthcare, we are coming to understand how difficult the safety problem is, in cultural, technical, clinical and psychological terms, not to mention its massive scale and heterogeneity. The second half of this book, beginning with this overview of clinical interventions and process improvement, covers the principal avenues of improvement and in later chapters addresses the complex task of integrating the human and technological changes that are needed. We have seen, in the analysis of individual incidents, just how many factors can contribute to the occurrence of an error or bad outcome. Yet still, at safety conferences, you will hear people saying 'it's the culture', 'the key is strong leadership', 'team building is the answer', 'if we just had good professional standards all would be well', 'we know we've got a problem, lets just get on and fix it' and so on. Of course all these things are important, and there are some things which can and should be 'just fixed', but one of the greatest obstacles to progress on patient safety is, paradoxically, the attraction of neat solutions, whether political, organizational or clinical. First, we must understand what a complex problem this is; only then will we be able to tackle all aspects of it effectively.

Patient Safety, 2nd edition. By Charles Vincent. Published 2010 by Blackwell Publishing Ltd.

Healthcare is an extremely diverse enterprise and the causes of harm, and the associated solutions, will differ according to the process under consideration. Some factors, such as leadership, culture and attitudes to safety, are generic and important in all environments. However, the kinds of specific solutions required to ensure high reliability in, for instance, blood transfusion services, will obviously differ from those aimed at reducing inpatient suicides. Improving safety requires some generic, cross-organizational action, coupled with some speciality and process specific activities.

At the clinical level, safety can be elusive, for all the specialist knowledge and experience available. There are multiple possibilities and lines of attack. Should we rely on team building, vigilance and awareness of hazards? Should we attack the numerous process problems, inefficiencies and frustrations that beset clinical staff, sapping their morale and precipitating error and patient harm? Perhaps, as in so many other industries, technology is the answer, getting the human being out of the loop? Or perhaps patient harm is best prevented by clinical innovations, for instance the development of new drugs and procedures to counteract the hazards of hospital acquired infection? All of these approaches are important but it is not easy to assess how much weight to give to any one of them in any specific circumstance. In this chapter and the next two we will examine technical solutions of various kinds with the aim of showing their essential features, advantages and limitations. First it is useful to sketch out the territory and consider some of the implicit, often unspoken, assumptions underlying approaches to improving safety.

Two visions of safety

A wealth of different techniques and approaches are available in the quest for safer healthcare, variously supported by theory, evidence and common sense, and it can be very difficult to discern underlying themes and directions. Underlying the plethora of approaches however, we can distinguish two broad approaches. These two visions of safety are seldom explicitly articulated, but are ever present themes in debates and discussions about patient safety.

The phrase 'Design, Technology and Standardization' encapsulates one vision of safety, which is closely linked to the engineering safety paradigm discussed in Chapter 5. In this view, human fallibility is to the fore and the aim is to simplify, standardize and improve basic processes and reduce reliance on people by automating or at least offering as much support as possible in those tasks for which people are necessary. Process improvement approaches are discussed in this chapter and the roles of design and technology in the next two. 'People create safety' encapsulates the second broad approach, discussed in later chapters. Woods and Cook (2002), following Rasmussen (1990) and others, have argued for an alternative to the rigid, proceduralized, technology driven view of safety and that more truly reflects the realities of clinical work. Underlying these two visions are two contrasting views of human ability and experience, the one stressing error and fallibility, the other stressing

Table 11.1 Two visions of safety

Replace or support human beings	Practitioners create safety
Emphasizes fallibility and irrationality	*Emphasizes expertise and skill*
Hindsight bias and memory failure	Flexibility and adaptability
Extreme over-confidence	Experience and wisdom
Vulnerable to environmental influences	Anticipation of hazards
Lack of control over thought and action	Recovery from error
Technical and procedural interventions	*New and enhanced skills*
Design and standardization	Culture of high reliability organizations
Protocols and guidelines	Mindfulness and hazard awareness
Information technology	Training in anticipation and recovery
Technical solutions	Teamwork and leadership

adaptability, foresight and resilience (Table 11.1). Adopting one or other of these positions, whether acknowledged or not, will determine the kind of practical steps taken to improve safety and so have important practical consequences. In practice, elements of both approaches may be needed to resolve particular problems, but distinguishing them is important as many discussions and debates about safety revolve around these two positions.

Design, technology and standardization

Many approaches to quality improvement in healthcare are rooted in a basic industrial model, in which the solutions to errors and defects rest in an increasing standardization usually coupled with a reliance on technology. Ideally, the human contribution to the process of care is reduced to a minimum, as in industrial production or commercial aviation. Careful design of the basic processes of care and appropriate use of technology overcomes human fallibility, vulnerability to fatigue and environmental influences. Examples of safety measures within this broad framework would include: simplification and standardization of clinical processes, more fundamental re-design of equipment and processes, computerized medication systems, electronic medical records and memory and decision support, whether computerized or in the form of protocols, guidelines, checklists and aide memoires. Note that even systems which explicitly acknowledge human fallibility, such as decision support systems, still require human ingenuity and expertise to use them. For instance, while support systems assist clinicians by reminding them of actions to be taken and recommending courses of action, they can only be useful if the clinician has the expertise to extract relevant information from the patient, use the system appropriately and so on. You need expertise in order to use decision support effectively.

We also need to distinguish two broad types of standardization and proceduralization. The first relates to systems which attempt to improve on existing systems of communication, such as the electronic medical record. There is no doubt that an electronic record could have immense advantages in terms of access to information, reliability of coding, standardization of information recorded and linkage to other systems. However, from the clinician's viewpoint, such systems may introduce other problems – for instance, problems of access when hardware fails, slowness of response, and other unanticipated problems. Nevertheless, most clinicians would agree that it is desirable to bring hospital information systems up to the standard of, for instance, the average supermarket chain.

A more important and contentious issue relates to the standardization of clinical practice itself, in the form of guidelines, protocols, decision support and structuring of tasks and procedures. Clinicians are sometime suspicious of these initiatives, suspecting that standardization is being imposed not to improve healthcare but in order to regulate, cut costs and otherwise constrain clinicians in their work. However, properly understood and implemented, such approaches are potentially a support to the clinical staff. Standardization and simplification of core processes should reduce the cognitive load on clinical staff – thus freeing them for more important clinical tasks that require human empathy and expertise.

People create safety

Proponents of the 'people create safety' view are, rightly, extremely impressed by how often outcomes are good in the face of extreme complexity, conflicting demands, hazards and uncertainty. Making healthcare safer depends on this view, not on minimizing the human contribution but on understanding technical work and how people overcome hazards. Cook, Render and Woods (2000) remind us how reliant safety is on clinicians and others looking ahead, bridging gaps, managing conflicts and, in effect, creating safety. A good illustration of this approach is in their recommendation that researchers study 'gaps', discontinuities in the process of care, which may be losses of information, losses of momentum or interruptions in the delivery of care. They suggest that safety will be increased by understanding and reinforcing practitioners' normal ability to bridge gaps.

While clinicians' ability to anticipate, react and accommodate to changing circumstances is crucial to effective and safe healthcare, we should not assume that safer care will be achieved solely by reliance on these human qualities. To begin with, this reliance on human expertise places an additional burden on those at the sharp end, returning us, oddly, to a reliance on training that systems thinking sought to free us from. True, it is training of a different kind (anticipation, flexibility), but training nonetheless. More importantly, it seems an odd response to gaps. Why should we not try to reduce the number of gaps in the first place, with more efficient systems and better design? This depends, of course, on the nature of the gaps and other problems that practitioners need to anticipate and address. Sudden changes in the patient's condition or an acute emergency require all the qualities that Cook and Woods rightly highlight. Anticipation is also used, however, to resolve organizational deficiencies, as when a surgeon has to improvise because notes are not available at the start of an operation, or telephones ahead to double check that equipment is available. However, notes and equipment that reliably turned up would reduce, if not obviate, the need for such anticipation. The real problem is to find a way to marry the two approaches, standardizing and proceduralizing where this is feasible and desirable, while knowing that this can never be a complete solution and simultaneously promoting human resilience and the 'creation of safety'. Before developing this theme however, we need to discuss the role of evidence based medicine in creating a safer healthcare system.

Clinical practices to improve safety

The first Institute of Medicine Report on patient safety, 'To err is human' (Kohn, Corrigan and Donaldson, 1999), called on all parties in healthcare to make patient safety a priority. To this end they recommended that the Agency for Healthcare Research and Quality (AHRQ) determine which patient safety practices were effective and produce a report to disseminate to all clinicians. The resulting report, produced by Kaveh Shojania and colleagues at the Evidence Based Practice Center in San Francisco with the assistance of numerous US experts, is a massive, wide ranging compendium of patient safety practices and an invaluable resource of clinical practices, which reduce the complications of healthcare (Shojania, Duncan and McDonald, 2001). The review followed, wherever possible, a standard approach to reviewing the literature on a specific topic, making a formal assessment of the strength of evidence available. For each safety practice, the authors of the relevant section were asked to examine:

- Prevalence of the problem targeted by the practice;
- Severity of the problem targeted by the practice;
- The current use of the practice;
- Evidence of efficacy and/or effectiveness of the practice;
- The practice's potential for harm;
- Data on cost if available;
- Implementation issues.

Shojania and colleagues acknowledged that this approach, more usually applied to specific clinical interventions, was difficult to apply to generic safety interventions, such as information technology or human factors work. Many of these practices were drawn from areas outside medicine and often little researched in healthcare. Some generic practices, such as clinical decision support, were separated out and described as techniques for promoting and implementing safety practices. The final list of 79 selected practices was roughly grouped according to the strength of evidence for each one and promising areas were highlighted for future research. Eleven practices (Box 11.1) were singled out as having very strong evidence of efficacy. A further 14 had good evidence for efficacy; these included such practices as using hip protectors to prevent injury after falls, localizing surgery to high volume centres, use of computer monitoring to prevent adverse drug reactions, improving information transfer at time of discharge, and multicomponent programmes to tackle pain management and hospital acquired delirium. In the summary, the authors emphasize that their report was a first attempt to organize and evaluate the relevant literature, which they hope will act as a catalyst for future work and not be seen as the final word on the subject.

BOX 11.1 Most highly rated patient safety practices from the AHRQ Report

- Appropriate use of prophylaxis to prevent venous thromboembolism (VTE) in patients at risk;
- Use of peri-operative beta-blockers in appropriate patients to prevent peri-operative morbidity and mortality;
- Use of maximum sterile barriers while placing central intravenous catheters to prevent infections;
- Appropriate use of antibiotic prophylaxis in surgical patients to prevent peri-operative infections;
- Asking that patients recall and restate what they have been told during the informed consent process;
- Continuous aspiration of subglottic secretions to prevent ventilator-associated pneumonia;
- Use of pressure relieving bedding materials to prevent pressure ulcers;
- Use of real-time ultrasound guidance during central line insertion to prevent complications;
- Patient self management for warfarin to achieve appropriate outpatient anticoagulation and prevent complications;
- Appropriate provision of nutrition, with a particular emphasis on early enteral nutrition in critically ill patients;
- Use of antibiotic impregnated central venous catheters to prevent catheter related infections.

(ADAPTED FROM: SHOJANIA KG, DUNCAN BW, McDONALD KM, ET AL., EDS. MAKING HEALTH CARE SAFER: A CRITICAL ANALYSIS OF PATIENT SAFETY PRACTICES. EVIDENCE REPORT/TECHNOLOGY ASSESSMENT NO. 43 (PREPARED BY THE UNIVERSITY OF CALIFORNIA AT SAN FRANCISCO–STANFORD EVIDENCE-BASED PRACTICE CENTER UNDER CONTRACT NO. 290-97-0013), AHRQ PUBLICATION NO. 01-E058, ROCKVILLE, MD: AGENCY FOR HEALTHCARE RESEARCH AND QUALITY. JULY 2001. AVAILABLE AT http://www.ahrq.gov/clinic/ptsafety/)

Preventing venous thromboembolism (VTE)

As an example of a safety practice with good evidence, we will consider the important topic of preventing thromboembolism. VTE refers to occlusion within the venous system, and includes deep vein thrombosis (DVT). VTE occurs frequently in hospital patients, with risk of VTE depending on multiple factors including age, medical condition, type of surgery and duration of immobilization. Without prophylaxis, DVT occurs after approximately 20% of all major surgical procedures and over 50% of orthopaedic procedures. Measures to prevent VTE can be pharmacological (heparin, warfarin, aspirin) or mechanical (elastic stockings, pneumatic compression). The authors of this section of the AHRQ report present extensive evidence for the efficacy, safety and cost-effectiveness of prophylaxis in a wide range of conditions and procedures. For instance, pooled results of 46 randomized trials have established that low dose unfractionated heparin (LDUH) reduces the risk of DVT after general surgery from 25 to 8%.

VTE is frequent, painful, dangerous, wastes time and resources and is sometimes fatal; it is, in many cases, preventable. In spite of this, prophylaxis is often underused or used inappropriately. Surveys of both general and orthopaedic surgeons in the United States, for instance, have found over 10% never use VTE prophylaxis, with rates of prophylaxis varying widely for different procedures. The use of appropriate prophylactic measures is undoubtedly a valuable clinical practice. The mystery is why, when the evidence is so strong, it is so often not used or used inappropriately. Educational programmes promoting guidelines and computerized decision support have improved the use of prophylaxis and there are now major campaigns in several countries, but adherence to these basic practices remains incomplete.

Evidence based medicine then provides the foundation of good practice but does not directly address the safety issue, which is why care known to be effective is not delivered to the patient. From our point of view, the most important point is that an evaluation of a clinical practice has led to questions of a psychological nature and towards core patient safety issues of error and human behaviour. These themes emerge more strongly in the next section, which addresses some criticisms of the report's approach to patient safety,

Evidence based medicine meets patient safety

Following the publication of the AHRQ report, Lucian Leape, Berwick and Bates (2002) wrote a powerful critique, in which they argued that the report had in various respects missed the point of patient safety. We will review their arguments, not to dismiss the undoubtedly useful report, but to highlight important issues about the nature of patient safety and the directions it should take in improving the safety of care.

In the first place, Leape and colleagues recalled that in the original Harvard study only about one-third of adverse events were not preventable with current practice. The remainder were due to error or more general problems in the process of care. The AHRQ report, they suggested, was targeting new therapies and techniques, and to some extent side-stepping the thorny issues of error and poor quality care. The primary reason for this, they suggested, was not that the AHRQ authors were reluctant to tackle these issues but simply that they followed the evidence and concentrated on areas where there was a substantial body of research. The upshot of this was that the report was heavily weighted towards individual safety practices and therapies and gave insufficient weight to the factors that determine what care patients actually receive. Leape and colleagues agreed that it was first necessary to identify practices with proven benefit, such as anticoagulation for VTE. However, the practical issues for patient safety practitioners were:

First how to ensure that every patient who needs anticoagulation receives it and second how to ensure that the medication is delivered flawlessly – on time, in the right dose, every time, without fail. Such systems are at the heart of patient safety but not addressed by the report.
(LEAPE *ET AL.*, 2002)

Leape and colleagues went on to argue that many established safety practices (i.e. sponge counts after an operation) had been omitted, simply because they are well established and, more importantly, that many promising avenues, such as systems for reducing medication errors, had not been given sufficient attention. They further questioned whether the standard evidence based approach was necessary where practices had obvious face validity or where sufficient evidence had accumulated in other environments (i.e. the impact of fatigue on performance and judgement).

Why were Leape and colleagues so concerned about the direction taken by this report? Essentially, it seems, because it might set a direction for patient safety that they regarded as misconceived. Even though the report does give some attention to human factors and systems issues, the weight given to specific clinical practices might suggest that the problems of patient safety could be effectively addressed with new therapies and careful evaluation. In fact, most patient safety practitioners are much more concerned about the fragmented, chaotic state of most healthcare systems and the frankly abysmal safety record in many areas. Resolving this requires a tenacious attempt to improve the basic processes and systems of healthcare as well as engaging all who work in healthcare in the endeavour. The remainder of this book addresses the various ways in which this colossal task is being attacked, beginning with the key issue of simplification and standardization.

Quality management and process improvement

Manufacturing industries have made huge gains in safety, efficiency and cost-effectiveness by close attention to the design, maintenance and performance of the processes used in factories. Rather than inspect products afterwards to identify defects, those concerned with quality control and management sought to build quality into the process. Much of the impetus for these improvements stemmed from the publication of W. Edwards Deming's 'System of Profound Knowledge', a title more suggestive of esoteric spiritual practices than the science of quality improvement. The intention of the book however, and the approach it describes, is resolutely practical. Deming, Joseph Juran, Kauro Ishigawa and others have described and documented the successful application of these approaches since the 1950s in Japanese and American industries (Langley *et al.*, 1996).

Doctors, nurses and others often find it hard to understand that approaches developed in manufacturing can have any relevance to healthcare. We deal with patients as individuals, how can we learn anything from companies that make cars? In fact, of course, cars and computers can now be completely customized and matched to individual needs and preferences. Healthcare is also full of processes, of varying degrees of complexity and incoherence, which are very akin to manufacturing processes: pharmacy, ordering test results, the blood service and so on. But the message of Deming and others is much more than that. Paul Batalden attended a series of lectures given by Deming in 1981. He recalls talking to the great man during the single hour that Deming allowed himself for dinner:

As we talked, he shared his views about the way the health system worked, what he observed. I realised he was used to 'seeing things' with different lenses. I went back to the lectures... I saw that he was not really talking about manufacturing; it was a theory of work which conceptualised the continual improvement of quality as intrinsic to the work itself. He didn't see a doctor then a nurse then a patient – he saw them as interdependent elements of a system and he looked for how that system could work better.
(BATALDEN, QUOTED IN KENNEY, 2008)

In 1983, the scope of quality control was expanded in systems that sought to extend the basic ideas to all the operations of a company, so that every function was oriented towards improving quality (Feigenbaum, 1983). Total quality management, driven particularly by Japanese industry, took this further still, emphasizing that the entire workforce needed to be involved in improving the quality of the organization and, through these efforts, in the quality of the final product. In healthcare this has become as aspiration, but not yet a reality. The report on the British NHS by Lord Darzi, for instance, puts quality at the centre of everything the NHS does and makes it clear that everyone should play their part in promoting and driving higher quality care for patients (Darzi, 2009).

The methods of quality management are well described in many books (i.e. Langley *et al.,* 1996; Nelson, Batalden and Godfrey, 2007). Quality methods are sometimes presented simply as a set of tools and techniques, but properly conceived the various systems aim at substantial and enduring organizational change based on principles and values that each organization must define for it. We cannot possibly review all the various approaches, but it is necessary to understand the importance of these approaches in promoting both safety and quality and the fact that improving some aspects of quality, for instance standardizing and simplifying processes, will also make care safer. Quality improvements approaches have also underpinned large-scale attempts to improve safety, such as the Safer Patients Initiative discussed in Chapter 19.

Simplifying and standardizing the processes of healthcare

Compared with manufacturing industry, healthcare has little standardization, comparatively little monitoring of processes and outcome, and few safeguards against error and other quality problems (Bates, 2000). Most healthcare processes were not designed, but just evolved and adapted to circumstances. A particular problem is that many healthcare processes are both long and complicated. Simply mapping the process that currently exists can be a major task, and performing a failure, modes and effects analysis on that process can be immensely time consuming, as we have seen. As Don Berwick points out, complex systems break down more often than simple ones, because there is more opportunity:

The statistics are quite simple. Imagine a system with, say, 25 elements each of which functions properly – no errors – 99% of the time. If the errors in each element occur independently of each other, then the probability that the entire system of 25 elements will function correctly is $(0.99)^{25}$ or about 0.78. With 50 elements, it is 0.61; with 100 elements, it is 0.37. Make the reliability of each element higher, say 0.999, and the overall success rates are 0.98 for 25 elements, 0.95 for 50 elements and 0.90 for 100 elements. We can, indeed, improve the reliability of a system by perfecting its parts and handoffs, but reducing complexity is even more powerful.
(BERWICK DM. "TAKING ACTION TO IMPROVE SAFETY: HOW TO IMPROVE THE CHANCES OF SUCCESS." PRESENTATION AT THE ANNENBERG CENTER FOR HEALTH SCIENCES CONFERENCE, *ENHANCING PATIENT SAFETY AND REDUCING ERRORS IN HEALTH CARE*, IN RANCHO MIRAGE, CALIFORNIA. NOVEMBER 8–10, 1998. REPRODUCED WITH PERMISSION FROM INSTITUTE FOR HEALTHCARE IMPROVEMENT)

The process of prescribing, ordering and giving drugs is a good example of complexity and lack of standardization. David Bates gives an example of the problems that he observed in his own hospital before a sustained attack on medication error and adverse drug reactions:

Take for example the allergy detection process used in our hospital several years ago, which was similar to that used in most hospitals at the time. Physicians, medical students and nurses all asked patients what their allergies were. This information was recorded at several sites in the medical record, though there was no one central location. The information was also required to be written at the top of every order sheet, although in practice this was rarely done. The pharmacy recorded the information in its computerised database, but it found out about allergies only if the information was entered into the orders, and often it was not. Checking by physicians, pharmacy and nursing staff was all manual. This information was not retained between the inpatient and outpatient settings, or from admission to admission. Not surprisingly, about one in three orders for drugs to which a patient had a known allergy slipped through.
(REPRODUCED FROM *BRITISH MEDICAL JOURNAL*, DAVID W BATES. "USING INFORMATION TECHNOLOGY TO REDUCE RATES OF MEDICATION ERRORS IN HOSPITALS". **320**, NO. 7237, [788–791], 2000, WITH PERMISSION FROM BMJ PUBLISHING GROUP LTD.)

Reading this description, it is hard to understand why, even before technological advances, this system had been allowed to continue for so many years: multiple sites of information; numerous, possibly conflicting sources of information; excessive reliance on human vigilance and memory; excessive complexity and potential for error at every stage. If you had been trying to design a system to produce errors you could hardly have done better. When you work in such a system, and we all do in one way or another, it is hard to step back and see the whole process and understand its flaws. Furthermore, in healthcare, very often no one person has responsibility or oversight of the whole system, which makes both monitoring and improvement very difficult.

The system Bates describes has now been replaced by one in which all allergies are noted in one place in the information system, drugs are mapped to 'drug families' (e.g. penicillin) so that they can be checked more easily, information is retained over time and checking for allergies is routinely performed by computers, rather than tired and fallible human beings. Many healthcare systems however, have not benefited from such an overhaul. Ordering and reading of X-rays, communication of risk information about suicidal or homicidal patients, informing patients and their family doctors about abnormal test results, booking patients in for emergency operations, effective discharge planning; all these and many more are vital for safe healthcare, yet day-to-day experience tells patients and staff that they are far from error free.

Waste, delay and rework

Successful businesses work constantly to reduce waste and delay and so constrain costs. Waste and delay in healthcare are obviously problems of quality and cost-effectiveness, but also indirectly impact on safety and patient experience; at its simplest, staff time spent on inefficient processes is staff time taken away from direct patient care. Every organization wastes time and resources to a varying degree, whether it is a home wasting food or a hospital wasting time and resources with complex, laborious and overly bureaucratic processes. Hospitals are repositories of the most unbelievable inefficiencies often sitting alongside feats of extraordinary ingenuity and efficiency. Many people work daily with a degree of disorganization in a drug cupboard that they would never tolerate in their own home – another bizarre example of how dangerous practices, which are right in front of us day after day, become invisible because 'that's how its always been.'

The elimination of waste and inefficiency is emphasized, particularly by the Toyota Production system, a complete philosophy of work and organization that has evolved over decades and is deeply embedded in the very fabric of the organization (Liker, 2004). 'Lean thinking' evolved from Toyota but developed independently in a variety of ways in different companies and industries always aiming to provide what the customer wants quickly, efficiently and with little waste. Obvious applications in healthcare would be minimizing or eliminating delays, repeated encounters, errors and inappropriate procedures and indeed any unnecessary work that takes staff away from work that contributes directly to patient care, whether at the bedside or elsewhere. Waste occurs in healthcare at every level (as in every other industry) but many delays and problems can be resolved by front line staff once they are given the freedom and encouragement to do so (Box 11.2).

BOX 11.2 Eliminating waste and delay in healthcare

In one hospital, on each shift nurses made an average of 23 searches for keys to the narcotics cabinet; this wasted 49 minutes per shift and delayed analgesia to patients. Administrators tested assigning numbered keys at the start of each shift, with safeguards to prevent loss or misuse. This procedure nearly eliminated searches for keys and saved 2895 nurse-hours yearly in a 350-bed hospital. Another hospital pharmacy used any deviations from procedures to reflect on the processes. Rather than accept workarounds they changed their systems. Without any technology investments, searches for missing medication decreased by 60% and stockouts fell by 85%.

(ADAPTED FROM THOMPSON, WOLF AND SPEAR, 2003; SPEAR AND SCHMIDHOFER, 2005)

A general internal medicine practice knew that the diagnostic testing process and reporting of test results to patients needed to be improved, because of long delays and frequent follow-up telephone calls from patients. Every member of the practice, doctors, nurses and administrators, completed an initial assessment of the process. After flowcharting the process, which revealed rework, waste, delay and long cycle times, the group brainstormed and then rank ordered the solutions. They then tested the solution of holding a short meeting at the beginning of the day to deal with all diagnostic test results at one time and decide on actions needed. Within two weeks patient phone calls for laboratory results had decreased, reflecting the fact that staff were now calling patients in a timely manner about their results

(*QUALITY BY DESIGN. A CLINICAL MICROSYSTEMS APPROACH*. NELSON, E. C., BATALDEN, P., & GODFREY, M. M. 2007, JOSSEY BASS, SAN FRANCISCO. REPRINTED WITH PERMISSION OF JOHN WILEY & SONS, INC.).

Reducing medication error

Designing and building simpler, standardized processes which rely less on human vigilance is therefore a powerful way of making at least some parts of healthcare much safer, as well as cheaper and more efficient. How is this to be done?

The Institute for Healthcare Improvement (IHI) has pioneered quality improvement in healthcare, drawing together ideas and practical experience from healthcare and many other sources. We will use their approach to reducing medication error as an overall framework to illustrate the potential of process improvement, addressing the particular role of technology in a later section.

IHI have led a number of collaborative projects to bring about rapid reduction in medication errors, drawing on the work of Lucian Leape, David Bates and many others and, importantly, also drawing heavily on the knowledge and expertise of people within the institutions taking part. These are genuine collaborative projects, not simply consultants coming in to advise or, at worst, 'asking to see your watch and then telling you the time'.

There are three basic elements to improving the safety of a medication process:
- Design the system to prevent errors occurring in the first place.
- Design the system to make errors more visible when they do occur.
- Design the system to limit the effects of errors so that they do not lead to harm.

Preventing errors is, broadly speaking, achieved by reducing the complexity of information that healthcare staff need, reducing the opportunity for mixing up different medications and trying to limit errors that occur because staff are trying to do too many things at once (Table 11.2). Errors can be made more visible by using a variety of additional checks, both by people (staff and patients) and by computers. For instance, having a pharmacist reviewing orders before dispensing, asking staff to repeat back verbal orders and careful use of laboratory monitoring systems are all means of detecting errors that may have occurred. Even with all these checks and system improvements, errors will sometimes occur, if only because of the enormous numbers of drugs given.

Table 11.2 Principles for reducing medication error

Reducing errors due to information complexity	Provide an information system that allows access to patient information for all staff and allows electronic prescribing Limit hospital formularies to essential drugs and doses Pharmacists on ward rounds to monitor and advise Briefing at handover and shift change on circumstances that increase risk of error, such as an unfamiliar disease, new staff or unusual drug regimens
Reducing errors due to complex or dangerous medication	Remove high risk medications, such as concentrated electrolyte solutions, from patient care areas Label high risk drugs clearly to indicate their danger Remove or clearly differentiate look alike or sound alike drugs
Reducing errors due to multiple competing tasks	Wherever possible reallocate tasks such as calculating, drawing up and mixing doses to pharmacy or the manufacturer Establish standard drug administration times and avoid interruptions at those times Assign one person to necessary double checks who does not have other duties at that time; use double checks sparingly and make them properly independent Standardize equipment and supplies, such as intravenous pumps, across all units Involve patients in active checks such as identifying themselves, checking drugs and allergies

(Adapted from Berwick DM. "Taking Action to Improve Safety: How to Improve the Chances of Success." Presentation at the Annenberg Center for Health Sciences conference, *Enhancing Patient Safety and Reducing Errors in Health Care*, in Rancho Mirage, California. November 8–10, 1998. Reproduced with permission from Institute for Healthcare Improvement.)

The final protection is to always be ready to mitigate the effects of any error, to assume in fact that errors will occur and to prepare for it. Anticipating error is a sign of a safe, rather than unsafe system. In this case keeping antidotes for high-risk drugs on hand at the point of administration is a key defence against harm to patients; staff also need to train and rehearse treatment of serious adverse reactions, such as anaphylaxis. Rehearsal of such routines is especially important if such reactions seldom occur, as that is when such skills are lost. These then are the general principles derived in years of experimentation, evaluation and practical application with many organizations. Let us see how this works in practice.

Reducing medication errors and adverse drug events at St Joseph's Medical Centre

St Joseph's Medical Centre is a 165-bed hospital in the heart of Illinois, providing a variety of services including open heart surgery and trauma care. The hospital has established a number of safety projects backed by a strong commitment to cultural change and backing from senior executives (Haig *et al.*, 2004).

In June 2001, a survey of records suggested an adverse drug event (ADE) rate of 5.8 per 1000. Flowcharting of the medication process proved it to be complicated, labour intensive and that it involved multiple members of staff from the time the order was written to the point where the patient received the medication. Common sources of errors included unavailable patient information, unavailable drug information, miscommunication of medication orders, problems with labelling or packaging, and drug standardization, storage, stocking and process flaws. By May 2003, ADEs were running at 0.50 per 1000, a 10-fold reduction, and the process of medication delivery had been hugely simplified and standardized. How was this achieved?

The broader commitment to safety and open reporting and discussion of errors provided the foundations for the programme; however, some very specific process improvements were the key to enduring change (Box 11.3), particularly medication reconciliation. Medication reconciliation is the process of comparing the medications the patient has been taking with the medications currently ordered. A common problem, for instance, is that when patients are discharged from hospital they do not return to the medication appropriate to their life at home. Medication reconciliation tackles this and related problems in three phases: on admission the home medications are compared to initial clinician's orders; on transfer between units, the medications on the previous unit are compared with those on the current unit; on discharge, hospital medication is compared with clinician orders for discharge medication and, if necessary, prescriptions from the general practitioner or family doctor. Any variances are then 'reconciled' by the nurse and pharmacist. In this thoughtful strategy, we can see first a mapping of the steps in the patient journey when errors may occur; second, the assumption that errors can and will occur; and third, a structured, standard process of checking to identify errors and problems and prevent actual patient harm.

> **BOX 11.3** Reducing medication errors in St Joseph Medical Centre
>
> - Added an adverse drug event hotline leading to a ten-fold increase in reporting of adverse drug events and medication errors;
> - Monthly reporting of medication data to hospital quality council;
> - Implemented use of a single heparin/enoxaparin nomogram;
> - Developed pre-printed heparin/enoxparin orders based on the nomogram;
> - Developed a single form that could be used for reconciliation of medications at both admission and discharge;
> - Separated sound-alike and look-alike medications in the pharmacy and on the nursing units;
> - Implemented daily rounds by a clinical pharmacist who compares medication orders to lab values;
> - Standardized intravenous drip concentrations;
> - Decreased the amount of stock medications kept on patient care units;
> - Eliminated the use of high-risk abbreviations;
> - Changed process for non-standard doses so that all are prepared and packaged in pharmacy;
> - Standardized epidural pumps and use yellow coloured tubing with these pumps.
>
> (SOURCE: INSTITUTE FOR HEALTHCARE IMPROVEMENT – IMPROVEMENT REPORT. *REDUCING ADES PER 1,000 DOSES: ORDER OF ST. FRANCIS — ST. JOSEPH MEDICAL CENTER (BLOOMINGTON, ILLINOIS, USA).* AVAILABLE AT: http://www.ihi.org/IHI/Topics/PatientSafety/MedicationSystems/ImprovementStories/ImprovementReportReducingADEsper1000Doses.htm)

Standardization of processes was a major feature of this programme, with particular attention paid to high-risk medications. For instance, all adult intravenous medications were standardized and a single, weight based, Heparin Nomogram was developed and used throughout the hospital. A particularly popular intervention was increasing the availability of pharmacists on nursing units to review and enter medication orders. This had the double benefit of saving nurse time, though at the cost of increased pharmacist time, and also giving the pharmacist the opportunity to identify potential dosage errors, drug interactions and so on. Finally, the patients themselves were engaged in the process. Each patient admitted to the hospital is given a Medication Safety Brochure that provides advice for them and a form on which to list their current medication. Patients are also actively encouraged to check with staff if they have been given unfamiliar medication. Technological innovations, in the form of automated medication dispensing machines, formed the next phase of the drive to further reduce errors.

While medication errors and medication processes have received most attention, achievements have not been confined to medication safety. Box 11.4 shows an example of a similarly sustained and radical change in the interpretation of radiographs. As so often happens, healthcare processes had evolved and adapted over time, rather than being designed to produce a certain standard of care. Looking at the examples quoted so far in this chapter, common themes emerge: data collection, defining the process, identifying weak points, simplification and standardization. We might also note that all these improvements took time, commitment and patience. An important lesson that healthcare needs to learn is that safety and quality require a much bigger investment of time and resources than it has been given so far. Producing major changes to systems may start with a few enthusiasts fitting in meetings around their other work, but sustained safety and quality requires committed staff with dedicated time and resources.

BOX 11.4 Reducing errors made by emergency physicians in interpreting radiographs

When Espinosa and Nolan began their initial improvement efforts, the average rate of clinically significant errors was 3%. Long delays in processing films were common. At this time, four separate radiology systems were in place, with the process and responsibility for interpreting varying with time of day and between weekdays and weekends. Initial improvement efforts left the basic system untouched, but brought a much stronger focus on reducing error. All staff reviewed clinically significant discrepancies at monthly meetings; a file of clinically significant errors was kept and used for training; study of this file was made mandatory for all new staff; patterns of errors for each physician and for the department as a whole were routinely reviewed and discussed. Over the subsequent two years, the error rate fell to 1.2%, essentially by a sustained focus on training, attention to error and collaborative work by the team.

To further reduce delays and errors, a more fundamental redesign of the process was then carried out by an interdisciplinary team. A system was developed for interpreting radiographs that would be followed, regardless of the day of the week or time of day. All standard radiographs were brought directly to the emergency physician for immediate interpretation; a radiologist provided a further interpretation within 12 hours as a quality check, with rapid recall of patients if necessary. The primary responsibility was clearly assigned to the emergency physician, reducing the confusion and ambiguously defined responsibilities of the previous system. A new form was designed to provide feedback about significant discrepancies, embedding feedback and training into the day-to-day running of the department. These further changes reduced the error rate to below 0.5. The authors stress the importance of cooperation between professional groups and the systemic nature of the intervention, relying both on individual and team effort and process improvement.

(REPRODUCED FROM *BRITISH MEDICAL JOURNAL*, JAMES A ESPINOSA, THOMAS W NOLAN. "REDUCING ERRORS MADE BY EMERGENCY PHYSICIANS IN INTERPRETING RADIOGRAPHS: LONGITUDINAL STUDY". **320**, NO. 7237, [737–740], 2000, WITH PERMISSION FROM BMJ PUBLISHING GROUP LTD.)

Positive personal characteristics can inhibit process improvement

Quality improvement techniques clearly have huge potential to transform healthcare, and indeed have already had a major impact, of which more evidence will emerge in later chapters. It would seem that the main challenge is to engage and train healthcare staff and to develop improvement projects. Naturally, there are barriers to overcome such as scepticism, shortage of time, conflicting organizational priorities and so on. However, there is another subtle and counterintuitive barrier to process improvement and indeed to wider organizational change. One might think that individual effort would always enhance organizational performance and enhance safety. As so often though with safety, there is a twist. The very ingenuity and resourcefulness, which are rightly admired in clinical staff and which produce immediate benefits for patients, can inhibit more fundamental organizational change.

In a fascinating study, Tucker and Edmondson (2003) carried out over 200 hours of observation of 26 nurses at 9 different hospitals in the United States, focusing on the problems the nurses encountered in their daily work. Problems were defined as disruptions in the worker's ability to carry out a prescribed task, either because something they needed was unavailable or because something else was interfering with the work. Examples of problems include missing supplies, missing medications or missing information, such as medical records or laboratory results. It is not uncommon for medical staff to spend a large amount of time looking for charts and equipment. Often each ward and unit has their own rules about the placement of charts and equipment. In addition, the organization of charts and equipment may vary within the hospital, making expeditious use of information or tools difficult for house staff who care for patients on multiple wards, especially in emergencies (Volpp and Grande, 2003):

Where is Mrs Tilly's chart? I can't remember where they keep the charts on this floor. I am covering her care for the regular resident and don't know her well. I was called to see her for respiratory distress, but I can't find the pulse oximeter or an Ambu-bag.
(VOLPP AND GRANDE, 2003)

Both nurses and doctors are extremely adept at dealing with these problems. They have to be or the system would have collapsed; working around system inefficiencies is part of the job:

By being able to get IV bags, clean linen or whatever else I need, it enables me to do my job and to have a positive impact on a person's life. And I am the kind of person who does not just get one set of linen, I will bring back several for the other nurses.
(TUCKER AND EDMONDSON, 2003)

Tucker and Edmondson call the approach this nurse describes first-order problem solving; being adaptable, flexible, responding to changes in demand

and fixing problems. Admirable, of course, and reminiscent of the qualities espoused in high reliability organizations. The problem is that this very resourcefulness can mean that nothing ever changes, as usually no one is informed that there were no IV bags. The IV bags are meant to be there in the first place and ideally the nurse should not have to waste their time looking for them. First-order problem solving is effective in the short term, but prevents problems surfacing as learning opportunities. In addition, first-order problem solving may create problems elsewhere in the organization, as supplies go missing from other areas of the hospital, leading to further organizational problems. Second-order problem solving on the other hand involves patching the immediate problem, but also letting the relevant people know that the problem has occurred. They cite an example of a nurse from intensive care calling a ward who had mistakenly kept an ICU bed after moving a sick child to their ward; she simply let them know what happened in order to prevent future problems.

Tucker and Edmondson emphasize that all the nurses they observed worked well beyond their allotted hours and were dedicated to patient care, yet the problems persisted. They argue that, while these problems are entrenched, many are relatively straightforward to resolve, given some time and commitment. The answer they suggest lies in the counterintuitive notion that positive personal and organizational attributes are preventing organizational change. First, individual vigilance and resourcefulness and the ability to solve problems, militates against change as we have discussed. Second, this is compounded and reinforced by a system which makes sure that nurses are constantly used to the full, which means that they only have time to care for patients and not to resolve wider organizational issues. Third, many quality improvement methods rely on empowering frontline workers, such as nurses, to resolve problems. This is certainly important for resolving immediate difficulties. The downside can be however, that the managers, who actually have the power to resolve these problems in the longer term, are not aware of them and not engaged to resolve them. It is clear, for instance, that each hospital should develop a single system for chart storage, placement of vital sign flow sheets, location and type of equipment, storage and composition of procedure kits, and examination-room layout so that valuable time is not lost looking for equipment or determining how to use unfamiliar equipment (Volpp and Grande, 2003). Instead, however, the system runs on adaptability and improvization, papering over the cracks rather than sorting out the processes.

The cardinal virtues and abilities of clinical staff are being squandered on administrative and organizational inefficiencies rather than put at the service of patients. In the longer term, wards and units who persistently have to battle against organizational inefficiency gradually cease to function effectively. Clinical staff maintain safety by adapting and working around these inefficiencies. If we truly want safer healthcare though, front line staff may have to complain more and demand action on behalf of themselves and their patients.

References

Bates, D.W. (2000) Using information technology to reduce rates of medication errors in hospitals. *British Medical Journal*, **320**(7237), 788–791.

Berwick, D.M. (1998) *Taking Action to Improve Safety: How to Increase the Odds of Success*, Rancho Mirage, California.

Cook, R.I., Render, M. and Woods, D.D. (2000) Gaps in the continuity of care and progress on patient safety. *British Medical Journal*, **320**, 791–794.

Darzi, A. (2009) *High Quality Care for All*, Department of Health, London.

Espinosa, J.A. and Nolan, T.W. (2000) Reducing errors made by emergency physicians in interpreting radiographs: longitudinal study. *British Medical Journal*, **320**(7237), 737–740.

Feigenbaum, A.V. (1983) *Total Quality Control*, McGraw Hill, New York.

Haig, K., Wills, L., Pedersen, P. *et al.* (2004) Improvement Report: Reducing ADEs per 1,000 doses. www.ihi.org.

Kenney, C. (2008) *The Best Practice. How the New Quality Movement is Transforming Medicine*, Public Affairs, New York.

Kohn, L., Corrigan, J. and Donaldson, M.E. (1999) *To Err is Human*, National Academy Press, Washington DC.

Langley, G.J., Nolan, K.M., Nolan, T.W. *et al.* (1996) *The Improvement Guide: A Practical Approach to Enhancing Organizational Performance*, Jossey-Bass Publishers, San Francisco.

Leape, L.L., Berwick, D.M. and Bates, D.W. (2002) What practices will most improve safety? Evidence-based medicine meets patient safety. *Journal of the American Medical Association*, **288**(4), 501–507.

Liker, J.K. (2004) *The Toyota Way. 14 Management Principles from the World's Greatest Manufacturer*, McGraw Hill, San Francisco.

Nelson, E.C., Batalden, P. and Godfrey, M.M. (2007) *Quality by Design. A Clinical Microsystems Approach*, Jossey Bass, San Francisco.

Rasmussen, J. (1990) The role of error in organising behaviour. *Ergonomics*, **33**, 1185–1199.

Shojania, K.G., Duncan, B.W. and McDonald, K.M. (2001) Making Health Care Safer: A Critical Analysis of Patient Safety Practices. Evidence Report/Technology Assessment No. 43: 2001.

Spear, S.J. and Schmidhofer, M. (2005) Ambiguity and workarounds as contributors to medical error. *Annals of Internal Medicine*, **142**(8), 627–630.

Thompson, D.N., Wolf, G.A. and Spear, S.J. (2003) Driving improvement in patient care: lessons from Toyota. *Journal of Nursing Administration*, **33**(11), 585–595.

Tucker, A.L. and Edmondson, A. (2003) Why hospitals don't learn from failures. Organisational and psychological dynamics that inhibit change. *California Management Review*, **45**(2), 55–72.

Volpp, K.G. and Grande, D. (2003) Residents' suggestions for reducing errors in teaching hospitals. *New England Journal of Medicine*, **348**(9), 851–855.

Woods, D.D. and Cook, R.I. (2002) Nine steps to move forward from error. *Cognition Technology and Work*, **4**, 137–144.

CHAPTER 12
Design for patient safety

The term 'design' has many meanings; most commonly one thinks of the design of a shape, form or structure. To designers however, the word conveys the broader meaning of 'creating and developing concepts and specifications that optimize the function, value and appearance of products and systems' (Ulrich and Eppinger, 1995). Design of a clinical process or technology therefore implies a fundamental review of a product or system. Rather than tinkering to affect some marginal improvement, a designer endeavours to envision the product afresh, drawing on an understanding of the way human beings naturally work and interact with technology. In contrast, the term 'process improvement' suggests that there are some underlying deficiencies but that, essentially, the process concerned is reasonably robust and sensible. Clearly though, some healthcare processes and systems have evolved in such a way that improvement is no longer an option. We saw, for instance, that one team abandoned the analysis of the medication system in their own hospital because it was so complicated that no one could actually understand it.

I approach design as a complete amateur, but I have had the good fortune to work alongside designers whose aim is to use design to improve the safety and quality of healthcare. Apart from the sheer fun of it, the most striking feature of their approach is their willingness to start with a blank sheet of paper, asking very basic but pointed questions like 'What are we trying to achieve?' 'What does this piece of equipment have to do?' and 'What's the best way for this team to achieve this task?' There are some wonderfully designed and constructed pieces of equipment in healthcare but, taken as a whole, the system has not benefited from the design and engineering disciplines that have informed other safety-critical industries. In a short chapter we cannot do justice to the depth of these approaches, but we can at least show the potential of thinking from the ground up and putting safety firmly into the design equation. In keeping with the objectives of the book, I have chosen examples from the minutiae of clinical processes through to attempts to bring design to every facet of an entire hospital system.

Patient Safety, 2nd edition. By Charles Vincent. Published 2010 by Blackwell Publishing Ltd.

Design and error

A good design is distinguished, in part, by the fact that the device is used in a way that seems quite natural and obvious to us. In contrast, when things go wrong, bad design can be all too apparent. John Reiling quotes the architect Bruce Mau who pithily summarizes this experience, while Don Norman provides the human examples (Box 12.1):

For most of us, design is invisible. Until it fails ... when systems fail, we become temporarily conscious of the extraordinary force and power of design. Every accident provides a brief moment of awareness of real life, what is actually happening, and our dependence on the underlying systems of design.
(REILING, 2006)

BOX 12.1 The psychopathology of everyday things

'The human mind is exquisitely tailored to make sense of the world. Give it the slightest clue and off it goes, providing explanation, rationalization, understanding. Consider the objects – books, radios, kitchen equipment, office machines and light switches – that make up our everyday lives. Well designed objects are easy to understand. They contain visible clues to their operation. Poorly designed objects can be difficult and frustrating to use. They provide no clues – or sometimes false clues. They trap the user and thwart the normal understanding.'

'If I were placed in the cockpit of a modern jet airliner, my inability to perform gracefully and smoothly would neither surprise nor bother me. But I shouldn't have trouble with doors. "Doors?" I can hear the reader saying, "You have trouble with opening doors?" Yes. I push doors that are meant to be pulled, pull doors that should be pushed, and walk into doors that should be slid. Moreover I see others having the same troubles – unnecessary troubles. There are psychological principles that can be followed to make these things understandable and useable.'
(FROM *THE DESIGN OF EVERYDAY THINGS* (NORMAN, 1988)

The formal study of error and design dates from the Second World War. Studies of aviation accidents revealed that some were caused by pilots incorrectly operating very similar or confusing controls. In a classic early example, nearly identical cockpit controls for retracting the flaps and retracting the landing gear were placed alongside each other in some aircraft, causing pilots to retract the landing gear after they had landed, with disastrous results. Engineers began to realize that they had to take the psychological characteristics of human beings into account as well as the technical issues. This gave rise to the discipline of ergonomics, sometimes called 'human factors':

Ergonomics (or human factors) is the scientific discipline concerned with the under-
standing of the interactions between humans and the other elements of a system, and the
profession that applies theory, principles and data and methods to design in order to
optimise human well-being and overall system performance.
(CARAYON, 2007)

For me, as a (biased) psychologist, much of ergonomics is psychology under
another name, as it concerns issues such as perception, cognition, human
performance, teamwork and organizations. Ergonomics however, has a particular focus on the interactions between human beings, technology and
organizations and a strong emphasis on practical applications. Ergonomics
was traditionally focused on the design of equipment and furniture (e.g.
appropriate chairs and lighting), which is indeed an important component,
but the definition makes clear that the cognitive and wider organizational and
systemic perspectives are also included in the overall approach. This leads to
an extraordinary range of activities and a huge amount of confusing terminology: human machine interfaces (hardware ergonomics), human computer
interaction (cognitive ergonomics), organizational issues (macroergonomics)
and so on.

Design for safer healthcare

Designers of healthcare equipment have to consider many different requirements and perspectives, but safety is often to the fore. For instance, a number of
safety features that have been designed into anaesthetic gas systems. Lines for
oxygen and nitrous oxide attach to a special port set in the wall or ceiling. These
lines are colour coded (in Britain, oxygen is white, nitrous oxide is blue) and
each pipe has a specific connector and collar that makes it impossible to attach
an oxygen pipe to a nitrous oxide port and vice versa. Spare oxygen and nitrous
oxide cylinders also have the same connectors and also a 'Pin Index System',
which ensures that only oxygen cylinders can be fitted to the space designed for
oxygen. These design features make it more or less impossible to miss-connect
gas pipes.

Just as medicine has increasingly adopted an evidence based approach to
treatment, designers and healthcare professionals have embraced evidence
based design and there is now a substantial and growing literature. This has
been recently reviewed and very effectively summarized by Roger Ulrich and
colleagues at the Centre for Health Design, University of Georgia, and we will
draw extensively on their review in this chapter. The involvement of designers
and architects who appreciate the healthcare context, and the potential
impact of design on safety and quality, has been given increased impetus by
the fact that the United States, and a number of other countries, are engaged
in a massive programme of hospital building. Many 1970s buildings have
become unsuited to modern healthcare and building a new hospital is often
more cost-effective than upgrading (Ulrich *et al.*, 2008). However, let us begin

with something rather more modest but equally critical – the design of labels and syringes.

Designing out medication error

Reducing medication error requires a multi-faceted approach involving computerized systems, simplification and standardization of clinical processes, education and training and wider cultural and organizational change. However, the design of labelling and packaging can be an important contributor to error and, by the same token, an important part of the solution. For instance, look-alike/sound-alike drug names are a serious problem in healthcare, accounting for 29% of medication dispensing errors. Confusion of drug names is a problem in about 20% of medication errors overall. Illegible handwriting, incomplete knowledge of drug names, new products and similarities in packaging and labelling, act as contributing factors to this problem.

Medication errors involving look-alike/sound-alike drug names can cause serious patient harm. For instance, a number of errors have been reported and published on the confusion between Lamisil® and Lamictal®. Reading these two names quickly, one can easily see how they could be confused, but re-design of the labels to highlight the differences rather than the similarities makes them markedly distinct (Figure 12.1).

The UK National Patient Safety Agency has drawn together a group of experts from healthcare and the pharmaceutical industry to draw up guidelines and to illustrate approaches to design that can reduce errors. As with any design for safety projects, they first identified the most common labelling related medication errors and then identified potential solutions or at least methods of reducing the likelihood of such errors (Boxes 12.2 and 12.3).

Some of these seem so simple as to be obvious, but all of them are relevant. Many medicines have packaging which is difficult to read, hard to open, with confusing methods of presenting information. Simple changes make crucial information stand out. For instance, anaesthetists in the United States, Canada, Australia and New Zealand developed a standardized colour coding for labels for the syringes of medications drawn up in the operating theatre; however, this has apparently not been universally taken up by the manufacturers (Berman, 2004). It is also important to realize that recommendations, while they take account of human psychology, are not absolute. We might all, for instance, agree that colour coding will be helpful in distinguishing different classes of drugs or different routes of administration, but unless there is co-ordination between manufacturers or an international standard, the potential for confusion remains. In addition, there are few studies as yet, either simulated or in clinical conditions, of the impact of changing packaging on error rates.

Although the attention given to these issues is very welcome, the pharmaceutical industry has not as yet put its weight behind patient safety, although

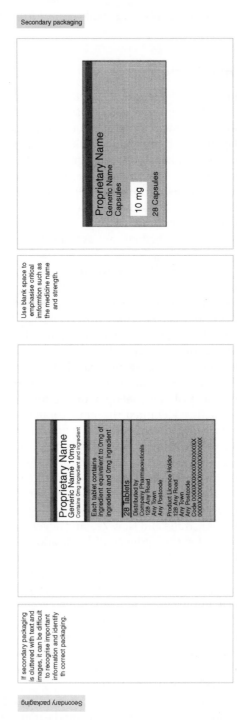

Figure 12.1 Distinguishing drug names through good design (Reproduced with permission of National Patient Safety Agency: www.npsa.nhs.uk).

BOX 12.2 Design implications of a medication error

A hospitalized geriatric patient was prescribed Lamisil 250 mg daily for 3 months to treat a fungal nail bed infection. The order was entered by a pharmacy technician into the pharmacy computer system as Lamotrigine. The error was discovered but four days after the Lamotrigine was discontinued, the patient developed a very severe total body rash with swelling of the face. The usual starting dose of Lamotrigine is 25 mg, and the patient had been taking 10 times this dose for 3 weeks.

Prescribing Recommendations:
- Include the indication for the medication on the prescription, that is, Lamisil for fungal infection;
- Lamictal for epilepsy/seizures;
- Label unit dose packages, individual prescription containers with the generic drug name followed by the brand name in parentheses for potentially confusing drug names or where the brand name is more familiar.

Design Recommendations
- Use warning flags next to drug names (generic and brand) in the computerized drug database to alert for potential mix-up in drug selection;
- Use tall-man lettering to distinguish look-alike/sound-alike drug names on manufacturer's bulk bottle labelling, prescription labels, medication administration records and in hospital and community pharmacy computer systems.
  LamiCTAL and LamiSIL

(*ISMP CANADA SAFETY BULLETIN*, "LOOK-ALIKE/SOUND-ALIKE DRUG NAMES: CAN WE DO BETTER IN CANADA?" **4**, NO.2, FEB 2004. REPRINTED WITH PERMISSION FROM ISMP CANADA)

BOX 12.3 Safe design of medication labels and packaging

- *Medicine name and strength obscured* – Allocate 70 × 35 mm white space for dispensing label;
- *Dispensing label and medicine name mismatched* – Position the generic name and medicine strength above or next to the space for the dispensing label;
- *Critical information does not appear in the same field of vision* – Put critical information in the same field of vision on at least three non-opposing faces
- *Difficult to recognize important information* – Use blank space to emphasize critical information;
- *Medicines with similar names confused for one another* – Use Tallman lettering to emphasize the difference between look-alike or sound-alike medicine names;

- *Easy to miss the decimal point in numbers with a trailing zero* – Do not add trailing zeros to numbers;
- *Small type size is difficult to read* – Body text in a minimum of 12 point;
- *Sentences in capital letters or italic type are hard to read* – Use upper and lower case.

there are some notable exceptions. For instance, in ophthalmology, where many patients naturally have poor vision, manufacturers have been using brightly coloured bottle tops to help patients identify eye drops and, because they often cannot read the labels, to prevent substitution errors between drugs. Similarly, after numerous problems and some deaths due to potassium chloride (where concentrated potassium chloride would be mistakenly injected instead of a weak sodium chloride solution), vials of potassium chloride in the United States now have a black top and are clearly labelled 'must be diluted' (Berman, 2004).

Re-designing the resuscitation trolley

If a patient's heart or breathing stops in hospital, an emergency 'crash' team of doctors and nurses is called to resuscitate the patient. Many studies have examined the success of resuscitation and have generally found that only 16 to 20% of patients survive the arrest to be discharged from hospital (Kalbag *et al.*, 2006; Sandroni *et al.*, 2007). The crash team uses a large array of medicines and medical devices such as a defibrillator, which are stored on a 'crash trolley'. This is permanently stocked and wheeled to the patient's side.

The first crash trolleys were introduced into hospital wards in the 1940s. Since cardiopulmonary resuscitation (CPR) was first described, there have been constant revisions and an evolution of the resuscitation process. This has not been echoed in the design of resuscitation trolleys, which are little more than modified tool trolleys. Though they fulfil the basic function of being mobile and providing space for equipment, they hinder rather than help the resuscitation team battling to save the patient in the few minutes they have available. At this most critical time, drawers often don't open properly, the wrong equipment is selected in error, the equipment may not be stored correctly and it is difficult for more than one person to access the trolley at any one time.

Resuscitation is also often hampered by poorly stocked trolleys being taken to the scene. Existing trolleys have all the equipment hidden away in drawers, often locked with a tamper seal. A daily check should be performed, which (if done at all) is done during a quiet time, often on a night shift. The procedure consists of removing equipment, item by item, and checking it against a list. This can be done in 20 minutes if the checker is experienced, but may take up to an hour, all of which takes time away from direct patient care.

In this project designers were teamed with clinicians, academics and psychologists, and were immersed in the clinical environment from the beginning. The team examined Advanced Life Support guidelines, attended courses on resuscitation, watched videos of resuscitations and experienced clinicians and resuscitation officers were interviewed and observed in numerous scenarios. This helped to build a detailed picture of the processes and associated errors throughout the resuscitation process. A Failure Mode and Effects Analysis (FMEA) was carried out to map what errors occurred, and at what point. Successive design ideas were developed and presented to clinical staff in a series of iterations and refinements. The clinicians were invited to talk through the benefits and drawbacks of each one, combining and rejecting functions as they saw fit. This led to a design prototype with the following features:

- The new trolley design has an open layout, similar to a shadow board in a workshop. This means that all the equipment can be seen at a glance, making access much easier and facilitating stock checks.
- The trolley can be split into three sections: one unit for managing the airway, one unit for drugs and intravenous care, and the final unit for miscellaneous items. This aids access and also helps to define team roles in an emergency.
- A Radio Frequency Identification (RFID) antenna was placed in the central unit to detect when items are removed, flashing up a warning on a touch screen when the stock is incomplete. This also facilitates the restocking process as the technology can display exactly what is missing, and the expiry date.

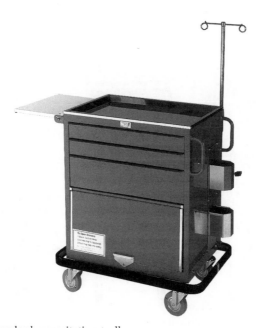

Figure 12.2 A standard resuscitation trolley.

(a)

(b)

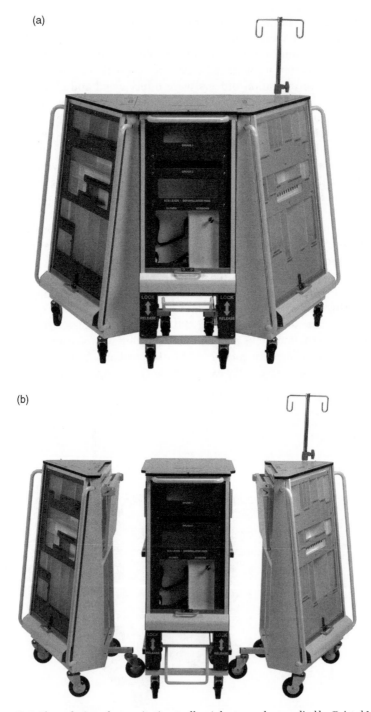

Figure 12.3 The redesigned resuscitation trolley (photographs supplied by Bristol Maid).

- The touch screen guides the leader of the resuscitation team through the necessary steps, and logs the actions of the team. This serves both as a prompt and as a means of recording and data collection, which is often difficult to capture in the aftermath of an emergency using current methods.

The prototype was taken to two virtual arrest scenarios, with responsive mannequins presenting with simulated conditions. Resuscitation teams were placed in the scenarios and told to use the new trolley which they had not seen previously. Scenarios were also run with existing trolleys as a control, and video feeds were recorded from hidden cameras. While the existing trolley produced many of the errors outlined previously, the team used the new design exactly as intended, with no training. At the time of writing, a third-generation prototype has been manufactured, and further simulations are being carried out preparatory to a full trial of the new equipment.

Designing out hospital acquired infection

As we have seen, hospital acquired infections are one of the main hazards to patients in hospital and a leading cause of death in many countries. Efforts to control infections partly rely on advances in treatment, isolation of patients, hand hygiene and other precautions on the part of both staff and patients. The environment can affect the likelihood of infection transmission, the behaviour of staff and patients and also the ease and thoroughness of cleaning raising the possibility that re-design of the environment could be an effective infection control strategy (Ulrich et al., 2008). Designers begin, however, with an analysis of the underlying problem, in this case the transmission of infection, which is briefly summarized here.

Generally speaking, infection transmission occurs via three routes: *contact*, *air* and *water*. Advances in molecular detection methods and sampling techniques for viruses, bacteria and fungi have enabled researchers to identify the exact strain and source of infections, and thereby develop a better understanding of transmission (Ulrich et al., 2008). Contact is widely considered the most frequent transmission route, but in practice all three routes may interact in the spread of nosocomial infections. Water borne transmission is a serious problem in some circumstances, but there are few studies on prevention and we will not consider it further here.

Airborne transmission refers to infections that are contracted from airborne micro-organisms such as dust, which can transmit spores of *Clostridium Difficile* or aerosol droplets which can hold tuberculosis or severe acute respiratory syndrome (SARS) (Ulrich and Wilson, 2006). Hospital air quality plays a decisive role in affecting the concentration of pathogens in the air, and thereby has major effects on the frequency of airborne infectious diseases such as tuberculosis, influenza and SARS. When ventilation systems are contaminated or break down, the consequences can be extremely serious. In one outbreak, for example, the ventilation grilles in two patient bays were found to be harbouring MRSA (Kumari et al., 1998). Whenever this ventilation system was shut down, it sucked air from the ward environment into the system, contaminating the outlet grilles, then it blew contaminated air back into the ward when the system was restarted.

Although airborne transmission poses serious safety risks, contact contamination is generally recognized as the principal transmission route of nosocomial infections, such as MRSA and *C. difficile*, which survive well on surfaces and other reservoirs (Bauer *et al.*, 1990; IOM, 2004). Healthcare workers' hands play a key role in both direct and indirect transmissions. A staff member may touch two patients in succession without washing his or her hands, or touch an environmental surface or feature after direct contact with an infected patient, which in turn contaminates the hands of someone else (Ulrich and Wilson, 2006). Because MRSA can survive for weeks on environmental surfaces, these surfaces can themselves become the source of new outbreaks.

The research literature strongly supports implementing several environmental approaches for controlling and preventing airborne infections: including installing effective filters; specifying appropriate ventilation systems and air change rates; and employing various control measures during construction or renovation. When state-of-the-art filters are combined with powerful ventilation systems, the impact on air quality can be dramatic; for instance the type of operating theatre ventilation system has been found to be an independent risk fact for sternal surgical site infections (Ulrich *et al.*, 2008)

A number of studies have shown that multifaceted interventions can significantly improve hand hygiene and reduce infections; a key component of the interventions is carefully positioned bedside alcohol-based hand-rub dispensers (Creedon, 2005; Pittet *et al.*, 2000; Randle, Clarke and Storr, 2006). The selection of appropriate furniture and floor coverings, and the ease of cleaning of surfaces have also been shown to impact on contact transmission. Design plays a key role in siting alcohol gel and washing facilities so that staff are constantly prompted to clean their hands but waste little time in doing so. Environmental changes are critical but clearly there are many other components to these interventions.

Single rooms and infection

C. difficile is a highly virulent infection spread mainly by contact, which causes more deaths than MRSA. Several deadly outbreaks of *C. difficile* in North American and European hospitals and thorough published investigations have underscored powerfully the threat to patient safety posed by multi-bed rooms. The infection is spread mainly by contact; infection rates are lower when there is very good air and water quality, and greater physical separation and space per patient. Several studies have shown that single rooms appeared to reduce or prevent MRSA infections compared to multi-bedded rooms in various healthcare settings, including 212 ICUs across Germany, 173 hospitals across Europe, a UK hospital with 1100 beds, and a NICU in the United States. We should note however, that if single rooms are to be effective, then they do need to be properly designed. Patients in single rooms in old buildings, which are hard to clean and without proper ventilation, may be as much at risk, or even at more risk, than patients in open wards.

Providing single rooms to patients has a number of very important advantages and influences all forms of infection transmission. First, single rooms enable the separation of patients upon admission and make it possible to prevent cross-infection. Second, they reduce airborne transmission by allowing filtration, ventilation and airflow control. Third, they are much easier to clean and decontaminate after a patient has been discharged. They may also influence hand washing behaviour, because each room is fitted with a sink and alcohol gel, raising the likelihood of reflex hand washing on the part of both staff and patients. One might think that there are also disadvantages, in terms of communication with staff and potential isolation. In fact, single rooms are much preferred by patients and they actually increase the number of family visits, social contacts and communication with staff (Ulrich *et al.*, 2008).

Whole system design

Even this brief sketch shows the potential of design to impact on some of the most problematic and deeply entrenched patient safety issues. There is evidence that many other design interventions have the potential to improve the safety and quality of care. When the time comes to build a new hospital, the opportunity arises to bring all the design solutions together to create a hospital with patient safety at its core. There are huge opportunities to reduce error, improve the patient experience, reduce stress and make the best use of the natural environment. This was the radical approach taken by St Joseph's Community Hospital, Wisconsin, where a new building was opened in 2005, on time and on budget. The process began with an unusual meeting in 2002 of engineers, architects, clinicians, researchers and others who together devised an approach to putting patient safety at the heart of the design of the new hospital. As John Reiling expresses it:

Derived from the learning lab was the collective belief that safe hospitals could be designed using a process that supports the anticipation, identification and avoidance of failure; by designing against the latent conditions and active failures which compromise physical and organisational defences; and by creating an organisational culture of safety. . . . In a systems approach, error reduction is achieved by strategically building defences, barriers and safeguards into the facility, equipment and processes that make up the system.
(REILING, 2006)

Through this process, the design team introduced a number of changes to the standard design process. Patients were involved right from the beginning in the design of rooms and facilities, with special attention being given to those most vulnerable to error and harm, such as the very sick, the very old or the very young. Most hospitals consider equipment at a late stage in the design process, fitting it into the building that has emerged; instead, this team planned for equipment, and future innovations in equipment, from the first day. Failure modes and effects analyses were carried out on many key processes. Mock-ups made at an early stage allowed simulations and thinking through the safety implications of each design solution. This evolution of the design process to put safety and patient welfare at its core led to many changes to the standard hospital design; these are some of the most striking:

The patient environment
Hospitals are extraordinarily noisy places, sometimes necessarily but often because of poor design and buildings that are ill equipped for sick people. If it was a hotel, you'd complain and tell your friends to avoid the place; as it's a hospital you have to put up with it. Noise, as we all know, disrupts sleep, which is particularly critical to recovery; it also increases stress and raises blood pressure. On the staff side, communication is harder, distractions are greater and concentration is poorer. The combination of quiet floor coverings, private rooms, good insulation, quiet ventilation and heating systems and quiet equipment can transform the environment. An ambience of monastic calm, rather than a downtown bus station.

Outside the hospital there is great scope for reducing stress levels by making the most use of the healing properties of the natural environment. For most sick people, trees and sunshine are a treatment in themselves; while we cannot all convalesce in the alpine splendour of the Magic Mountain, much can be done to bring nature into the hospital. Studies have suggested that patients are greatly soothed by the sight of trees and grass from the windows as compared with walls and buildings and there is some evidence of reduced length of stay when recovery takes place in healing environments.

Standardization
Follow a doctor or nurse around, especially if they are new to a hospital, and see how much time they spend just looking for things. More seriously, watch them looking at an unfamiliar infusion pump to see how this particular panel relates to the eventual speed and strength of the dose. Remember too that sick and vulnerable patients are using some of these devices. Much of this can be resolved, or at least considerably eased, by good design and standardization.

The St Joseph's team took the lesson of standardization to heart. Rooms have a standard layout, standard placement of switches, charts, controls and equipment; even latex gloves are stored in the same place in each room. Medication processes and systems are standardized as far as possible and they are moving towards standard IV lines, beds, monitors and other equipment. For both patients and staff everything is predictable and in its place, which reduces error and waste and frees time for direct patient care.

BOX 12.4 Designing around precarious events

Operative/Post-Operative Complications and Infections
Locate sinks in every patient care area so they are visible to patients; standardize visibility and location of sanitizer dispensers.

Inpatient Suicides
Implement patient room features to reduce suicide attempts.

Correct Tube–Correct Connector–Correct Hole/Oxygen Cylinder Hazards
Standardize connectors; standardize head walls in every room in the hospital; segregate tanks in storage room in central plan; standardize medical air throughout the facility.

Wrong-Site Surgery
Standardize operating room (OR) suites; install proper lighting; install cable for access to digital images and photographs of surgery site along with X-rays.

Events Relating to Medication Errors/Transfusion Related Events
Make certain that proper wiring/cabling is included in all 'non-traditional' areas where medication may be dispensed or delivered; technology applications such as pharmacy decision support, bar-coding, computerized physician order entry (CPOE), or electronic medical records (EMR) should be integrated with 'appliances' such as IV pumps.

Deaths of Patients in Restraints
Consider visibility of patients in design phase; provide comfortable space for family members to stay with patient.

Patient Falls
Develop bed exit technology to notify caregivers when patients are attempting to get out of bed.

MRI Hazards
Create a three-zone MRI suite; use hand-held metal detectors at point of entry; colour code any MRI compatible equipment; consider computer chip technology.
(ADAPTED FROM REILING, 2006)

Bringing services to the patient: reducing transfers and handovers

Any transfer or handover represents vulnerability in a system. As soon as you move a patient or transfer information between people, there is increased risk of error, infection and falls. By designing spacious patient rooms, equipment can be brought to the patient; minor procedures and investigations can be carried out without moving the patient to a special facility. By having lifts on every floor, patients can be moved in their own beds and not transferred by wheelchair. By having access to bar coding technology and the electronic record within the patient's room, the chances of medication errors are substantially reduced.

Many of the design themes contribute to a number of potential patient problems, which is seen most clearly in St Joseph's focus on designing around 'precarious events', which are essentially well-known sources of risk and harm to patients (Box 12.4). Once the building had been completed, the principles of design and early testing were carried over into the transfer from the old hospital to the new with early testing and a two-month period in which staff simulated caring for patients to test systems and iron out problems. The new building opened on time and on budget in 2005. By all accounts, the hospital is a marvellous environment, which has its effect on both patients and staff. As John Reiling expresses it, 'we changed our building and afterwards, our building changed us.'

References

Bauer, T.M., Ofner, E., Just, H.M. *et al.* (1990) An epidemiological study assessing the relative importance of airborne and direct contact transmission of micro-organisms in a medical intensive care unit. *Journal of Hospital Infection*, **15**(4), 301–309.

Berman, A. (2004) Reducing medication errors through naming, labeling, and packaging. *Journal of Medical Systems*, **28**(1), 9–29.

Carayon, P. (ed.) (2007) *Handbook of Human Factors and Ergonomics in Health Care and Patient Safety*, CRC Press, New York.

Creedon, S.A. (2005) Healthcare workers' hand decontamination practices: compliance with recommended guidelines. *Journal of Advanced Nursing*, **51**(3), 208–216.

Institute of Medicine (2004) *Keeping Patients Safe: Transforming the Work Environment of Nurses*, National Academies Press, Washington DC.

Kalbag, A., Kotyra, Z., Richards, M. *et al.* (2006) Long-term survival and residual hazard after in-hospital cardiac arrest. *Resuscitation*, **68**(1), 79–83.

Kumari, D.N., Haji, T.C., Keer, V. *et al.* (1998) Ventilation grilles as a potential source of methicillin-resistant *Staphylococcus aureus* causing an outbreak in an orthopaedic ward at a district general hospital. *Journal of Hospital Infection*, **39**(2), 127–133.

National Patient Safety Agency (2007) *Design for Patient Safety*, www.npsa.nhs.uk

Norman, D.A. (1988) *The Design of Everyday Things*, Basic Books, New York.

Pittet, D., Hugonnet, S., Harbarth, S. *et al.* (2000) Effectiveness of a hospital-wide programme to improve compliance with hand hygiene. Infection Control Programme. *Lancet*, **356**(9238), 1307–1312.

Randle, J., Clarke, M. and Storr, J. (2006) Hand hygiene compliance in healthcare workers. *Journal of Hospital Infection*, **64**(3), 205–209.

Reiling, J. (2006) Safe design of healthcare facilities. *Quality and Safety in Health Care*, **15**(Suppl. 1), i34–i40.

Sandroni, C., Nolan, J., Cavallaro, F. and Antonelli, M. (2007) In-hospital cardiac arrest: incidence, prognosis and possible measures to improve survival. *Intensive Care Medicine*, **33**(2), 237–245.

Ulrich, K.T. and Eppinger, S.D. (1995) *Product Design and Development*, 2nd edn, Irwin McGraw Hill, Boston.

Ulrich, R.S. and Wilson, P. (2006) Evidence based design for reducing infections. *Public Service Review: Health*, **8**, 24–25.

Ulrich, R.S., Zimring, C., Zhu, X. *et al.* (2008) A review of the research literature on evidence-based design, Center for Health Design, College of Architecture, Georgia Institute of Technology, United States.

CHAPTER 13

Using information technology to reduce error

Modern healthcare is hugely reliant on technology and new technologies are continually pushing the boundaries of what can be achieved in investigations and treatment. The advent of PET, CAT and MRI and scanners allows unprecedented diagnostic access in ways that were unthinkable 20 years ago. Advances in surgical technologies have transformed some operative procedures. For instance, treatment for an aortic aneurysm was formerly carried out by opening the abdomen, clamping and replacing a section of the aorta with a synthetic graft (a tube to replace and support the damaged aortic tissue). An open repair of an aortic aneurysm is a long, complex operation with high morbidity and mortality and, when successful, a long and slow recovery for many patients. Advances in both technology and technique mean that this procedure can now be carried out via a minimally invasive endovascular approach, by passing small instruments into arteries in the groin, which manoeuvre the stent-graft into place within the aorta. New advances, such as fenestrated stents that are customized to the patient's particular anatomy, and the use of robotic surgical techniques allow even greater precision and control in what was previously a frankly dangerous, though potentially life-saving, operation (Bicknell *et al.*, 2009; Riga *et al.*, 2009). Advances in surgical techniques and technology have dramatically altered the balance of risk and benefit for the patient.

Some technologies, particularly information technology, are directly targeted at the reduction of error and the improvement of safety. Of course, the principal motivation for their introduction may be cost control and greater efficiency, but safety is an increasingly important driver. The use of information technology is inevitably accompanied by some degree of standardization and reduction in the variability of provision provided by human beings. Such standardization, when in the form of guidelines and protocols, can be criticized as being overly prescriptive and not taking a patient's particular circumstance and constellation of symptoms into account. Computers however, when provided with the appropriate information, can completely tailor their guidance to the individual patient. In other, less complex industries, such as computer manufacturing, this is referred to as 'mass customization', the

Patient Safety, 2nd edition. By Charles Vincent. Published 2010 by Blackwell Publishing Ltd.

efficient and reliable customization of a product to fit the specification of the individual consumer. Thus technology potentially provides a marriage between the need for standardization, with the clinician's rightful insistence that treatment is tailored to the individual patient.

Bates and Gawande (2003) identify a number of ways in which information technology can reduce error: improving communication, making knowledge more readily accessible, prompting for key pieces of information (such as the dose of a drug), assisting with calculations, monitoring and checking in real time, and providing decision support. We will examine the role of information technology in reducing medication errors, improving communication, providing reminders, electronic records and decision support. Be aware, however, that this is a very limited discussion of an enormous topic. Before we turn to the information technology and its potential for enhancing safety, it is worth reminding ourselves why we need it, with a brief discussion of the respective strengths and fallibilities of computers and human beings.

The limits of memory

The sheer quantity of medical information, even within a single speciality, is often beyond the power of one person to comprehend. People, that is, the human brain, simply cannot cope with the amount of information that they need to function safely and effectively. For instance, more than 600 drugs require adjustment of doses for multiple levels of renal dysfunction; an easy task for a computer, but one which will inevitably be performed poorly by a person (Bates and Gawande, 2003). Machines can therefore act as a kind of extended memory, which we can access at will, to overcome the transience and limitations of human memory storage. However, these are not the only problems of memory; there are other limiting factors which are not always appreciated.

In his review of memory's strengths and imperfections, Daniel Schachter (1999) identified 'seven sins' of memory, each of which has application and relevance to clinical work. The first three are sins of omission, the next three instances of distortion or inaccuracy and the final one concerns memories we would rather forget. I have added examples of how these 'sins' might manifest in a clinical environment:

- *Transience*, meaning that information fades over time, or is at least less accessible. A doctor might forget that a patient has poor renal function when prescribing.
- *Absent-mindedness*, meaning inattention and consequent weak memory traces. A nurse might read and remember 500 when the label says 50.
- *Blocking*, temporary inaccessibility of memories, the so-called tip of the tongue phenomenon. A doctor might be unable to recall a drug dosage even though they had given the drug many times before.
- *Misattribution* involves attributing a recollection or idea to the wrong source, such as thinking that a particular scene from a film came from another with a

similar theme. When seeing a patient in a clinic, a doctor might recall and act on a medical history that in fact applies to a different patient.

- *Suggestibility*. Studies of eye witness testimony have shown that we easily, and unknowingly, adjust our memories to accord with new information and become convinced that our new 'memories' are veridical. An example would be unintentionally convincing your patient that they had had an angiogram, even though they did not.
- *Bias* involves retrospective distortions and unconscious inferences that are related to current knowledge and beliefs; we adjust our memory of events to accord with our current experience, whether good or bad. For instance, remembering incorrectly that you had noticed previously that a cancer patient showed early signs of the disease consistent with your current diagnosis.
- *Persistence* refers to pathological memories: information or events we wish we could forget but cannot. The distressing memory of your worst mistake that comes to mind at unexpected moments.

Our memory then, while generally highly effective and efficient in daily life, may lead us astray in a number of ways. An example of an instance in which relying on memory led to disaster is shown in Box 13.1. There are, of course, many other lessons to be taken from this story of wrong site surgery, particularly about personal responsibility, hierarchy and communication. However, the fallibility of memory is a core theme; relying on remembering that the biopsy was taken from the right side in the face of evidence from the medical record that it came from the left is, to put it charitably, not entirely sensible. Schachter points out though that we should not necessarily conclude that memory is hopelessly flawed. Most of these features which make us fallible in some circumstances are also adaptive. Forgetting unnecessary information, such as where you parked your car the day before yesterday, is highly adaptive. Jorge Luis Borges' story, *Funes the Memorious*, imagines a man who forgets nothing; Funes is paralysed by reminiscence. Real life examples exist of mnemonists with perfect recall who are unable to function at an abstract level through being inundated with detail. A perfect memory in a computer is marvellous; in a person it could be a liability.

BOX 13.1 Hemivulvectomy for vulvar cancer: the wrong side removed

A 33-year-old female with microinvasive vulvar carcinoma was admitted to a teaching hospital for a unilateral hemivulvectomy. After the patient was intubated for general anaesthesia, the trainee reviewed her chart and noted that the positive biopsy was from the left side. As the trainee prepared to make an incision on the left side of the vulva the attending surgeon stopped him and redirected him to the right side. The trainee informed the attending surgeon that he had just reviewed the chart and learned that the positive biopsy had come from the left. The attending surgeon informed the trainee that he himself performed the biopsies and recalled that they were taken from the right side. The trainee complied and performed a right hemivulvectomy.

The next day, the Chief of Pathology called the trainee to enquire about the case. The specimen he received was labelled 'right hemivulvectomy' and did not reveal any evidence of cancer. The pre-operative biopsies the pathologist had reviewed had been positive, however they were labelled 'left vulvar biopsy'. He wondered if there had been a labelling error.

The trainee informed the pathologist that the right side had been removed, and then informed the surgeon about the error. The attending surgeon denied that any error had been made; he insisted that the original biopsies had been mislabelled. The surgeon did not inform the patient of the error. When the patient returned for routine follow-up the surgeon performed a vulvar colposcopy and biopsied the left side. Microinvasive cancer was noted in the biopsies. Shortly thereafter, the patient underwent a second hemivulvectomy to treat her vulvar cancer.

(REPRODUCED FROM *BRITISH MEDICAL JOURNAL*, DAVID W BATES. "USING INFORMA-TION TECHNOLOGY TO REDUCE RATES OF MEDICATION ERRORS IN HOSPITALS". **320**, NO. 7237, [737–740], 2000, WITH PERMISSION FROM BMJ PUBLISHING GROUP LTD.)

Judgement and decision making

The fallibility of memory is an everyday experience, which is generally not too embarrassing to admit. Using devices to compensate, whether a shopping list, a diary or a computer, comes easily to us. Our judgements and decisions however, are more precious to our self esteem and there is much more resistance to allowing guidelines and protocols, whether on paper or instanti-ated in software, to take over human decisions. This was memorably expressed by François, Duc de al Roche Foucauld in 1666 in his *Maximes*, when he pointed out that 'Everyone complains about their memory, but no one complains about their judgement'

In other spheres, such as navigation, judgement has given way to measure-ment and calculation and now to computation. My grandfather, flying in the First World War, navigated by compass and flying along railway lines, dipping down to inspect the countryside from time to time. My father, flying a Sunderland flying boat in the Second World War, made careful calculations of direction, wind speed and compass bearing, taking into account the discrep-ancy of true and magnetic north and the error introduced in the compass reading by the metal hull of the aeroplane. Today, an onboard computer just sorts it all out.

Research on judgement (weighing the options) and decision making (choos-ing amongst the options) has yielded different perspectives on human abilities. On the one hand, the naturalistic decision-making school, most powerfully and persuasively represented by Gary Klein (1998), has shown how experts can rapidly assess a dangerous situation and, far from analysing and choosing, seem to just 'know' what to do. A firefighter can just see that the fire is in the basement and the building above is about to collapse; a physician takes one look at a patient and sees that they are dangerously hypoglycaemic. Klein describes this as 'recognition primed decision making', rapid, adaptive and effective. This is the classic image of the expert physician who assesses a complex set of symptoms and immediately perceives the correct diagnosis. It is difficult, though not impossible, to imagine replacing this kind of intuitive brilliance with the stolid, systematic approach of a computer. In principle, these decisions could be handled by a machine; in practice, the time spent entering the relevant data might be the limiting factor.

Consider, however, some other common medical scenarios, such as assessing the risk of suicide. A psychiatrist must consider past history, diagnosis, previous attempts at self harm, declared intention and family support available, then weigh all these factors and decide whether the patient can return to the community. Or, consider a paediatric cardiac surgeon weighing up the risks of operating on a tiny baby: anatomy of the heart, pulmonary artery pressure, findings from the echocardiogram and a host of other features may be considered to assess the likely short- and long-term outcomes for the child of operating now, operating in six months or not operating at all. Both of these decisions involve complex calculations, weighing of different factors and combining them to produce a judgement between two or more choices. People must assemble the information, but would a machine or an algorithm make a better decision? In fact, numerous studies have shown that we vastly overestimate our power to make such judgements and that we also overestimate the number of factors that we take into account. Using statistical methods and models is nearly always superior to using unaided human judgement (Box 13.2) (Hastie and Dawes, 2001). This phenomenon, of the superiority of statistical over clinical and other expert judgement, was first documented by Paul Meehl in 1954. In the most recent update of his findings, (Grove and Meehl, 1996), Meehl concluded that empirical comparisons show that the mechanical (statistical, whether computer or calculated) method is almost invariably equal or superior to the human judgement.

BOX 13.2 Clinical and statistical prediction

A world expert on Hodgkin's disease and two assistants rated nine characteristics of biopsies taken from patients and assessed 'overall severity' as a predictor of longevity. In fact, when experts judged the disease to be more severe, patients actually lived slightly longer; the judgement trend was in the wrong direction. In contrast, a multiple regression model based on the same nine characteristics showed a clear, though not strong, reliable association between actual and predicted longevity.

30 experienced psychologists and psychiatrists predicted the dangerousness of 40 newly admitted psychiatric patients. The experts were provided with 19 cues, mostly derived from the judgements of psychiatrists

who interviewed the patients on admission. The human judges predicted the likelihood of violent assault on another person in the first week of hospitalization with an accuracy of 0.12; the most accurate human judge scored 0.36. In contrast, a linear statistical model achieved an accuracy of 0.82 with the same data.

(REPRODUCED FROM HASTIE R. & DAWES R.M. *RATIONAL CHOICE IN AN UNCERTAIN WORLD: THE PSYCHOLOGY OF JUDGMENT AND DECISION MAKING*, 2001, WITH PERMISSION FROM SAGE PUBLICATIONS INC, CALIFORNIA)

The field of judgement and decision making is vast and the issue of human ability and fallibility much debated. My intention is simply to show that, in some instances at least, there is good reason for thinking that the computational aspects of some medical decisions might be more consistently and accurately carried out by a computer than by a person, however expert. Decision support therefore may, if used appropriately, have a major impact on patient safety.

One of the key problems for the future then will be discovering where technology can help and where we need to rely on human judgement. As Bates *et al.* (2001) point out, human beings are erratic and err in unexpected ways, yet we are also resourceful and inventive and can recover from errors and crises. In comparison, machines, at least most of those currently in use, are dependable but also dependably stupid. An almost perfect instruction, quite good enough for any human operator, can completely disable a machine. Human beings also have the capacity to respond to an 'unknown unknown', that is an event that could not have been predicted (Bates *et al.*,2001).

At the moment it seems safe to say that there is excessive reliance in healthcare on human memory and other fallible processes; computers, memory and decision aids of all kinds are grossly underused. The boundaries of the human machine interface will change over time, as we develop more powerful and sophisticated systems and accept that clinical expertise, essential though it is, does not necessarily bring reliability and consistency to routine operations. In some areas however, there have already been considerable advances; a notable example is the use of computerized systems in the process of medication administration.

Using information technology to reduce medication errors

Medication errors arise from a variety of causes. Almost half result, in some degree, from clinicians lacking information about the patient or the drug. This may be because they do not know the information themselves, because test results are missing or because other patient or drug specific information is not available. Other common problems are that handwritten orders are illegible, do not contain all necessary information, are transcribed incorrectly or contain errors of calculation (Bates, 2000). Several medication technology systems have been addressing these and other problems, operating at various stages of

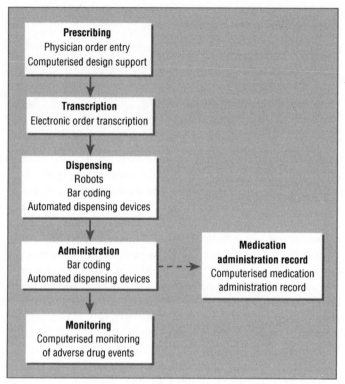

Figure 13.1 Role of automation at each stage of the medication process (from Bates (2000)).

the medication and delivery process (Figure 13.1). They show great promise but, as David Bates warns, are not a panacea:

Information technologies . . . . may make some things better and others worse; the net effect is not entirely predictable, and it is vital to study the impact of these technologies. They have their greatest impact in organizing and making available information, in identifying links between pieces of information, and in doing boring repetitive tasks, including checks for problems. The best medication processes will thus not replace people but will harness the strengths of information technology and allow people to do the things best done by people, such as making complex decisions and communicating with each other.
(BATES, 2000)

The system that has probably had the largest impact on medication error is computerized physician order entry (CPOE), in which medication orders are written online. This improves orders in several ways. First, they are structured, so they must include a drug, dose and frequency; the computer, unlike a person, can refuse to accept any order without this information. They are always legible, and the clinician making the order can always be identified if there is a need to check back. Finally, all orders can be routinely and automatically checked for allergies, drug interactions, excessively high or low doses and whether the dosage is appropriate for the patient's liver and kidney function. Clinical staff may fear that these advantages may be offset by the time lost in typing rather than writing orders. However, Hollingworth *et al.* (2007) found that increases were only marginal (12 seconds per order) and there was little disruption to workflow. We should also note that the overall effect on the system, as opposed to the individual prescriber, could well be greater efficiency because fewer orders have to be corrected and fewer adverse drug events occur.

Bates *et al.* (1998) showed that the introduction of a computerized order entry system resulted in a 55% reduction in medication errors. This system provided clinicians with information about drugs, including appropriate constraints on choices (dose, route, frequency) and assistance with calculations and monitoring. With the addition of higher levels of decision support, in the form of more comprehensive checking for allergies and drug interactions, there was an 83% reduction. Other studies have shown, for instance, improvement of prescribing of anticoagulants, heparin and anti-infective agents and reductions in inappropriate doses and frequency of drugs given to patients with renal insufficiency (Kaushal, Shojania and Bates, 2003). Evidence of the value of CPOE continues to accumulate. In a recent meta-analysis of complex prescribing in vulnerable patients, Floor van Rosse *et al.* (2009) reviewed 12 studies in paediatric and adult intensive care settings and found that CPOE reduced medication errors but that the impact on clinical outcomes remained equivocal. In a review of CPOE, Kaushal, Shojania and Bates (2003) caution that while these systems show great promise, most studies have examined 'home-grown' systems, and have only considered small numbers of patients in specific settings. Much more research is needed to compare different applications, identify key components, examine factors relating to acceptance and uptake and anticipate and monitor the problems that such systems may induce.

Another critical safety issue is that there can be a discrepancy between the drugs that patients are meant to be receiving and those that they are actually taking. Medicines reconciliation refers to the process of producing a definitive list of the drugs the patient should be taking and then checking them against the drugs they are actually taking; as you might imagine, points of transition, such as discharge from hospital, are particularly vulnerable to errors of this kind. Schnipper *et al.* (2009) looked for discrepancies between preadmission medication, medication during admission and medication at discharge. They found an average of 1.4 potential adverse drug events per admission – not very good odds for the patient. This rate was reduced by a third after the introduction of a Web-based computerized medicines reconciliation system, which enabled clinical staff to view and compare medication information from ambulatory (out of hospital) settings with hospital medication. The team also clarified responsibility for medicines reconciliation at different time points, reduced multiple history taking and used cross-checking between staff to increase compliance with the new systems, so there was much more to this intervention than simply the technology.

Looking further ahead, it is possible to envisage the use of many other technologies in the process of medication delivery. Most of these are in the early stages of development, are relatively untested and sometimes delayed by external constraints. Bar coding for instance, widely used in supermarkets, could be enormously useful but cannot be implemented until drug manufacturers have agreed common standards (Bates, 2000). Considerable advances have been made however, in the reliability and efficiency of blood sampling and blood transfusion (Box 13.3).

BOX 13.3 Bar coding and blood transfusion

The transfusion process is long, complex and laborious. Clinical staff are vulnerable to fatigue, distraction and error. The single most important factor in blood transfusion incidents is mis-identification of the patient. Observations showed that staff were frequently distracted whilst checking blood, by having to answer the phone or respond to questions from colleagues. The programme of improvement evolved in four distinct stages:

Blood sample collection and the pre-transfusion bedside check
The first stage addressed two bedside processes previously: blood sample collection for compatibility testing and pre-transfusion checking. A hand-held bar code device was introduced, which checked all stages of the process. For instance, staff had to scan the bar coded patient identity tag before proceeding to the next stage. The results of the implementation of the electronic transfusion process were dramatic, reducing the number of process steps and bringing sustained and significant improvements in blood sample collection and pre-transfusion checking. For example, correct verbal identification of patients rose from 11.8 to 100%.

Bar coding the transfusion process
Baseline observations revealed high error rates at almost every step of the transfusion process. Bar coding checks to the transfusion process brought significant improvements. These included an increase from 8 to 100% in checking that the pack was in date and the blood group and unit number on the blood pack matched the compatibility label. Similar significant improvements were found in blood sample collection, the collection of blood from blood refrigerators, and the documentation of transfusion; the time taken to collect a blood unit reduced from an average of 3 minutes to 1 minute per unit.

Electronic remote blood issue
The issue of red cell units was traditionally carried out within the blood transfusion laboratories. Electronic remote blood issue (ERBI) allowed

blood to be released to specific patients at blood refrigerators in wards, theatres and other sites. The results showed that ERBI reduced the time to make blood available for surgical patients and improved the efficiency of hospital transfusion. Before it took 24 minutes to get blood to the patient; afterwards 59 seconds. Unused requests for blood reduced significantly and the process significantly reduced the workload of both blood transfusion laboratory and clinical staff.

Implementation of the electronic transfusion process in three acute hospitals

The electronic transfusion processes were implemented across three acute hospitals, with 1500 inpatient beds between them. The implementation was planned in 10 phases, involving 6 or more clinical areas per phase each of 4 weeks duration. Careful advance planning made it feasible to provide the necessary infrastructure in stages (e.g. wristband printers, handhelds) and to provide intensive training to small groups of staff. The task of training all the staff was huge, involving 1300 doctors, 3200 nurses, as well as phlebotomists and porters. At the end of the first year of the implementation stage, the electronic process was being used for taking 88% of samples for the blood transfusion laboratory and for administering 83% of transfusions, later rising to 95% of both samples and transfusion. Reduction of red cell usage and reduction in the rate of sample rejection have produced significant savings.

(*TRANSFUSION*, MURPHY, M. F., STAVES, J., DAVIES, A., FRASER, E., PARKER, R., CRIPPS, B., KAY, J., & VINCENT, C. "HOW DO WE APPROACH A MAJOR CHANGE PROGRAM USING THE EXAMPLE OF THE DEVELOPMENT, EVALUATION, AND IMPLEMENTATION OF AN ELECTRONIC TRANSFUSION MANAGEMENT SYSTEM". **49**, NO. 5, 829–837, 2009. REPRODUCED WITH PERMISSION FROM WILEY-BLACKWELL)

Communication and alerts

A particularly dangerous time for loss of essential information, particularly for patients who are very sick and whose condition is fluctuating, is at the handover, or sign-out, when one member of staff takes over from another. Handover, when verbal, is frequently rushed, casual, and sometimes absent altogether:

I just got called by the nurse about Mrs Davis, who is hypotensive. All I know about her is that she is an 82-year-old woman with a urinary tract infection who is due to go home tomorrow.
(VOLPP AND GRANDE, 2003)

At the Brigham and Women's Hospital in Boston, a computerized sign-out system automatically includes up-to-date information on drug allergies, current medications, results of recent tests and relevant medical history. Doctors covering the wards are expected to update the medical history each day with details of changes in clinical condition and current treatment plan. All this information is available to other clinical staff. Furthermore, the electronic process of sign-out and the transfer of pagers ensure there is no ambiguity about who is on duty at any one time.

Information technology can also detect and transmit information about laboratory abnormalities as soon as the result is available. For instance, a dangerously low serum potassium level requires urgent action, but the information may be delayed while a ward clerk sorts the results and may not reach the relevant doctor until some time later. With an alert system coupled to a handheld PDA or mobile phone, an instant alert can be generated and transmitted. In a controlled trial, such a system reduced response time by 11% and reduced the duration of dangerous conditions in patients by 29% (Bates and Gawande, 2003). Such systems can be especially valuable when trying to assemble patient information in a timely fashion over a wide geographical area. A marvellous example of the effective use of technology in a relatively poor environment is provided by Joaquin Blaya and colleagues, who introduced PDAs for the collection of tuberculosis results in the Peruvian healthcare system. A controlled trial showed the processing times for cultures were reduced from 23 to 8 days. Highly dangerous long delays in processing of over three months, which previously occurred in 11% of cases, were almost eliminated (Blaya *et al.*, 2009).

Forcing functions and corollary orders

Forcing functions are reminders or constraints that suggest or require a certain response from the person using the machine. When you use your debit card to obtain money from a cash machine, the screen prompts you to remove your card before issuing any money (Nolan, 2000). This is a classic use of design to overcome human absent mindedness and the previously common situation of removing the cash, which is the focus of your attention, and leaving the card in the machine. You meant to take the card, but you were talking to your friend, took your money, turned away and left the card in the machine. Similarly, clinicians placing certain drug orders usually intend, but quite often forget, to order the necessary tests that routinely accompany the medication.

Overhage *et al.* (1997) call these basic medical decisions corollary orders. Ordering gentamicin should, almost always, trigger ordering gentamicin levels; angiotensin converting enzyme (ACE) inhibitors require serum creatine levels; insulin means blood glucose monitoring and so on. Although the decision to carry out a corollary order is simple, they are frequently missed. Various strategies have been used to combat these omissions, such as monitoring adherence using chart review and mounting educational programmes. These can be successful but are difficult to maintain in the long term. Paper based reminders placed in the chart are partially effective but not always available to the clinician at the time they write the order. A computerized reminder however, linked to an electronic medical record system, allows an immediate prompt. Overhage *et al.* (1997), in a six month trial, showed that clinicians ordered the suggested corollary orders in 46% of cases when prompted, compared with 22% in a control group. Clinicians discriminated amongst the suggested orders, rejecting some while accepting others, and it is reasonable to assume that the additional orders were necessary ones that the clinicians, once reminded, considered important.

Electronic medical records

The introduction of an effective electronic medical record should improve basic communication and co-ordination of patient information. Staff have access to a common database of medical information, including the results of investigations and tests, notes on outpatient visits and hospitalizations, records of drug allergies and recent medical history. Some healthcare systems, such as the Veterans Affairs, have already transferred to electronic records giving access to the record to all relevant staff wherever the patient is in the United States. British general practice has also used electronic records and computerized prescribing for many years. The impact of these systems once embedded has not always been fully assessed but few users long for a return to loosely bound heaps of paper records, even though paper always retains some advantages; for instance, you can scribble a diagram on it very easily. Implementation of such systems in ambulatory (outpatient) settings in the Kaiser Permanente system has reduced visits to doctors' offices by 10%. The main reason for this seemed to be the increase in scheduled telephone calls to patients, made more effective by the regular availability of the full clinical record and, very probably, the increased use of decision support embedded in the electronic record (Garrido *et al.*, 2005). While the technological and standardization problems of implementing such systems are formidable, particularly when covering a whole healthcare system such as the British National Health Service, there is clearly scope for massive increases in efficiency, avoidance of duplication of investigations and treatment, and reduction of errors caused by crucial information not being available.

Pioneering centres, such as the Cleveland Clinic in Ohio, have gone a step further in giving patients access to their medical records. Cleveland has created 'MyChart', which allows, indeed encourages, patients to access their record and to find medical research on relevant conditions. Doctors must record all examinations, test results, prescriptions and diagnoses for patients to review, offering almost complete transparency of the medical process. Patients can now check the record, point out errors and also be reminded of important events, such as when they need a follow-up or vaccination. Cleveland are now going a step further, working with Google to make the record available to the patient wherever they are in the world.

Decision support

Decision support encompasses a vast range of tools with different names, foci and outputs and with widely differing levels of technological input (Wears and Berg, 2005). For example, an automatic prompt could be described as decision support, as it reminds the clinician to take the decision to order a test. Clinicians have always used decision support in the form of pocket guides to drugs, personal lists and reminders of ward practices and so on. Decision support systems include: paper based guidelines giving general guidance and objectives; more specific paper based algorithms that assist diagnosis or calculations of appropriate drug dosages; computer based systems that prompt possible diagnoses; right through to systems which could potentially supplant human judgement (Morris, 2002).

Computer based decision support has a major advantage over almost all paper based general protocols and guidelines; it can be patient specific to a degree that is almost impossible to achieve in a paper based guide. A computer based system can remind you when to act, suggest courses of action, perform necessary calculations, monitor the output and take any number of patient specific clinical variables into account. Far from being cookbook medicine, this opens up the possibility of treatment being individualized and customized to a much greater degree. The majority of systems are prototypes, being tested and evaluated in particular local circumstances and have not yet achieved full clinical integration. Increasingly however, systems are being developed which have not only been shown to improve decision making but have been adopted as an essential part of routine practice (Box 13.4).

BOX 13.4 Some examples of computerized decision support

Computerized mechanical ventilation protocols for Acute Respiratory Distress Syndrome

In an intensive care unit, measures of intravenous flow, intravenous drug administration and physiological indicators are continually monitored and integrated with other data entered by the clinician. The decision support system generates warnings and offers recommendations for action. In a trial in 10 hospitals, physicians objected to only 0.3% of generated suggestions for action over 32 000 hours of application. Patients treated in units with decision support experienced significantly fewer barotraumas and overall survival was similar.

(ADAPTED FROM MORRIS, 2002)

Implementing antibiotic practice guidelines through computer assisted decision support

In the treatment of infections, decision support programmes provide information on the presence of resistant pathogens, untreated infections, an incorrect dose, route or interval and the need for serum levels and cost effective alternatives to current treatment. Over seven years, 63 000 patients were studied. The proportion of patients receiving antibiotics increased from 31.8 to 53.1%, though overall costs decreased. Treatment with appropriate prophylactic antibiotics before surgery increased from 40 to 99.1%. Antibiotic related adverse drug events decreased by 30%.

(ADAPTED FROM EVANS, PESTONIK AND CLASSEN, 1998)

Major reviews of the impact of decision support have concluded that there is positive, though mixed support for its implementation. A review of 100 studies by Amit Garg *et al.* (2005) found that 64% of the interventions produced positive effects, though noted that there was so far little evidence of any impact on outcomes. A still larger review of 257 studies by Chaudhry *et al.* (2006) examined the more general question of the impact of health information technology, mostly decision support and electronic records. They found evidence for increased adherence to guidelines, better surveillance and monitoring of disease and reduced medication errors, but few studies assessed the impact on efficiency and cost. They also noted that almost a quarter of the studies were carried out in just four centres in the United States, raising doubts about the extent to which such technologies could be implemented in poorer environments (Einbinder and Bates, 2007).

Garg *et al.* (2005) divided the decision support systems into four broad categories: systems for diagnosis; reminder systems for prevention; systems for disease management; and systems for supporting prescribing and drug dosing (discussed previously). Diagnostic systems were the least studied, in that only ten formal studies were identified; four showing an advantage in performance but none demonstrating clear clinical benefits. However, systems for identifying cardiac ischaemia in the emergency department reduced unnecessary admissions by 15%. Systems for disease prevention provided reminders for screening, counselling, vaccination, testing, medication use and the identification of at risk behaviours, prompting the doctor or nurse to ask about the relevant issue or order relevant tests. Three-quarters of these trials showed improvements in, for instance, the ordering of mammography, screening for bowel cancer and vaccinations. While most studies were restricted to a single site, a small number showed widespread take-up across multiple sites. Forty systems aimed to improve the management of chronic diseases, particularly diabetes and cardiovascular disease, with a combination of automatic reminders, forcing functions and formal decision support in the form of specific recommendations. The majority of trials of diabetes care and a number of those for cardiovascular disease showed improvements in compliance. Overall, 23 of the 37 studying practitioner performance reported improvements, but only a small number found concomitant changes in clinical outcomes.

Patients' response to decision support

How will patients react to the increasing use of decision support? The computer by the intensive care bedside monitoring physiology and the drugs given could be seen as a support, even a comfort, to a patient, perhaps allowing the nurses more opportunity to care for very sick and vulnerable people. But would you want to go to your surgeon and find that they use a computer to decide whether to operate or not? Would the use of a computer destroy trust and degrade the doctor–patient relationship?

Decision support will become more important to patients as they increasingly participate in treatment decisions and have to face the same complexities as clinicians. Do I watch and wait with possible prostate cancer and put up with the symptoms? Do I opt for radiotherapy and its attendant risks or do I prefer radical surgery, potential complete cure but with possible loss of sexual function? In part, this decision will depend on the weighing of options and in part on personal values and preferences, and the key to the proper use of decision support lies in separating these two aspects. Decision support can, and should, be placed at the service of the doctor–patient relationship, handling what one might call the 'calculative' aspects of the decision while allowing the doctor and patient to explore the human side, the personal and emotional consequences of each course of action. The preferences of the patient, and the doctor, are separated from the preferred mode of judgement and decision making and no longer conflated as they are in a more traditional clinical scenario. Doctor and patient first explore what the patient feels is most important; the doctor has assessed the clinical factors and the full clinical interview is still conducted; the machine, or other decision aid, weights the options on the basis of the information and presents the likely outcomes. In the end though, the patient still decides (Dowie, 2001).

The implementation of information technology

In a thoughtful editorial accompanying the Garg review, Wears and Berg (2005) sought to put the findings into perspective:

Behind the cheers and high hopes that dominate conference proceedings, vendor information and large parts of the scientific literature, the reality is that systems that are used in multiple locations, that have satisfied users, and that have effectively contributed to the quality and safety of care are few and far between.
(WEARS AND BERG, 2005)

Wears and Berg pointed out that, although the review was valuable in providing an overview of the field, it raised as many questions as it answered. A huge range of different types of systems had been considered under the general rubric of decision support and it was not possible to discern the reasons for success or failure. Systems might fail because of poor design, poor implementation, inappropriate use by clinicians or for many other reasons. They argued for a broader evaluation and assessment in which the aim of decision support is conceived in terms of improving the performance of the wider healthcare system rather than in narrow technological terms. They pointed out that there is often a mismatch between the implied conception of clinical work embedded in the technology, which assumes problems are constrained and clear cut, and the real world of clinical work, which is interpretative, multitasking, collaborative, opportunistic and reactive. In saying this, they were not arguing against decision support, but pointing to the need to consider the real context of clinical work from the earliest stages of development to the final evaluation (Wears and Berg, 2005).

So what makes one system succeed and another fail? This critical question was addressed in a review of 70 studies of decision support systems, which examined 15 different features of those systems (Kawamoto *et al.*, 2005). Just under 70% of the systems showed positive results. There were four critical determinants of success. The most powerful factor was that the system automatically provided decision support as part of the clinician workflow. Decision support did not have to be provided by a computer; for instance, in one study, diabetes care recommendations were attached to relevant paper records by support staff. Other determinants of success were that the system provided actual recommendations of what should be done, rather than simply an assessment or presentation of options, that the decision support was provided at the time the decision was being made and that the support was provided by a computer. In summary, a system will succeed if it is easy to use and provides clear recommendations at the time the clinician needs them.

Even if the technology is effective and meets the needs of users, the implementation process is fraught with innumerable hazards and needs to be carefully thought through. Trish Greenhalgh and colleagues have shed light on this process in their examination of the introduction of the summary electronic health records in Britain, in a study which involved 1500 hours of ethnographic observation, interviews with 170 staff and review of a mass of documentation. The ease of use, functionality and benefits of the technology were obviously critical to its success. However, people who had to use the new system were also influenced by champions and opinion leaders and by previous experience of innovation in the workplace. As you might imagine, organizations needed time, resources and technical expertise but also a willingness to take some risk in the hope of longer-term benefits. In summarizing the findings of their study, Greenhalgh *et al.* write persuasively of the need to shift from a technology push model to a sociotechnical model of change:

The predominant change model adopted for the summary care record programme was one of 'technology push' – centrally driven, rationalistic, with a focus on documentation and reporting, and oriented to predefined, relatively inflexible goals... Nevertheless, coexisting with Connecting for Health's technology push model were occasional initiatives such as away-days, networking events, and consultations that resonated with more contemporary models of change built around theories of co-evolution and knowledge creation, and which reflect a 'socio-technical pull' model. Our data ... suggest that as the programme expands further movement in this socio-technical direction is likely to improve its chances of success.
REPRODUCED FROM *BRITISH MEDICAL JOURNAL*, TRISHA GREENHALGH, KATJA STRAMER, TANJA BRATAN ET AL. "INTRODUCTION OF SHARED ELECTRONIC RECORDS: MULTI-SITE CASE STUDY USING DIFFUSION OF INNOVATION THEORY". **337**, NO. 1 (OCT 23), [1786], 2008, WITH PERMISSION FROM BMJ PUBLISHING GROUP LTD.

The push model is essentially one of project management in which the programme is planned and controlled centrally and then rolled out in the relevant areas. Success is measured primarily in terms of the adoption of the programme without much regard for its wider impact; the programme is an end in itself. In contrast, those at the receiving end, including patients, are much more interested in the programme's impact on their own work and on patient care. Moving to a sociotechnical change model means keeping these wider aims in view and being conscious of the need to work collaboratively with all those influenced by the programme.

The unintended consequences of information technology

Studies of the problems associated with technology in healthcare are few and far between, though anecdotes are easy to come by. The shutdown of an automatic drug dispensing system in an Emergency Department for instance, led to delays in giving urgent drugs and a near disaster; subsequently nurses took to carrying adrenalin around in their pockets in case the problem recurred. In another example, staff took to sticking reminder notes on the computer screen, because the software did not allow them to input the reminders they needed. These classic 'workarounds', while understandable, clearly creates the potential for other kinds of errors. They stem not so much from technology *per se*, but from technology designed and implemented without sufficient understanding or regard for the way clinical work is actually carried out. A particularly unfortunate problem is that automation can take over tasks that humans do quite well, leaving residual tasks that humans find very challenging; this is one of the ironies of automation.

The ironies of automation

The increasing use of technology, and the rapid increase in computer power, has allowed many systems to operate with little or no intervention from human beings. The classic exemplar of such systems is the flight deck of a modern commercial airliner, in which the pilot's role has, apparently at least, progressively been diminished. The aircraft of the future, so the story goes, will be flown by a single pilot and a dog; the dog is there to bite the pilot if he touches anything. In fact, the pilot needs greater skills with such a highly automated system; they must be able to both fly the plane and understand the automated system, which becomes steadily more difficult as automation increases.

Such systems are, of course, always vulnerable to both hardware and software breakdowns, but their very sophistication and level of automation produces new problems for the human operator and new vulnerabilities. These are, in Lisanne Bainbridge's elegant phrase, the ironies of automation (Bainbridge, 1987). In a classic paper, she outlined some of the principal ironies, summarized here as:

- Many systems successfully automate the routine elements of a process, yet leave the supposedly unreliable human operator to carry out tasks which the designer could not think how to automate – most notably recovering from system breakdown.
- In highly automated systems, the main task of the human being is to monitor the systems and check for any abnormalities. Yet, vigilance and monitoring over long periods are notoriously difficult for human beings.

- When systems break down only rarely, the human operators have little chance to practice recovering from the breakdown or of using their own skills to take over control. Skills such as these degrade when not used, which inevitably happens when a machine takes over.
- The systems which are most highly automated paradoxically require the highest level of skill and training to deal with their complex, sometimes opaque modes of operation.

Few healthcare systems are near this level of automation, though it may apply to some laboratory processes. Bainbridge's cogent analysis does, however, point to the fact that we can expect the increasing use of information technology, even if clearly beneficial overall, to produce its own problems.

Inflexibility and rigidity

Ash, Berg and Coeiera (2004), in a paper entitled 'The unintended consequences of technology', have begun to outline some of the principal forms of error that healthcare technology introduces. Computerized systems may be inflexible, insufficiently adaptable to the complexities of real, individualized patient treatment; if urgent medication is required, and cannot be released before the full authorization and data input, dangerous delays may be introduced; transfers from Emergency to a ward can similarly be delayed while the admitting system demands key information which is not available. Computer interfaces with easy, pull down menus or other quick ways of entering data can lead to substitution errors, especially when people are distracted:

I was ordering Cortisporin, and Cortisporin solution and suspension comes up. The patient was talking to me, and I accidentally put down solution, then realized. . . . I would not have made that mistake if I had been writing it. (ASH ET AL., 2004)

Such examples show why technology is never a panacea, in the sense that whenever one introduces a technology to reduce one kind of error, one is likely to introduce the possibility of new kinds of error. Extensive road testing in real settings is the only way to reveal these vulnerabilities and points again to the need to keep the realities of the clinical world constantly in mind during development.

Integration within the work process

Failing to study the nature and flow of the work prior to implementation can lead to more serious problems. In one British hospital, laboratory results were telephoned to the wards, direct to physicians, thus allowing rapid communication of urgent results. When this system was replaced by entering results into a computer system, physicians had to remember to log on and check the laboratory results; the new system had advantages in terms of clinical workload and time management, but it led to delays in receiving urgent information and some results that were missed entirely (Ash et al., 2004).

In a careful qualitative study of the introduction of a bar coding system for medication, Emily Paterson and colleagues (Patterson, Cook and Render, 2002) noted five main types of unanticipated side effects of the system. First, there were occasions where the nurses were simply confused by the system, particularly when it dropped medication orders simply because they had been delayed. Second, it sometimes led to a decrease in communication between physicians and nurses. Third, it reduced checking, in that physicians would previously have a quick glance at the (paper) medication records, but would generally not check the computer system because it was slower. In addition, there were problems with scheduling activities, as the system demanded very precise timings, delaying other clinical work that should have taken priority, and there were difficulties in entering unusual, non-standard medication regimens. Finally, they observed the ingenuity of the nurses in getting round the system with workarounds when they were short of time or otherwise pressured. Rather than scan the wristband on the patient's wrist, they might type in the code number, scan the patient ID card instead or take the wristband off and scan it on the table. Scanning of multiple medications at the same time saved time, as did delaying documentation of medications that would not scan at the time. In all these workarounds, we can see the trade off between needing to get things done and bypassing the systems at the cost of a greater likelihood of making a mistake by, for instance, typing in a code number rather than scanning the bar code.

A false sense of security

A final problem relates to the achievement of very high levels of safety in any system. When errors and problems occur all the time, then people become used to dealing with them, are continually on the lookout for error and develop ways of recovering. The system may be error prone but it is also resilient. However, when errors are very rare, we can become lulled into a false sense of security, particularly with apparently 100% reliable technology. Bates *et al.*, 2001 quotes an example of this phenomenon in the highly reliable setting of radiation therapy. Macklis, Meier and Weinhaus (1998) examined the safety record of a system that double-checked radiation treatments. The system had an error rate of only 0.18%, and all the errors that did occur were minor in nature. However, about 15% of the errors that did occur related to the way operators used the system. Because they believed it was so reliable, they tended to believe 'the machine had to be right', even in the face of conflicting evidence. Thus over reliance on technology, indeed on any highly reliable system, can increase the possibility of certain kinds of errors through reduced vigilance.

Information technology, especially computerized decision support, is still not widely accepted and not in routine use. Many barriers remain to be overcome, some financial, as considerable investment is needed for large-scale change, some practical, such as the lack of standards for representation of data, and some cultural, in that neither the research nor the use of decision support are fully accepted in clinical circles (Bates and Gawande, 2003). Nevertheless, harking back to the discussion of human memory and decision making, it is clear that much greater use of information technology is needed if healthcare is ever going to attain even reasonable standards of reliability and safety. The fact that the implementation of technological solutions can lead to errors and unanticipated hazards does not mean that we should stop implementing information and other technology to improve safety. Rather, we need to be alert in design, implementation and usage to the unanticipated consequences and side effects.

References

Ash, J.S., Berg, M. and Coiera, E. (2004) Some unintended consequences of information technology in healthcare: the nature of patient care information system-related errors. *Journal of the American Medical Informatics Association*, **11**, 104–112.

Bainbridge, L. (1987) The ironies of automation, in *New Technologies and Human Error* (eds J. Rasmussen, K. Duncanand J. Le Plat), John Wiley & Sons, Ltd, London.

Bates, D.W. (2000) Using information technology to reduce rates of medication errors in hospitals. *British Medical Journal*, **320**(7237), 788–791.

Bates, D.W. and Gawande, A.A. (2003) Improving safety with information technology. *The New England Journal of Medicine*, **348**(25), 2526.

Bates, D.W., Leape, L.L., Cullen, D.J. *et al.* (1998) Effect of computerized physician order entry and a team intervention on prevention of serious medication errors. *Journal of the American Medical Association*, **280**(15), 1311–1316.

Bates, D.W., Cohen, M., Leape, L.L. *et al.* (2001) Reducing the frequency of medication errors using information technology. *Journal of the American Medical Informatics Association*, **8**, 299–308.

Bicknell, C.D., Cheshire, N.J., Riga, C.V. *et al.* (2009) Treatment of complex aneurysmal disease with fenestrated and branched stent grafts. *European Journal of Vascular and Endovascular Surgery*, **37**(2), 175–181.

Blaya, J.A., Cohen, T., Rodriguez, P. *et al.* (2009) Personal digital assistants to collect tuberculosis bacteriology data in Peru reduce delays, errors, and workload, and are acceptable to users: cluster randomized controlled trial. *International Journal of Infectious Disease*, **13**(3), 410–418.

Chaudhry, B., Wang, J., Wu, S. *et al.* (2006) Systematic review: impact of health information technology on quality, efficiency, and costs of medical care. *Annals of Internal Medicine*, **144**(10), 742–752.

Dowie, J. (2001) Decision analysis and the evaluating of decision technologies. *Quality and Safety in Health Care*, **10**, 1–2.

Einbinder, J.S. and Bates, D.W. (2007) Leveraging information technology to improve quality and safety. *Yearbook of Medical Informatics*, **46**, 22–29.

Evans, R.S., Pestonik, S.C. and Classen, D.C. (1998) A computer assisted management program for antibiotics and other anti-infective agents. *New England Journal of Medicine*, **338**, 232–238.

Garg, A.X., Adhikari, N.K.J., McDonald, H. *et al.* (2005) Effects of computerized clinical decision support systems on practitioner performance and patient outcomes: a systematic review. *Journal of the American Medical Association*, **293**(10), 1223–1238.

Garrido, T., Jamieson, L., Zhou, Y. *et al.* (2005) Effect of electronic health records in ambulatory care: retrospective, serial, cross-sectional study. *British Medical Journal*, **330**(7491), 581.

Greenhalgh, T., Stramer, K., Bratan, T. *et al.* (2008) Introduction of shared electronic records: multi-site case study using diffusion of innovation theory. *British Medical Journal*, **337**, 1040–1044.

Grove, W.M. and Meehl, P.E. (1996) Comparative efficiency of informal (subjective impressionistic) and formal (mechanistic, algorithmic) prediction procedures: the clinical – statistical controversy. *Psychology, Public Policy and Law*, **2**, 293–323.

Hastie, R. and Dawes, R.M. (2001) *Rational Choice in An Uncertain World. The Psychology of Judgement and Decision Making*, Sage Publications, California.

Hollingworth, W., Devine, E.B., Hansen, R.N. *et al.* (2007) The impact of e-prescribing on prescriber and staff time in ambulatory care clinics: a time motion study. *Journal of the American Medical Informatics Association*, **14**(6), 722–730.

Kaushal, R., Shojania, K.G. and Bates, D.W. (2003) Effects of computerized physician order entry and clinical decision support systems on medication safety: a systematic review. *Archives of Internal Medicine*, **163**(12), 1409–1416.

Kawamoto, K., Houlihan, C.A., Balas, E.A. and Lobach, D.F. (2005) Improving clinical practice using clinical decision support systems: a systematic review of trials to identify features critical to success. *British Medical Journal*, **330**(7494), 765.

Klein, G. (1998) *Sources of Power. How People Make Decision*, MIT Press, Boston.

Macklis, R.M., Meier, T. and Weinhaus, M.S. (1998) Error rates in clinical radiotherapy. *Journal of Clinical Oncology*, **16**, 551–556.

Morris, A.H. (2002) Decision support and safety of clinical environments. *Quality and Safety in Health Care*, **11**(1), 69–75.

Murphy, M.F., Staves, J., Davies, A. *et al.* (2009) How do we approach a major change program using the example of the development, evaluation, and implementation of an electronic transfusion management system. *Transfusion*, **49**(5), 829–837.

Nolan, T.W. (2000) System changes to improve patient safety. *British Medical Journal*, **320**, 771–773.

Overhage, J.M., Tiernery, W.M., Zhou, X. and McDonald, C.J. (1997) A randomized trial of 'corollary orders' to prevent errors of omission. *Journal of the American Medical Informatics Association*, **4**(5), 364–375.

Patterson, E.S., Cook, R.I. and Render, M.L. (2002) Improving patient safety by identifying side effects from introducing bar coding in medication administration. *Journal of the American Medical Informatics Association.*, **9**(5), 540–553.

Riga, C.V., Bicknell, C.D., Wallace, D. *et al.* (2009) Robot-assisted antegrade *in-situ* fenestrated stent grafting. *Cardiovascular and Interventional Radiology*, **32**(3), 522–524.

Schachter, D.L. (1999) The seven sins of memory. Insights from psychology and cognitive science. *American Psychologist*, **54**, 182–203.

Schnipper, J.L., Hamann, C., Ndumele, C.D. *et al.* (2009) Effect of an electronic medication reconciliation application and process redesign on potential adverse drug events: a cluster-randomized trial. *Archives of Internal Medicine*, **169**(8), 771–780.

van Rosse, F., Maat, B., Rademaker, C.M.A. *et al.* (2009) The effect of computerized physician order entry on medication prescription errors and clinical outcome in paediatric and intensive care: a systematic review. *Paediatrics*, **123**(4), 1184–1190.

Volpp, K.G.M. and Grande, D. (2003) Residents' suggestions for reducing errors in teaching hospitals. *The New England Journal of Medicine*, **348**(9), 851.

Wears, R.L. and Berg, M. (2005) Computer technology and clinical work: still waiting for Godot. *JAMA: The Journal of the American Medical Association*, **293**(10), 1261–1263.

People Create Safety

CHAPTER 14
Creating a culture of safety

The term culture is used in many different ways in discussions of safety in healthcare and many different claims are made for its importance. Consider these two apparently contradictory reflections on safety culture:

Join us in converting a culture of blame that hides information about risk and error into a culture of safety that flushes information out and enables us to prevent or quickly recover from mistakes before they become patient injuries.
LEAPE *ET AL.* (1998)

A somewhat lethal cocktail of impatience, scientific ignorance and naive optimism may have dangerously inflated our expectations of safety culture.
(COX AND FLIN, 1998)

Both these statements are true but they point to different roles that culture can play in the struggle for safer healthcare. When Lucian Leape and others talk about changing the culture, they reflect a deeply held belief and commitment to a fundamental change in the way error and safety are approached and an equally deeply felt conviction that until the culture changes, nothing else will. However, there is in fact comparatively little hard evidence that changing the safety culture has any direct impact on safety. As Cox and Flin (1998) point out, a naïve belief in the concept has far out-stripped the evidence for its utility. We will see that these two viewpoints can be reconciled once we distinguish culture as a necessary foundation for change from culture as a force for change in its own right. But first we must examine the concept a little more closely.

The many facets of safety culture in healthcare

Anyone who begins to examine the safety literature comes across a bewildering array of descriptors applied to the word culture, each of which is supposed to illuminate some essential facet of the all important safety culture. No blame culture, open and fair culture, flexible, learning, reporting, generative, resilient, mindful . . . the list goes on and on. In part, this reflects that safety culture is not fully understood and that people have not rallied around a single definition

---

Patient Safety, 2nd edition. By Charles Vincent. Published 2010 by Blackwell Publishing Ltd.

or set of concepts. However, it also reflects the fact that there are a number of important facets to a culture of safety, as can be seen in the various examples of absent or inadequate safety culture (Box 14.1).

BOX 14.1 Safety culture in healthcare

'There is too often a blame culture. When things go wrong, the response is to seek one or two individuals to blame, who may then be subject to disciplinary measures or professional censure. That is not to say that in some circumstances individuals should not be held to account, but as the predominant approach this acts as a significant deterrent to the reporting of adverse events and near misses' (Department of Health, 2000, p. 77).

Increasingly patients and physicians in the United States live and interact in a culture characterized by anger, blame, guilt, fear, frustration and distrust. The public has responded by escalating the punishment for error. Clinicians and some healthcare organizations generally have responded by suppression, stonewalling and cover-up. That approach has been less than successful (Leape *et al.*, 1998: p. 1446).

Absence of safety culture. A young boy died after failing to recover from a general anaesthetic administered at a dental practice. A fatal accident enquiry concluded that the boy's death could have been prevented if a number of reasonable precautions had been in place. There was no agreement with a local hospital for rapid transfer of patients in emergencies, no heart monitor was attached when the anaesthetic was given, the anaesthetist lacked a specialist qualification and all staff lacked training in medical emergencies (Department of Health, 2000; p. 36).

A culture developed within the hospital that allowed 'unprofessional, counter therapeutic and degrading – even cruel – practices to take place. These practices went unchecked and were even condoned or excused when brought to the attention of the hospital. Some staff interviewed did not even recognize the abuse, which had taken place, as unacceptable practice. (Report of UK Commission for Health Improvement following an investigation into physical and psychological abuse of elderly patients 2000.)

The examples of poor culture first show the importance attached to culture by experienced clinicians and safety experts. They also illuminate, to some extent, the different facets of culture and the different senses in which the word is used. The first two quotes are primarily concerned with the reaction to errors after they have occurred and the authors are rightly critical of unthinking, heavy handed reactions both inside healthcare organizations and in the wider society; we are therefore concerned with the culture of both healthcare organizations and wider social mores. Another theme apparent here is that excessive blame prevents recognition of error and impedes learning and effective action to improve safety. The principal theme of the third example on the other hand, while also concerned with error, concerns anticipation rather than response. Here safety culture implies that the people concerned should maintain good standards of practice but also be alert to the possibility of error and take steps to reduce or eliminate that possibility. The final example reveals another facet of safety culture, or rather its absence. In a deeply pathological culture, the difficulty is not so much blame, as that problems are denied or not even acknowledged. As is sometimes said, the hardest problems to resolve are those where no one recognizes anything is wrong. Here the abuse referred to seems to have become normal, and therefore unnoticed by the staff concerned. Gradually, little by little, in a group isolated from mainstream clinical practice, behaviour that is unthinkable to begin with can become first tolerated, then routine and finally invisible.

All these examples supposedly concern the culture of safety; it seems to be a pretty broad, ill-defined and all encompassing concept. Does this matter? Well, yes it does. If our challenge is to change the culture, as so many commentators urge, then we need to understand what safety culture is, or at the very least decide what aspects to highlight, and bring as much precision to the definition as can be mustered. First though, we need to see how the concept emerged.

Organizational culture

The word culture has several different, but related meanings. We are accustomed to thinking of culture in terms of the literary and artistic heritage of a people or the prevailing values and ethos of a particular nation. In medicine, culture has another meaning, as an environment in which bacteria or other organisms reproduce. This latter meaning could be seen as a metaphor for safety culture – provide the right culture and the required attitudes and behaviours will flourish. In a business environment, the structural school of thought argue that authority, clear hierarchy and rules are the primary determinants of good functioning organizations; the cultural perspective on the other hand considers attitudes, values and norms to be fundamental (Huczynski and Buchanan, 1991). In the safety context, the contrast would be between relying on rules and regulations to produce safety and trying to engender a culture of safety.

While organizational culture has been studied for decades, it came to prominence as an explanatory concept during the 1980s. Rather than look at the particular structures and management practices, management gurus such as Peters and Waterman (1982) emphasized the cultural attributes and the clear guiding values of high performance organizations. Given that quite a few of these companies have now gone to the wall, it may be that the importance of culture was overstated, but nevertheless the concept of culture as a determinant of organizational performance remained. The person who most clearly articulated the idea of organizational culture was Edgar Schein in a book called

'Organisational Culture and Leadership' (Schein, 1985). The link with leadership will be discussed further below, but what interests us now is the clarity of Schein's conceptualization of culture. Weick and Sutcliffe (2001) summarize this as:

Schein says that culture is defined by six formal properties: (1) shared basic assumptions that are (2) invented, discovered or developed by a given group as it (3) learns to cope with its problem of external adaptation and internal integration in ways that (4) have worked well enough to be considered valid and therefore (5) can be taught to new members of the group as the (6) correct way to perceive, think and feel in relation to those problems. When we talk about culture therefore, we are talking about assumptions that preserve lessons learned; values derived from those assumptions that prescribe how the organisation should act; and visible markers and activities that embody and give substance to the espoused values.
(WEICK AND SUTCLIFFE, 2001)

So, in a healthcare setting, one basic assumption for all clinicians is that colleagues will always respond to a true emergency call; the priority of patient care in such situations is a core value, overriding all others. Locally however, culture takes specific forms. Consider the experience of moving to a new hospital or a new ward to work. Very quickly one senses the differences in, for instance, how formal people are, how easy it is to speak up in meetings and whether it is possible to challenge or question senior staff; all these reflect the culture of that particular organization or group. In primary care, different practices organize themselves in different ways, with differing levels of availability to patients, differing degrees of shared responsibility and mutual support and so on. In short culture is, as has often been said, 'the way we do things round here'.

Organizational culture and group culture

Culture, as noted above, is how we do things round here. Notice however, that 'here' can be a small group, part of an organization, a group of professionals or an entire, huge organization like the British National Health Service, the largest employer in Europe. (The Chinese army is apparently larger worldwide, though I do not have definitive figures.) Ideally, members of an organization share the same values and commitment, whether in a university, a business or a nuclear power plant. Safety, one would hope, would be a value on which everyone could agree and attitudes and values cohere. However, the safety culture within an organization may vary markedly in different areas and in different groups. For instance, in a survey of employees in the nuclear industry, Harvey *et al.* (2002) found that managers had largely positive views of their own commitment to safety and saw themselves as taking responsibility for safety issues. Shop floor workers, on the other hand, generally had more negative views about management commitment to safety and management's ability to listen and respond to safety concerns. The divergence in views of managers and shop floor workers may possibly sound familiar to anyone who works in healthcare.

Healthcare is particularly complex because of the large number of professional groups, each with their own culture and ways of doing things. Nursing, for instance, tends to have a much stricter disciplinary code and harsher attitude to errors, than medicine. Substantive nursing errors are often followed by formal warnings or sanctions, to a much greater extent than other professional groups. National culture may also be influential, as Bob Helmreich's work has elegantly shown in the context of aviation (Helmreich and Merrit, 1998). Efforts to train cockpit teams in more open styles of communication for instance, have had to contend with widely varying cultural attitudes to seniority and hierarchy. Some cultures, particularly Asian nations, have a much greater 'power gradient' than most European countries; there is greater deference to authority, and unwillingness to challenge senior figures; in this case, cockpit attitudes reflect wider social mores. As we begin to explore the attitudes and experiences of patient safety in different countries, these differences are likely to emerge in healthcare.

Safety culture

Safety culture is one aspect of the wider culture of the organization. In this section, we will define safety culture and consider some of the most important aspects, those relating to openness, blame, reporting and learning.

The UK Health and Safety Commission (1993) quotes the following definition in many of its documents, which was originally provided by the Advisory Committee on the Safety of Nuclear Installations. It succinctly captures the essential features:

The safety culture of an organisation is the product of the individual and group values, attitudes, competencies and patterns of behaviour that determine the commitment to, and the style and proficiency of, an organisation's health and safety programmes. Organisations with a positive safety culture are characterised by communications founded on mutual trust, by shared perceptions of the importance of safety, and by confidence in the efficacy of preventative measures.
(VINCENT, 2006)

A safety culture is therefore founded on the individual attitudes and values of everyone in the organization. A strong organizational and management commitment is also implied; safety needs to be taken seriously at every level of the organization. The Chief Executive needs to provide clear and committed leadership, communicated throughout the organization, that gives the safety of patients and staff a priority. The cleaner on the wards must be conscious of infection risks, nurses are alert for potential equipment problems and drug hazards and managers are monitoring incident reports. Finally, as the ACSNI committee indicates, producing and maintaining a *safety culture* is a long-term, systematic and continuing process. There is never a time when the job of enhancing and maintaining a safety culture is finished. Safety, like trust, is a highly perishable commodity with, as Richard Cook likes to say, the half life of adrenaline.

An open and fair culture

The tendency for excessive, immediate and unreasoning blame in the face of patient harm, both from within and outside healthcare organizations, has led some to call for a 'no-blame' culture. This, if taken literally, would appear to remove personal accountability and also remove many social, disciplinary and legal strictures on clinical practice. A culture without blame would therefore seem to be both unworkable and to remove some of the restrictions and safeguards on safe behaviour. A much better objective is to try to develop an open and fair culture, which preserves personal responsibility and account-ability but requires a much more thoughtful and supportive response to error and harm when they do occur.

The tendency to blame people for errors that have severe outcomes, satisfying as it may be in the short term, is often unwarranted and certainly not in the long-term interests of patient safety. Yet it takes a very cool headed and thoughtful clinical leader or chief executive to take a systems view when faced with some awful incident, particularly when they may be under consid-erable pressure from relatives, the media, even government. Regulatory and professional bodies also face these pressures and equally have to decide whether a clinician's behaviour is deserving of censure and disciplinary action. It's no good simply appealing to systems thinking and a just culture; a call has to be made one way or the other and some action taken.

Assessing culpability: the incident decision tree

In order to give form and structure to these decisions about culpability, Boeing developed a decision aid for maintenance error, in which the psychological principles involved in the occurrence of such error were given flesh in the form of a step-by-step decision aid examining the nature of the error, the influence of context and contributing factors, health and pressures and so forth. James Reason (1997) outlined a more general 'culpability matrix', which in turn was adapted by the UK National Patient Safety Agency to produce their 'Incident Decision Tree'.

The structure of the NPSAs Incident Decision Tree is shown in Figure 14.1. Essentially, after the incident has been investigated and some thought given to its causes, a series of questions is asked. Were the actions intentional? If, yes, was there an intention to cause harm or not? Is there any evidence of a medical condition? Was there a departure from agreed protocols and so on. Suppose, for instance, a staff nurse gives a dose of diamorphine to an elderly patient in severe pain without waiting for a prescription to be written. Is this justified? Poten-tially, if there is no other option. Suppose, however, she has made no attempt to contact the relevant doctor. In this case her actions were clearly intentional,

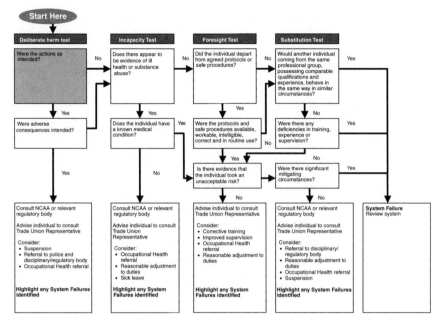

Figure 14.1 Incident Decision Tree adapted from UK National Patient Safety Agency.

the violation of protocols deliberate and without justification. In other cases, protocols and procedures may still have been ignored, but in circumstances that mitigate the error. The NPSA gives examples of a midwife who failed to notice discrepancies in a foetal heart reading through having been on duty 15 hours without a break to cover absent colleagues. Finally, there are areas of particular difficulty when the 'correct' action is not clear cut, when a judgement must be made as to whether the risks outweigh the benefits. The decision aid commendably makes this an explicit issue:

A surgical patient is receiving opiate analgesia via a syringe pump. A senior nurse, who has just come on duty, realises the pump has been set up to run much too fast and the patient's breathing is slow and shallow. The charge nurse urgently summons medical staff assistance but there is no response. The patient stops breathing. The nurse decides there is no option but to deliver a naloxone injection himself to try and save the patient's life. In doing so, he knowingly breached trust protocols (which were generally clear, workable and in routine use) and his own profession's standards of accountability. However, the nurse was faced with a life or death situation and the risk to the patient of waiting for medical help was much greater than the nurse taking on what was properly a medical decision.

(WWW.NPSA.NHS.UK)

Using the incident decision tree requires an initial analysis of the case and some reflection on the web of causes and contributory factors and the intentions and circumstances of the people involved. Deciding whether someone should be supported, praised or disciplined is never easy, but the formal decision process should make the eventual judgement more explicit, fairer to the staff involved and more in the interests of future patients in that healthcare organization.

A culture of learning

One my favourite aphorisms is that practice, in many different areas, is just 'one mistake after another'. This is partly a rueful acceptance of the humiliating and frustrating nature of the acquisition of any skill; learning the piano, for example, is inevitably an experience of fumbled notes, incomprehension and strident discords each time one advances to a more difficult piece. More importantly though, this phrase brings out the idea that people, and indeed organizations, learn through noticing and reflecting on errors. The Total Quality Management gurus go as far as to say that every error is a treasure, which may be a step too far for some, but certainly errors can be highly informative. Organizations can advance and evolve by the recognition of error or, conversely, decay and become unsafe by suppressing information about error and safety and adopting an ostrich-like 'head in the sand' approach to the landscape of error and hazard.

The nature and mechanisms of reporting systems were discussed in Chapter 4, and some of the reasons why people do and do not report. Returning to this theme again we are more concerned, in the cultural context, with the attitudes and values that underlie a willingness to report and, more importantly, to reflect and learn. This means not just acknowledging error, but sometimes even celebrating its successful resolution. There is a famous story about Werner von Braun, the rocket scientist (and inspiration for Dr Strangelove) presenting a bottle of champagne to a NASA engineer who had brought a major problem to his attention. Don Berwick provides a more recent example showing that this tradition continues (Box 14.2).

BOX 14.2

The Titan rocket was powered by liquid oxygen and hydrogen. The design of the rocket required great precision in the use of fuel – every drop had to be consumed before engine shutdown, completely emptying the tanks. To ensure the liquid emptied completely, four small metal baffles were placed at the bottom of the tank to stop the liquid swirling round the exit from the tank. Unfortunately, the fitted baffles were a little too big and an expensive, but necessary fix was organized. The tanks were drained and a man lowered on a harness in a diving suit to trim the baffles. Four bolts and metal fragments had to be removed and collected; if metal was left in the tank, it would be sucked into the high-pressure pump and the rocket would explode.

The problem arose when the engineer who did the trimming, Jerry Gonsalves, returned, emptied the cloth sack to find only three bolts. They returned, looked carefully for the missing bolt, could not find it and concluded that there must only have been three. That night, Gonsalves could not sleep for thinking about the missing bolt. He returned to the tank, looked down to see if there were any places the bolt could be hidden. He found two, and called the Director of Safety, Guy Cohen. The next morning they all assembled again, emptied the tank at huge expense, and lowered another engineer to check. He went to the first of the two hiding places Gonsalves had identified, and found the bolt.

Guy Cohen asked me a question at this stage in the story. 'Suppose it had been a nurse,' he asked, 'and we were talking about a serious drug error. What would happen in one of your hospitals?' I knew the answer very well. 'An incident report,' I said. 'And the nurse would probably have had some sort of warning put in her file. If the patient had died, she would probably be fired or worse.'

'Then you'll never be safe,' he said. 'That's not what we did. We saved that bolt and had it gold plated and mounted on a plaque. And we had the NASA administrator come to the launch of that rocket a couple of days later. And in full view of everyone there, we gave the plaque to Jerry Gonsalves, and we dedicated the launch to him.'

(ADAPTED FROM BERWICK, 1998)

The key phrase for me in the story of the Titan rocket, the fulcrum on which it turns, is 'then you'll never be safe'. The attitude and understanding expressed here is that punishing people for honest error is not simply unfair and pointless; it is in fact, dangerous. Why is it dangerous? Because the effect of mindless sanctions is to suppress the very information you need to create and maintain a state of safety. The matrix of reward and punishment is handled entirely differently in the case of the nurse and the engineer; the nurse is punished for the error, but the engineer is rewarded for his 'safety behaviour', in this case his continuing anxiety and honesty in the face of having made an error. The response of Cohen, and indeed the wider organization, was not to castigate him for the error, but to act on the safety information and check the rocket once again. In considering Don Berwick's story, we can see that the people involved are expressing something more than an operational policy of collecting error information. The organization is guided by a core principle that safety information must be valued, analysed, understood and communicated; this is the culture of understanding and learning.

Flexibility and resilience: the culture of high reliability

Throughout this book we have used case studies of clinical scenarios to achieve a better understanding of the nature of error and safety. Case studies have also been used to bring a better understanding of the culture and practices of organizations, including those which, in the face of extraordinary levels of hazards, manage to achieve high levels of both safety and performance. These 'high reliability organizations' (HROs), which include nuclear power plants, aircraft carriers and air traffic control, have been rigorously examined by a mixture of observations, interviews, questionnaires and archival analysis (Roberts, 1990; La Porte, 1996). Many authors believe that the culture and practices of these organizations can inform the changing business and health-care environments (Waller and Roberts, 2003).

To begin with, we can get a flavour of life in an HRO from a US Navy veteran's description of life on board a carrier, quoted by Karl Weick and Kathy Sutcliffe:

Imagine that it's a busy day, and you shrink San Francisco airport to only one short runway and one ramp and one gate. Make planes take off and land at the same time, at half the present time interval, rock the runway from side to side, and require that everyone who leaves in the morning returns the same day. Make sure the equipment is so close to the envelope that it's fragile. Then turn off the radar to avoid detection, impose strict controls on the radios, fuel the aircraft in place with their engines running, put an enemy in the air and scatter live bombs and rockets around. Now, wet the whole thing down with sea water and oil and man it with twenty year olds, half of whom have never seen an airplane close up. Oh, and by the way, try not to kill anyone.
(WEICK AND SUTCLIFFE, 2001)

Weick and Sutcliffe go on to ask, in the context of addressing business leaders, 'Can you think of another environment that is quite this full of the un-expected?' Well, yes, in healthcare maybe we can. Here is my paraphrase description of a central London Accident and Emergency department:

Imagine that it's always a busy day and you shrink the entire hospital to one department and one entrance. Patients come and go every minute or two, wanting to be seen immediately. Any kind of illness may present, in a person of any age, physical and mental conditions; many patients do not speak the language of the doctors and nurses. Some are drug addicts, often HIV positive, posing real dangers to staff. Then impose severe constraints on the time available for diagnosis and investigation, the availability of back-up staff and beds, fill the area with dangerous drugs, add the threat of violence from a good proportion of the patients attending and the frequent presence of the police. Now, add a few cases of major trauma, staff the place with twenty-five year olds who are completely new to this kind of environment and make sure the experienced staff are tied up with administration. Oh, and by the way, try not to kill anyone.

The similarities between HROs and some aspects of healthcare are at least superficially persuasive. Previous attempts to import lessons on quality and safety from manufacturing have sometimes been resisted because the routine, production line processes seem to have little in common with the dynamic, hands on, highly variable and adaptive nature of much work in healthcare. HROs seem to offer a better model because their procedures and practices have evolved specifically to deal with the dynamic, the variable and the unexpected. We should, however, inject a note of caution here. Much of healthcare is routine and largely predictable. Some aspects, such as pharmacy distribution or the supply of blood products, are much more like manufacturing processes than HROs. It is perhaps worth remarking that there is a certain appeal in comparing one's own work to that of fighter pilots and those who operate nuclear carriers, but this can be overplayed; much harder to think that healthcare might have something to learn from the communication and information systems at the local coffee shop franchise. (Though not always. Pat Croskerry, an emergency physician in Canada, laments that the information technology used to support his morning coffee purchase is far superior to the imperfect systems he uses to keep his patients alive).

The lessons of high reliability organizations (HRO)

Many of the HROs studied are military or at least have many military personnel and built very solidly on strict training, discipline and adherence to procedures, protocols and routine (Reason, 1997). The qualities that are identified as particularly characteristic of HROs only come into play at certain times. Clinicians, in contrast, might be faulted for being unwilling to adhere to basic routines, introducing variability into practice when it is neither necessary nor desirable. While there is certainly hierarchy and discipline, sanctions and rewards, there are also shared values and attitudes which cannot be wholly engendered by rules and regulations. Weick and Sutcliffe (2001) argue that, as surveillance at all times by managers and senior staff is obviously impossible, shared understanding has to be mediated by culture, in essence by an acceptance of common ways of working and shared assumptions and values. Weick and Sutcliffe make the crucial point that the shared understanding and common view allows a flexible approach when it is required; in HROs, the very acceptance and adherence to standardization and procedures is what permits a decentralized approach when necessary. Flexibility can be tolerated and utilized because when the need for it is over the organization can return to routine operation without being threatened by the temporary relaxation of hierarchy and procedure. The routine, discipline and standardization inherent in the HROs are not usually emphasized in healthcare, where people prefer the excitement of learning about dealing with crisis.

The aspect of HROs that has received most attention is their response to the unexpected, to crisis and change. Weick and Sutcliffe identify five hallmarks of high reliability in organizations (Table 14.1). The relevance of each of these characteristics to healthcare could be examined in detail, and we can only pick out some key features. By preoccupation with failure, Weick and Sutcliffe point to what James Reason refers to as chronic unease, ceaselessly watching for unexpected or disconfirming information. On a personal level, a clinician may become suspicious about a sudden rise in the patient's temperature; at an organizational level the risk manager may react to a flurry of reports about equipment from the Intensive Therapy Unit. Reluctance to simplify is being

Table 14.1 Five processes for collective mindfulness in organizations

Mindfulness is '… the combination of ongoing scrutiny of existing expectations, continuous refinement and differentiation of expectations based on newer experience, willingness and capability to invent new expectations that make sense of unprecedented events, a more nuanced appreciation of context and ways to deal with it, and identification of new dimensions of context that improve foresight and current functioning.' Weick and Sutcliffe, 2001: p. 42	
Preoccupation with failure	• Operational errors, no matter how small, are reported and analysed promptly. • Reporting of errors is encouraged through an open and fair culture. • An open team-working climate exists in which individuals can actively monitor and question others actions and interpretations.
Reluctance to simplify	• HROs make few assumptions regarding the current state of the system and encourage people to actively seek. • A rich and varied picture of warning signs and potential consequences is built. • Selection practices that promote diversity, frequent job-rotation and re-training.
Sensitivity to operations	• Staff actively seek information about the state of the system and future status. • Real-time, up-to-date information is made available on how critical actions are progressing. • Frequent operations meetings and situational assessments permit early identification of problems.
Commitment to resilience	• Staff have the ability to detect and contain errors through anticipation, intelligent monitoring, reaction and recovery. • HROs recognize the limitations of formalized procedures in certain conditions. • Training through simulated scenarios allow staff to practice recovery.
Deference to expertise	• In high-demand situations, control and decision authority can be transferred to front line staff. • Comprehensive training ensures that front line staff operators are capable of assuming responsibility for operational control. • Staff are prepared to act autonomously to interrupt operations if they determine a safety risk.

Adapted from Weick and Sutcliffe, 2001

willing, at an organizational level, not to accept the most obvious interpretation at face value. In an analysis of the failures at the Bristol Royal Infirmary, Weick and Sutcliffe (2003) identified a mindset in which poor results in cardiac surgery were explained away by reference to patient characteristics, rather than trying to see the more challenging and complex reality of a catastrophic breakdown in organizational and clinical processes. The commitment to resilience is seen in the attention given to small errors and problems, in the knowledge that if not corrected they can lead to larger problems and an organization-wide attempt to deal with problems as they arise. It also encompasses an ability to anticipate and recover from error and crisis at both an individual and organizational level.

Deference to expertise is a most important concept and one with immediate and clear relevance to healthcare. Weick and Sutcliffe explain that, for various reasons, rigid hierarchies have their own special vulnerability to errors. If only senior staff are mandated to act, and those lower down have to wait for orders, this can be fatal in a fast changing, hazardous situation. Junior doctors, for instance, are expected to act as best they can in an emergency if no senior help is available. Deference to expertise however is more subtle, allowing junior staff to take the lead even when senior staff are present. In hazardous, crisis situations, senior commanders will defer to those with knowledge of the immediate environment, often, in the military, non-commissioned officers or enlisted men. At these times open communication and negotiation of differences of view, as opposed to a blind following of orders, become critical (La Porte and Consolini, 1991).

This is a crucial issue in healthcare, when hierarchies within professions tend to be rigid and relationships between professions and specialties complicated by issues of power and status. Deference to expertise is a concept that, ideally, cuts across hierarchy to point to action in the patient's best interests. Will the senior physician visiting the ward on his rounds rely on their own necessarily brief assessment of the patient or listen to the views of the young nurse who has watched their deterioration through the night? Will a young doctor take advice from a senior nurse with 20 years more experience than he has? Will the psychiatrist be persuaded by her team that this patient is more dangerous than she had previously thought? Many of these negotiations and conversations happen successfully in medicine, being managed thoughtfully and without fuss by people who know and respect each other. What the HROs tell us is that we perhaps need to go further, that deference to expertise needs to be discussed, the circumstances in which it is necessary outlined, and a greater respect for informal communication inculcated.

Reflections on high reliability research

We have only scratched the surface of the nature of HROs and their relevance to healthcare. This is a complex issue and, while these organizations display some fundamentally important characteristics, an uncritical adoption of high reliability practices into healthcare could be a mistake in some settings. While the original descriptive studies of HROs are inspiring pieces of research, it is difficult to identify clear lessons for other contexts such as healthcare, in that the parallels with other types of activities are not always clear, the lessons and observations are varied and the findings of detailed ethnographic field studies not easily generalizable.

Almost 20 years on from the publication of the original HRO studies, there are potentially a number of inherent limitations in the way the literature has developed (Vincent, Benn and Hanna, 2010). First, the original studies drew attention to a very wide range of characteristics said to be important to reliable performance and different authors stressed different aspects; it is not clear which characteristics are really fundamental. Second, subsequent authors, however insightful, have compounded these problems by selectively addressing whichever aspects they considered most important and in addition have offered new interpretations and terminology. The range of alleged high reliability concepts is now enormous. Third, very few empirical studies have been carried out since those of the original Berkeley group; theoretical abstractions abound, with little empirical development to drive the emergence of a consensual model of high reliability factors. Fourth, the field has remained resolutely descriptive with little attempt to operationalize or measure HRO characteristics, though there are some exceptions to this tendency. Fifth, although the original studies were carefully and thoughtfully conducted, they are largely descriptive in nature and there is little hard evidence that these characteristics are associated with safety or, in healthcare, with excellent clinical outcomes. Sixth, the conceptual diversity and lack of empirical foundation mean that this potentially important literature offers very little in the way of a practical guide for enhancing safety. Put simply, reading the HRO literature offers a great deal of inspiration, but little idea of what to do in practice to enhance safety.

Later in this book we will discuss the need for organizations to be prepared before embarking on a programme of safety and quality improvement: leadership, financial stability, basic structures and process and awareness of the need for action all have to be in place. Rene Amalberti (2001) has pointed out, in the context of aviation, that the kind of safety measures needed in an organization relate to the degree of safety it has already achieved. Remember the extent of the proceduralization that underlies the flexibility of HROs; they can be flexible because they can also return to hierarchy and procedure. Trying to graft high reliability characteristics into a healthcare organization too early in its safety evolution, when it really needs better standards and procedures, could be destabilizing rather than safety enhancing. The wider cultural aspects of HROs have their counterpoint in individual behaviour, and we shall address both the need to follow rules and the need to depart from them in a later chapter.

Measuring safety culture

Safety culture, as can be seen from our overview, has multiple facets and, less agreeably, seems to have multiple meanings. Sharpening the concept and assessing its validity requires first measuring it and second seeing if safety culture does indeed relate to other indices of safety, such as rates of error or incidents. In industrial settings, some progress has been made on both these objectives, although there is still no solid consensus on the key characteristics of safety culture.

We must first note that outside healthcare the term 'safety climate' is generally used when discussing measures of the underlying safety culture. The reasons for this are complex, and relate to debates in organizational theory, but the basic idea is that safety climate is the surface manifestation of safety culture. A survey, whether by questionnaire or interview, can only tell you about the safety culture at that particular moment. As Cox and Flin (1998) express it, safety climate is a snapshot of the state of safety, providing an indicator of the underlying safety culture of a work group, plant or organization. In healthcare people generally talk about measuring the safety culture, but the term safety climate is also used.

Flin *et al.* (2006) reviewed 18 different measures of safety climate in various industrial settings. Common features identified concerned management attitudes to safety, the presence of safety systems and policies, perceptions of risk and sometimes information on work pressures and competence: a fairly mixed bag of concepts variously subsumed under the general term 'safety climate'. Some of these instruments had been validated, in that measures of safety climate had been related to accident rates. This group went on to examine 12 different instruments in use in healthcare, most of which did not meet basic psychometric standards for questionnaire design. A huge range of issues were covered, which varied between the different measures. They identified Nieva and Sorra's 'Hospital Survey on Patient Safety' (Box 14.3) as one of the best developed questionnaires, although this has not been used as widely as some other instruments. Some of these studies showed that ratings of culture were associated with clinicians' reports of safe behaviours, but only two tried to relate safety culture to actual incidents, and only one of these concerned injuries to patients. For all the enthusiasm for safety culture there is, as yet, little hard evidence that a positive safety culture is indeed associated with reduced harm to patients.

BOX 14.3 Hospital survey on patient safety

42 items, covering the following issues:
- Supervisor/manager expectations and actions promoting patient safety
- Organizational learning and continuous improvement
- Teamwork within units
- Communication and openness
- Feedback and communication about error
- Non-punitive response to error
- Staffing levels
- Hospital management support for patient safety
- Teamwork across hospital units
- Hospitals handoffs and transitions.

(REPRODUCED FROM *QUALITY & SAFETY IN HEALTH CARE*, V F NIEVA, J SORRA. "SAFETY CULTURE ASSESSMENT: A TOOL FOR IMPROVING PATIENT SAFETY IN HEALTHCARE ORGANIZATIONS". **12**, NO. SUPPL 2, [17–23], 2003, WITH PERMISSION FROM BMJ PUBLISHING GROUP LTD.)

Safety culture surveys have also been used simply to push forward the safety agenda and engage clinicians and leaders. Peter Pronovost and colleagues at John Hopkins used short surveys of safety culture and strategies for leadership as a baseline for their attempts to improve patient safety (Pronovost *et al.*, 2003). Senior managers perceived safety to be better developed than members of the patient safety committee, and front line staff perceived that their immediate supervisors were more concerned with safety than were senior managers. Singer *et al.* (2003, 2009) have also found that healthcare management have much more positive attitudes and experiences than front line clinical staff. They suggest this could be because front line staff and middle managers tend to gloss over safety problems when briefing senior staff, which would make it very difficult for senior executives to understand the true state of their organizations and the extent of action needed on safety. Alternatively, the results could imply that senior executives have a genuine commitment to safety which is not being communicated to front line staff. These surveys highlighted that senior leaders needed to become more visible to front line staff in their efforts to improve safety, that there was a need for much more proactive strategic planning and also a need to educate clinicians about patient safety. This prompted the development of such a strategy and a hospital wide programme of action on patient safety.

Can we change the culture?

Mark Twain famously remarked, on the subject of the weather in England, that everyone complains about it, but no one does anything about it. Is culture like the weather, something we have to tolerate and adapt to, or can culture be developed and changed over time? Organizational theorists of different persuasions have different views on this question. Some, of a more anthropological orientation, see culture as a product of personal values and attitudes, deeply rooted in the history of a nation or an organization. Others, with a more business orientation, see culture as something that can be encouraged, developed and perhaps even manipulated. Changing national culture or the social mores of a society is a dangerous business and, arguably, an intrusion on personal freedom and values. Attitudes to safety and risky behaviour however, can and do change, often for the better. Think, for instance, of attitudes to driving while drunk or wearing of seat belts in cars, which have changed hugely, albeit slowly, in the last 20 years. With safety, we are hoping to change specific work related attitudes and values rather than deeply held personal beliefs.

Rules, regulations, sanctions and rewards certainly play a part in defining a safety culture. If you are rewarded for reporting a safety issue, you are more likely to do it again next time than if you were disciplined. Above all though, culture is socially mediated, a product of the relationships between people in the organization, particularly those who are influential in virtue of the position they hold or the respect they receive (ideally both). Weick and Sutcliffe (2001),

in discussing how leaders can encourage a mindful approach to high performance, explain the emergence of a high reliability culture as:

*What you need to do is to modify what people expect from each other . . . This modification
is not just a change in how people think, as important as that is, but a change in how
people feel. You need people to absorb the lessons of mindfulness at an emotional level so
that they will express approval when others hold certain beliefs and act in certain ways.
For example, people need to feel strongly that it's good to speak up when they make a
mistake, good to spot flawed assumptions, good to focus on a persistent operational
anomaly. They need to expect praise for these acts when they do them, and they need to
offer praise when they spot someone else doing them. Likewise you need to attach
disapproval to people believing and acting in ways that undermine mindfulness. For
example, people need to agree among themselves and feel strongly that it's bad to refrain
from asking for help, bad to let success go to their heads, bad to ignore lower-ranking
experts. They need to express key values by making clear what is disapproved as much as
by praising what is approved. When people make these kinds of changes, a new culture
begins to emerge. The culture takes the form of a new set of expectations and a new
urgency that people will live up to them.*
(WEICK AND SUTCLIFFE, 2001)

Culture therefore is maintained and manifests in social processes and interactions. Everyone in an organization contributes, consciously or not, to its
culture. What emerges may be positive and safety conscious or, over time, drift
to a relentless negativity in which all manner of dangerous behaviour is
tolerated or even encouraged. Maintaining a safety culture, indeed any kind
of culture, requires leadership and ongoing work and commitment from
everyone concerned.

And if we can change the culture, will patients be any safer?

A positive safety culture seems like a good idea. Surely to have a safety aware
workforce, imbued with safety attitudes, open about error and so forth must be
helpful? But is there any evidence that changing the culture is likely to improve
the quality of healthcare or the safety of patients? A few years ago the answer
to this was simply no, or at best only indirect evidence. Now however, a cadre of
brave researchers undaunted by conceptual and methodological minefields
have begun to address this issue. But it is difficult and there are no simple
answers.

Before examining some of the relevant research, we need to reflect on some
of the difficulties. First, you will recall that culture is 'how we do things round
here'. Well, what do we mean by 'here'? This could be a small team, a unit, or an
entire hospital. We can examine culture on all these different levels and relate
to clinical processes and outcomes at each of these different levels. We might,
for instance, find that culture at unit level relates to patient outcomes, but the

culture of different hospitals bears little relation to their overall performance. Second, there is a host of possible clinical processes and outcomes that might be affected by culture, that is, by the attitudes and behaviour of staff. Reporting rates for instance, might be strongly related to culture, whereas infection rates might not. Third, even if there is a relationship, could we find it? Just think, from the case analyses earlier in the book, how many factors seem to interact when a patient is harmed. Clinical outcomes are determined by a multitude of factors, of which culture is only one, and fairly intangible at that. Finally, even if we find a relationship, it is not clear that changing culture produces a change in clinical outcomes; it is also possible that working in a unit with good outcomes produces a positive culture. So, if the research and the conclusions seem a little tentative, bear in mind the difficulty and complexity of the enterprise (Gaba, Singer and Rosen, 2007; Clarke, 2006).

The relationship between safety culture, or more accurately, safety climate, as expressing a measure of culture at a particular time, has been studied extensively outside healthcare. Researchers have found a link between safety climate and lower accident or injury rates in chemical and nuclear processing, the military, construction and manufacturing and service industries. The nature of this relationship has been examined in a review and meta-analysis of 32 studies by Sharon Clarke (2006), of which only two were hospital based. She confirmed the link between safety climate and accident involvement, which was reassuringly stronger for predictive studies which measured climate and then tracked accidents in the following months. Safety compliance in the sense of adhering to rules and regulations, and following safety procedures conscientiously, predicted lower accident rates. However, safety participation, which assessed proactive initiative, positive efforts to improve safety and help colleagues promote safety, was a more powerful predictor. This suggests, tentatively, that complying with rules gives a good foundation for safety but active participation and engagement are critical to a good safety record.

Turning to healthcare, there is preliminary evidence that safety climate aggregated at an institutional level is related to some measures of safety. Singer *et al.* (2003) sent surveys to 92 hospitals as part of the American Hospitals Association 2004 annual survey; surveys went to 100 senior managers, 100 doctors and a 10% sample of other employees. Response rate was 52% but, as usual, a lower response for doctors. Findings from this survey were examined for their association with 20 patient safety indicators, derived from standard discharge summaries covering potentially preventable inpatient complications and adverse events. Results showed that hospitals with higher scores on safety climate were less likely to have patient safety indicator events; the effect was small but, in a sample of over 18 000, strongly significant. Further analyses showed that the presence of fear of blame and shame, rather than the more organizational aspects of culture, were critical to explaining the relationship with the indicators. Moreover, the relationship was mostly accounted for by a reduction in pressure sores and ulcers, perhaps the most visible and most susceptible to the attitudes and practices of individual staff.

In subsequent analyses, Singer and colleagues examined the extent to which responses could be identified as 'problematic', indicating a poor safety culture, on each of the dimensions. The average rate of problematic responses was 17.6%, but varied between 10.9 and 26.6%, suggesting that differences between hospitals can be quite marked. Emergency department personnel perceived worse safety climate and personnel in non-clinical areas perceived better safety climate than workers in other areas. Nurses were more negative than physicians regarding their work unit's support and recognition of safety efforts, and physicians showed marginally more fear of shame than nurses. For other dimensions of safety climate, physician-nurse differences depended on their work area (Singer *et al.*, 2009).

Safety climate can, as discussed, also be examined at a unit level, where it can vary markedly both within and between hospitals. For instance, Makary *et al.* (2006) developed a surgically specific safety climate scale and showed massive variation between surgical units, ranging from 100% of staff reporting a good climate to only 17%. Hofman and Mark (2006) used a large ongoing project on nursing outcomes as a basis for a study of 1127 nurses across 81 medical and nursing units in 42 different hospitals. Their safety climate scale was strongly orientated to attitude and openness about error and willingness to reflect and learn from errors. The nursing outcomes, already validated and obtained from reviewing records, included both patient outcomes (urinary tract infections and medication errors) and injuries to staff (back and needle stick injuries), as well as patient experience indices. A positive safety climate was associated with a reduction in all these indices, except needle stick injuries. However, in a similar study in a surgical context, Daniel Davenport *et al.* (2007) failed to find a relationship between either team or safety climate scale and risk adjusted surgical outcomes; better outcomes were, however, associated with staff reporting higher levels of communication and collaboration.

These studies illustrate the complexity of the potential relationships between safety climate and clinical processes and outcomes. Both research and practical efforts to improve safety culture are still evolving, so it is too early to come to definitive conclusions. Certainly there is some evidence that a good safety climate is associated with lower injury rates, both outside and within healthcare. However, this relationship will vary according to the way safety climate is assessed and the clinical context, and it may be mediated in a number of ways. Safety climate has, for instance, been shown to predict likelihood of reporting incidents which might have an indirect effect on the overall safety consciousness of a unit. Some aspects of safety climate though, such as willingness to actively intervene when a patient is at risk, might reflect much more direct influences on clinical practice. A safety culture is therefore certainly a necessary foundation for improving safety and quality, but relying only on changing attitudes, values and culture may only have limited effects.

References

Amalberti, R. (2001) The paradoxes of almost totally safe transportation systems. *Safety Science*, **37**(2–3), 109–126.

Berwick, D.M. (1998) Taking action to improve safety: How to increase the odds of success, Rancho Mirage, California.

Clarke, S. (2006) The relationship between safety climate and safety performance: a meta-analytic review. *Journal of Occupational Health Psychology*, **11**(4), 315–327.

Cox, S. and Flin, R. (1998) Safety culture. Philosopher's stone or man of straw. *Work and Stress*, **12**, 189–201.

Davenport, D.L., Henderson, W.G., Mosca, C.L. *et al.* (2007) Risk-adjusted morbidity in teaching hospitals correlates with reported levels of communication and collaboration on surgical teams but not with scale measures of teamwork climate, safety climate, or working conditions. *Journal of the American College of Surgeons*, **205**(6), 778–784.

Department of Health (2000) An Organisation with a Memory: Learning from Adverse Events in the NHS, The Stationery Office, London.

Flin, R., Burns, C., Mearns, K. *et al.* (2006) Measuring safety climate in healthcare. *Quality and Safety in Health Care*, **15**(2), 109–115.

Gaba, D.M., Singer, S.J. and Rosen, A.K. (2007) Safety culture: is the 'unit' the right 'unit of analysis'? *Critical Care Medicine*, **35**(1), 314–316.

Harvey, J., Erdos, G., Bolam, H. *et al.* (2002) An analysis of safety culture attitudes in a highly regulated environment. *Work and Stress*, **16**(1), 18–36.

Health and Safety Commission (HSC) (1993) Organizing for safety, ACSNI Human Factors Study Group, The Stationery Office, London, 3.

Helmreich, R.L. and Merrit, A.C. (1998) *Culture at Work in Aviation and Medicine: National, Organisational and* Professional *Influences*, Ashgate, Aldershot.

Hofman, D.A. and Mark, B. (2006) An investigation between safety climate and medication errors and other nurse and patient outcomes. *Personnel Psychology*, **59**, 847–869.

Huczynski, A. and Buchanan, D. (1991) *Organisational Behaviour*, 2nd edn, Prentice Hall International, Hemel Hempstead UK.

La Porte, T.R. (1996) High reliability organisations: Unlikely, demanding and at risk. *Journal of Contingencies and Crisis Management*, **4**, 60–71.

La Porte, T.R. and Consolini, P.M. (1991) Working in practice but not in theory – theoretical challenges of high reliability organisations. *Journal of Public Administration Research & Theory*, **1**, 1–21.

Leape, L.L., Woods, D.D., Hatlie, M.J. *et al.* (1998) Promoting patient safety by preventing medical error. *Journal of the American Medical Association*, **280**(16), 1444–1447.

Makary, M.A., Sexton, J.B., Freischlag, J.A. *et al.* (2006) Patient safety in surgery. *Annals of Surgery*, **243**(5), 628–632.

Nieva, V.F. and Sorra, J. (2003) Safety culture assessment: a tool for improving patient safety in healthcare organizations. *Quality and Safety in Health Care*, **12**(Suppl. II), ii17–ii23.

Peters, T.J. and Waterman, R.M. (1982) *In search of excellence*, Harper and Row, New York.

Pronovost, P., Weast, B., Holzmueller, C.G. *et al.* (2003) Evaluation of the culture of safety: a survey of clinicians and managers in an academic medical center. *Quality and Safety in Health Care*, **12**, 405–410.

Reason, J.T. (1997) *Managing the Risks of Organisational Accidents*, Ashgate, Aldershot.

Roberts, K.M. (1990) Some characteristics of high reliability organisations. *Organisation Science*, **1**, 160–177.

Schein, B. (1985) *Organisation Culture and Leadership*, Jossey Bass, San Francisco CA.

Singer, S.J., Gaba, D.M., Geppert, J.J. *et al.* (2003) The culture of safety: results of an organization-wide survey in 15 California hospitals. *Quality and Safety in Health Care*, **12**, 112–118.

Singer, S.J., Gaba, D.M., Falwell, A. *et al.* (2009) Patient safety climate in 92 US hospitals: differences by work area and discipline. *Medical Care*, **47**(1), 23–31.

Vincent, C.A. (2006) *Patient Safety*, 1st edn, Elsevier, Edinburgh.

Vincent, C.A., Benn, J. and Hanna, G.B. (2010) High reliability and healthcare. *British Medical Journal*, **340**, 225–226.

Waller, M.J. and Roberts, K.H. (2003) High reliability and organizational behavior: finally the twain must meet. *Journal of Organizational Behavior*, **24**, 813–814.

Weick, K. and Sutcliffe, K.M. (2001) *Managing the Unexpected. Assuring High Performance in an Age of Complexity*, Jossey Bass, San Francisco CL.

Weick, K. and Sutcliffe, K.M. (2003) Hospitals as cultures of entrapment: A re-analysis of the Bristol Royal Infirmary. *California Management Review*, **45**(2), 73–84.

CHAPTER 15

Patient involvement in patient safety

Patient safety, you would think from the name, has the patient's interests at heart and so it does in many respects. However, this has seldom extended to actually involving the patient in the quest for safer care. Safety is addressed and discussed in multiple ways, and lessons are sought from all manner of other industries and experts, from the disciplines of psychology, ergonomic, engineering and many others. Yet the one source of experience and expertise that still remains largely ignored is that of the patient.

One might argue that patients do not have much to contribute; after all, many people fly, but aviation safety does not rely on the passengers for safe operation. In healthcare however, unlike aviation, the patient is a privileged witness of events both in the sense that they are at the centre of the treatment process and also that, unlike clinical staff who come and go, they observe almost the whole process of care. The patient may not, of course, understand the technical and clinical issues at stake, but they do observe and experience the kindnesses, the small humiliations, the skilfulness of a line insertion, the inconsistencies in care, the errors and sometimes the disasters. In the case of people with chronic illnesses, they become experts not only on their own disease but on the frailties, limitations and unintentional cruelties of their healthcare system. The trouble is that, for all this potential knowledge and insight into the frailties of the healthcare system, they find it astonishingly difficult to make their voice heard, particularly where errors and safety are concerned.

Even an experienced senior doctor can find it hard to make their voice heard when dealing with hospital staff caring for themselves or their family. Don Berwick has movingly described his experiences of being with his wife Ann during her treatment for a serious autoimmune condition (Box 15.1). In his account, Don stresses the good will, kindness, generosity and commitment of the healthcare staff but, even after two decades of grappling with the quality and safety of healthcare, was appalled at the operation of the healthcare systems. Notice especially his last remark about migrating to the edge of being a difficult patient; drawing attention to the deficiencies in your care does not necessarily make you popular and the last thing any patient wants to do, in hospital at least, is to alienate the staff who may literally have your life in their hands.

Patient Safety, 2nd edition. By Charles Vincent. Published 2010 by Blackwell Publishing Ltd.

BOX 15.1 Being and feeling unsafe in hospital

Above all, we needed safety; and yet Ann was unsafe . . . The errors were not rare; they were the norm. During one admission, the neurologist told us in the morning, 'By no means should you be getting anticholinergic agents,' and a medication with profoundly anticholinergic side effects was given that afternoon. The attending neurologist in another admission told us by phone that a crucial and potentially toxic drug should be started immediately. He said, 'Time is of the essence.' That was on Thursday morning at 10.00 a.m. The first dose was given 60 hours later. Nothing I could do, nothing I did, nothing I could think of made any difference. It nearly drove me mad. Colace was discontinued by a physician's order on Day 1 and was nonetheless brought by the nurse every single evening throughout a 14-day admission . . . I tell you from my personal observation: No day passed – not one – without a medication error. Most weren't serious, but they scared us.

We needed consistent, reliable information, based, we would have hoped, on the best science available. Instead we often heard a cacophony of meaningless and sometimes contradictory conclusions. . . . Drugs tried and proven futile in one admission would be recommended in the next as if they were fresh ideas. A spinal tap was done for a test for Lyme disease, but the doctor collected too little fluid and the test had to be repeated. During a crucial phase of diagnosis, one doctor told us to hope that the diagnosis would be of a certain disease, because that disease has a benign course. That same evening, another doctor told us to hope for the opposite, because that same disease is relentless, sometimes fatal. Complex, serial information on blood counts, temperature, functional status and weight – the information on the basis of which risky and expensive decisions were relying – was collected in disorganized, narrative formats, embedded in nursing notes and narrative forms. As far as I know, the only person who ever drew a graph of Ann's fevers or white blood cell count was me, and the data were so complex that, short of a graph, no rational interpretation was possible. As a result, physicians often reached erroneous conclusions, such as assuming that Ann had improved after a specific treatment when, in fact, she had improved before it or not at all.

The experience of patient-hood, or patient spouse-hood, as the case may be, was one of trying to get the attention of decision makers to correct their impressions or assumptions. Sociologically, this proved very tough, as we felt time and again our migration to the edge of the label 'difficult patient'.

(ADAPTED FROM BERWICK DM. "TAKING ACTION TO IMPROVE SAFETY: HOW TO IMPROVE THE CHANCES OF SUCCESS." PRESENTATION AT THE ANNENBERG CENTER FOR HEALTH SCIENCES CONFERENCE, *ENHANCING PATIENT SAFETY AND REDUCING ERRORS IN HEALTH CARE*, IN RANCHO MIRAGE, CALIFORNIA. NOVEMBER 8–10, 1998. REPRODUCED WITH PERMISSION FROM INSTITUTE FOR HEALTHCARE IMPROVEMENT)

Patients as active participants in their care

Patients are usually thought of as the passive victims of errors and safety failures, but there is considerable scope for them to play an active part in ensuring their care is effective, appropriate and safe. Angela Coulter (1999) has argued that instead of treating patients as passive recipients of medical care, it is much more appropriate to view them as partners or co-producers with an active role. For instance, patients have a vital role to play in providing an accurate and relevant clinical history. Unfortunately, they are often not permitted to tell their story. When allowed to speak without interruption, and with simple encouragement, most people in outpatient consultations only seem to need about 90 seconds to present their story before spontaneously saying something like 'That's all, doctor' (Langewitz, Denz and Keller, 2002). In practice, however, doctors frequently interrupt before the story has been told. In a study in the United States, patients were allowed to speak for only 23 seconds before being interrupted by their doctor, with the result that important information was often missed (Marvel, Epstein, Flowers and Beckman, 1999).

Patients contribute to their own care at every stage through provision of diagnostic information, participation in treatment decisions, choice of provider, the management and treatment of disease and the monitoring of adverse events and other ways (Box 15.2) (Vincent and Coulter, 2002; Coulter and Ellins, 2007). Patients also need to actively intervene to protect themselves from errors or to avoid delays; for instance, patients frequently provide repeat histories to compensate for missing notes, relay information between clinicians, remind nurses of tests that should be done and chase test results. Unruh and Pratt (2007) nicely describe this as the 'invisible work' that patients do in a healthcare system and provide some apposite examples of the ways in which cancer patients monitor and actively intervene to ensure they receive the correct treatments (Box 15.3).

BOX 15.2 Ways that patients can participate in the safety of healthcare:

- Making informed choices about providers;
- Helping to reach an accurate diagnosis;
- Sharing decisions about treatments and procedures;
- Contributing to safe medication use;
- Participating in infection control initiatives;
- Checking the accuracy of medical records;
- Observing and checking care processes;
- Identifying and reporting treatment complications and adverse events;
- Practising effective self-management (including treatment monitoring);
- Shaping the design and improvement of services.

(REPRODUCED FROM *BRITISH MEDICAL JOURNAL*, ANGELA COULTER, JO ELLINS. "EFFECTIVENESS OF STRATEGIES FOR INFORMING, EDUCATING, AND INVOLVING PATIENTS". 335, NO. 7609, [24–27], 2007, WITH PERMISSION FROM BMJ PUBLISHING GROUP LTD.)

BOX 15.3 The invisible work of patients

Detecting Procedural Errors

Noticing that an IV drip had finished before it should have done: 'It's obvious. The nurse said that it would take 20 minutes, but it starts beeping after 8 minutes (indicating the end of the infusion bag). It turned out to be the confusion of a 50 ml bag with a 100 ml bag.'

Co-ordinating Treatment Tasks

Preventing adhesive being applied to an area of skin that had been irradiated: 'I'm not sure but, because of the radiation, I don't think I'm meant to have a dressing there.'

Handing Over to New Staff and Maintaining Continuity of Care

Breast cancer patient with history of Hodgkins' disease and previous removal of spleen, with consequently raised risk of pneumonia. When seeing an unfamiliar nurse: 'I come in to the infusion clinic saying to a new nurse 'Would you listen to my lungs as well?' Because I really want to keep track of that, because I don't have a spleen and I'm at great risk of pneumonia and things like that. You know, I really have to watch out for that.'

Checking That Key Information is Known

I get hives from alcohol. The regular infusion nurse remembers it, but if there's a new one, I make sure the new nurse doesn't swab me down with alcohol.'

(REPRINTED FROM *INTERNATIONAL JOURNAL OF MEDICAL INFORMATICS*, KENTON T. UNRUH AND WANDA PRATT. "PATIENTS AS ACTORS: THE PATIENT'S ROLE IN DETECTING, PREVENTING, AND RECOVERING FROM MEDICAL ERRORS". **76**, [236–244], 2007, WITH PERMISSION FROM ELSEVIER)

The degree to which patients can be involved will vary considerably, depending on the nature and complexity of the treatment and the degree of technical knowledge required to understand the treatment process. Most importantly, it will depend on the extent to which each person feels willing and able to play a more active. At the one extreme are those people who prefer, whether from temperament or custom, to leave all decisions to their doctor and take a passive role. At the other extreme are those who wish to be involved in the minutest details of their treatment. Both these approaches can be appropriate in particular circumstances: for an acute medical emergency the sensible patient leaves almost all immediate decisions to the staff. In the case of a long-term chronic illness, the actively involved, enquiring patient is more likely to cope more effectively and receive appropriate treatment.

The patient's role in patient safety

To encourage patients to take a more active stance, some organizations have produced leaflets setting out what patients can do to make their own care safer. The US Joint Commission on Accreditation of Healthcare Organizations (JCA-HO) for instance, has campaigned for patient to 'speak up' to prevent errors in their care (Box 15.4). Their openness about the possibility of error and the

---

BOX 15.4 Speaking up

Speak up if you have questions of concerns, and if you don't understand, ask again. It's your body and you have a right to know:
- Don't be afraid to ask about safety. If you're having surgery, for example, ask the doctor to mark the area that is to be operated on, so that there's no confusion in the operating room.
- Don't be afraid to tell the nurse or doctor if you think you are about to receive the wrong medication.

Pay attention to the care you're receiving. Make sure you're getting the right treatments and medications. Don't assume anything:
- Notice whether your caregivers have washed their hands. Hand washing is the most important way to prevent the spread of infections. Don't be afraid to gently remind a doctor or nurse to do this.
- Make sure your nurse or doctor checks your wristband or asks your name before he or she administers any medication or treatment.

Educate yourself about your diagnosis, the medical tests you are undergoing and your treatment plan:
- Ask your doctor about the specialized training and experience that qualifies him or her to treat your illness.
- Write down important facts your doctor tells you, so that you can look for additional information later. And ask your doctor if he or she has any written information you can keep.

Ask a trusted family member or friend to be your advocate:
- Ask this person to stay with you, even overnight, when you are hospitalized. You will be able to rest more comfortably and your advocate can help to make sure you get the right medications and treatment.
- Review consents for treatment with your advocate before you sign them and make sure you both understand exactly what you are agreeing to.

Know what medications you take and why you take them. Medication errors are the most common healthcare mistakes:
- If you do not recognize a medication, verify that it is for you. Ask about oral medications before swallowing and read the contents of intravenous (IV) fluids. If you're not well enough, ask your advocate to do this.
- If you are given an IV ask the nurse how long it should take for the liquid to 'run out'. Tell the nurse if it seems to be dripping too fast or too slow.

(ADAPTED FROM *SPEAKING UP*. LEAFLET ISSUED BY JOINT COMMISSION FOR ACCREDITATION OF HEALTHCARE ORGANISATIONS)

active involvement of patients in some specific activities must certainly be welcomed. Encouraging patients to ask questions about their medication to make sure they understand, not to take medication unless they are clear about its purpose and to be responsible for their own contribution to their treatment seem reasonable and useful precautions although, if followed to the letter on all occasions, could take up a great deal of staff time.

Encouraging patients to ask questions is straightforward enough and would be accepted by most patients and staff, though attitudes to such questioning vary considerably in different countries. Much more difficult is the suggestion that patients might actively challenge a health professional. Patients are meant to observe whether their identification band has been checked, tell the staff if they think they might be being confused with another patient and remind nurses and doctors to wash their hands. Although well intentioned, this is a considerable extension of the patient's role and, arguably, an abdication of responsibility on the part of healthcare staff.

Patient involvement is potentially attractive on several counts; involving patients in safety problems, such as poor hygiene and infection, may well be very worthwhile. It accords with government policy, or at least with government rhetoric, in many countries striving to give the patient a greater voice in healthcare. These initiatives are also attractive because they seem cheap and straightforward. However, even the brief reflections above show us that these interventions are not as simple as they seem. Will sick people, or their advocates, be able and willing to be actively involved in safety? How will such involvement be received by staff? Is such a shift in responsibility acceptable and ethically justified? We are not yet in a position to fully answer these questions, but some important studies are now emerging, which shed light on these issues.

Patient involvement in patient safety: fundamental issues

What role can patients play in patient safety? This seemingly simple question hides some rather complex issues, which we must unpack before we can sensibly address the relevant issues. The first stage is to set out the underlying issues and the factors that may influence patient involvement. My colleague Rachel Davis (2009) has pointed out in her systematic review that there are a number of prerequisites for patient involvement:

- Patients, or their family or advocates, must be knowledgeable. They must know something of the clinical process and how to act or intervene.
- Patients, or advocates, must be able to intervene. If they are very sick, have limited cognitive capacity or are in a very frail state, it is clearly unreasonable to expect active involvement.
- Patients must also be willing to participate. This depends on personal values and preferences and on a broader ethical assessment of responsibility for healthcare processes and outcomes.
- Healthcare professionals must actively encourage and appreciate patient involvement.

Knowledge, ability to act and willingness to participate will vary for different patients and in different circumstances. Will older people, for instance, brought up at a time when a doctor's authority was seldom questioned, be able to ask questions about error and safety? In addition to age, cultural and social attitudes to authority may make patient involvement very difficult in some countries. When I gave a talk about patient involvement in one European country, an entire conference audience was completely incredulous at the idea that a patient might be encouraged to check that their operation was being carried out at the correct site.

Assuming a basic knowledge and willingness, a further set of questions arise that concern the nature of the involvement. Willingness to participate will depend on what is being asked. Is it just checking? Does it involve challenging someone? Knowledge of processes will vary from patient to patient and across different arenas of healthcare. A person with chronic diabetes may well be expert on all aspects of their diabetic care, but have little to contribute when they are admitted for surgery. Having laid out some of the principal conceptual and practical issues, we can now turn to research which has illuminated some of these issues.

Patients' willingness to engage in safety practices

Since the publication of patient information sheets encouraging participation in safety practices, a small number of studies have assessed patients' willingness to speak up and otherwise check on hospital procedures. We will consider three representative studies focusing respectively on consumers (i.e. people not in hospital), recently discharged patients and patients in hospital.

William Marella and colleagues surveyed 856 people in Pennsylvania in a telephone survey about 10 hospital orientated safety practices. The respondents were not in hospital, but nevertheless gave an opinion on what they thought they would do. The likelihood of action varied considerably; for instance, 85% of people said they would question the reason for a procedure in hospital, whereas only 45% were prepared to consider refusing care, such as a radiograph or the taking of blood that they had not been told about. Admittedly the latter are minor procedures, but this does show the difficulty many people have in standing up for themselves while in hospital; one cannot imagine, for instance, passively acquiescing to repairs on one's car for instance, without even asking why they were necessary.

A similar telephone survey was carried out by Waterman, Gallagher and Garbutt (2006), who spoke to 2078 patients who had been recently discharged from hospitals in the mid-West of the United States. Over 90% were prepared to ask a nurse about the purpose of medication, though only 75% did so when they had the opportunity. Many fewer patients (75%) would have been prepared to help staff with marking a surgical site, and fewer still (45%) would have considered asking medical personnel whether they had washed their hands. When patients had the opportunity to assist with site marking, only

17% did so and fewer still (4.6%) asked staff about hand washing. Admittedly, these patients had probably not been specifically asked to help with site marking or engage with a hand washing campaign, but we can see that there may be a considerable gap between intending to check on procedures and actually doing so.

Even doctors and nurses can be surprised at how vulnerable they feel when they or a relative is admitted to hospital; previously assertive people can feel surprisingly passive when ill, partially clothed and confined to a hospital bed. To what extent do patients who are actually in hospital feel able to question healthcare about safety and quality issues? This was the question explored by my colleague Rachel Davis on a surgical ward (Box 15.5). This study confirmed that many patients in hospital could not contemplate challenging staff, especially doctors, on matters such as hand washing. Men were less inclined to ask questions than women, as were those who were unemployed or not educated to degree level. Willingness to question could be increased substantially however, if that patient had been personally asked to question staff. For example, patients were much more likely to react positively to 'If instructed to by a doctor, would you ask a doctor: Have you washed your hands?' than to 'Would you ask a doctor: "Have you washed your hands?"' Davis, Koutantji and Vincent (2008) argue that patient safety initiatives involving patients will

---

BOX 15.5 Patients' willingness to ask safety questions

Factual Questions:

Would you ask a doctor/nurse: How long will I be in hospital for?

Would you ask a doctor/nurse: When will I return to my normal activities?

Would you ask a doctor/nurse: What signs should I be looking for to tell me that my wound may not be healing as it should?

Would you ask a doctor/nurse: How long will the pain last?

Would you ask a doctor: How long will I have to be off work after the operation?

Would you ask a doctor: What are the alternatives to surgery?

Would you ask a doctor: How is the procedure done?

Challenging Questions:

Would you ask a doctor/nurse: Why are you removing that piece of monitoring equipment?

Would you ask a doctor/nurse: Who are you and what is your job?

Would you ask a doctor/nurse: I don't think that is the medication I am on, can you check please?

Would you ask a doctor/nurse: Have you washed your hands?

Would you ask a doctor: How many times have you done this operation?

(REPRODUCED FROM *QUALITY & SAFETY IN HEALTH CARE*, R E DAVIS, M KOUTANTJI, C A VINCENT. "HOW WILLING ARE PATIENTS TO QUESTION HEALTHCARE STAFF ON ISSUES RELATED TO THE QUALITY AND SAFETY OF THEIR HEALTHCARE? AN EXPLORATORY STUDY". **17**, NO. 2, [90–96], 2008, WITH PERMISSION FROM BMJ PUBLISHING GROUP LTD.)

have to be carefully tailored to different needs and contexts and will also have to involve staff if they are to be successful. If patients feel that they are being burdened by challenging questions and responsibilities, they are highly unlikely to engage and may well feel resentful. If, on the other hand, staff and patients are engaged in a collaborative effort to promote hand hygiene, then the response if likely to be very different.

In summary therefore, these studies suggest that people, whether in, out or recently discharged from hospital, feel more able to ask factual questions of doctors and nurses than to challenge them on procedures. We cannot therefore rely on patients (and why should we?) to actively challenge staff, even when the procedures are designed to protect them from the dangers inherent in hospitalization. The practical implications are well summarized by Marella and colleagues, who suggest that if patients are potentially willing partners in the quest for safer care, they need to be helped and educated in the practices that will promote their own safety. In addition:

Patients must not be required . . . to challenge the skill, competence, or good intentions of their caregivers. When patients engage in these practices, they should receive an automatic 'Thank you for reminding me' or 'I'm glad you asked' as positive reinforcement.
(MARELLA *ET AL.*, 2009)

Patients reporting of adverse events

One of the challenges of understanding and improving safety and quality is to capture the full range of events that occurs during a patient's journey through healthcare. Clearly a complete description is not feasible, but we would at least like to capture the most important experiences and incidents. Medical records contain some of this information but are only a summary of key events and decisions. Interviews with staff can produce more detail but, as they have lives to lead and need to sleep periodically, they too have only a partial picture. The hospitalized patient on the other hand is there all the time, with little to do except watch and wait. Potentially therefore, they are an ideal observer.

In the real world of course, it is not so simple. People by virtue of illness, education, motivation or culture may not be inclined or willing to report incidents and few patients have the knowledge or technical understanding of the staff around them. Fortunately we can go beyond speculation and examine some studies of this important issue. Two studies in particular have greatly illuminated the question of patient reports of adverse events, both by Saul Weingart and his colleagues at Dana Farber Cancer Institute in Boston (Weingart, 2005; Weissman, Schneider and Weingart, 2008). In the first, they interviewed 229 patients in hospital, who were both willing and able to participate, asking them three general questions:

- Do you believe that there were any problems with your care during this hospitalization?
- Do you believe that you were hurt or stayed in the hospital longer than necessary because of problems with your care?
- Do you believe that anyone made a mistake that affected your care during this hospitalization?

The first thing to note is that it was possible to ask patients very blunt and direct questions about safety without destroying their trust in the hospital. Dana Farber is admittedly one of the leading proponents of openness and patient involvement, but even so, this was a step beyond simply consulting patients. These questions essentially mirror those asked in the classic adverse event studies discussed in Chapter 4.

From these simple five-minute interviews, patients identified a host of process failures such as problems with diagnosis, medication, procedures, clinical services (such as radiology, phlebotomy and laboratory) and service quality. All of these were reviewed by doctors, and classed as adverse events, near misses or simply errors or process problems; 17 patients (8%) experienced 20 adverse events, with 11 of these being confirmed in the medical record. This suggests that patients can and do identify key safety issues and that at least some of these can be verified in the medical record. The study also suggests, though cannot confirm, that patients might be able to provide an additional perspective to that found in the medical record. This was examined further in a second study nicely subtitled 'Do patients know something that hospitals do not?'

In a second study, Weissman *et al.* (2008) interviewed 998 recently discharged patients using a carefully structured survey addressing common types of hospital treatment such as medicines, diagnostic tests and surgery. In addition to general questions, they also asked about 11 specified complications and injuries, including heart attack, stroke, uncontrolled bleeding, rash and others. This study, however, went beyond just checking patient reports; they carried out a parallel review of the medical records of all the patients they interviewed. Patient reports were formally reviewed and only classified as adverse events if they met standard criteria. Patient reports then were not simply accepted at face value, but scrutinized and assessed for their validity.

Record review revealed a by now familiar finding: 11% of patients suffered an adverse event, with about a tenth (11 cases) of these being serious and preventable. However, 23% of patients reported an adverse event and there was little concordance between the two methods. Patient reports revealed an additional 21 serious and preventable events (Table 15.1), in addition to the 11 found in medical records, thus tripling the rate revealed by record review. The true rate of incidents potentially reportable by patients may be higher still, as some interviews took place several months after discharge and patients who died or were very sick post discharge were excluded from the study. As the examples show, many of the incidents reported by patients were serious untoward events that should have been described in the medical record.

Table 15.1 Examples of serious and preventable adverse events reported by patients only

Timing and Type of Event	Description
During hospital stay	
Operative vessel injury	Patient bled after laparoscopic gallbladder surgery and needed additional surgery to stop the bleeding
Operative nerve injury	The patient suffered numbness and weakness of the hand after lung resection for cancer
Adverse drug event	After receiving new medications in the hospital, the patient became disorientated and confused for 24 hours
Hospital-acquired pneumonia	The patient developed postoperative pneumonia after a surgical procedure
Hospital-acquired deep venous thrombosis	After a knee replacement, the patient developed deep venous thrombosis in the lower leg
Post discharge	
Wound infection	After back surgery, the patient returned to the hospital with an infection requiring reopening of the wound
Wound infection	The patient had surgery on the arteries of his legs. He developed a wound infection requiring a return to hospital for additional surgery and treatment
Wound infection	After surgery for a broken leg, the patient developed a *Staphylococcus aureus* infection and was readmitted for additional surgery and treatment
Operative organ injury	The patient developed a bile leak after laparoscopic gallbladder removal and returned to the hospital for a further operation and pain control

Adapted from Weissman *et al.* (2008)

Clearly patients reported many more adverse events than were found in the medical records; however, record review also revealed incidents and adverse events that were not reported in interviews. Weissman and colleagues suggest that neither record review nor patient reports can provide a gold standard, but that both are necessary to obtain a reasonably complete picture of the harm from healthcare.

Safety interventions: collaboration between patients and professionals

Anyone who has had a serious or chronic illness, or been involved in the care of someone seriously ill, knows that it is sometimes necessary to monitor and co-ordinate the care given in an effort to compensate for the deficiencies of the healthcare system. Don Berwick has provided us with a dramatic, and painful, example of this. His perspective is clearly much more informed than the average patient; most of us would be unable to monitor drug effects and inter-actions for instance. The question is whether this active engagement can be harnessed and systematically employed to increase safety. The hope and implication of much of the literature advocating patient involvement is that patients can actually improve the safety of their own care and, potentially, also the safety of care generally. Given the rhetoric and wide promotion of these ideas, in some circles there are surprisingly few studies evaluating these claims. We will examine two key safety issues: patient identification and hand hygiene.

Patient identification

Patients routinely and necessarily confirm their own identity in all healthcare settings, but particularly in hospital. In North America, Britain and elsewhere, this identification is supplemented by wearing identification bracelets, which provide a name, hospital or other number and potentially more complex information in the form of bar codes. However, this is not routine in much of Europe or the rest of the world and, surprisingly, patients who have not been accustomed to identity bracelets are not uniformly in favour of wearing one. Cleopas, Kolly and Bovier (2004) surveyed 1411 patients discharged from Geneva University Hospital, where identity bracelets were not in use; 84% of patients thought that the hospital should introduce bracelets, rising slightly when examples of possible mis-identification were given; over 90% agreed to wear one if they were introduced; however, this still left a substantial number of patients who variously argued that bracelets were indiscreet, rendered them too anonymous, were only necessary for certain patients or who disliked any compulsory procedure. Given the acceptance of identity bracelets elsewhere, it is likely that these objections could be overcome, but it is salutary to see that even obvious and useful safety measures can be resisted by some patients.

Patients are, of course, necessarily and routinely involved in identification, if only when giving or confirming their name when arriving for an appointment. Many of the advice leaflets however, suggest a much more active involvement in checking that identification is actually correct. Christopher DiGiovanni and colleagues set out to assess the viability of such an approach by asking patients having orthopaedic surgery at a private clinic to assist with identity checking. All had given consent and discussed the operation with the surgeon. In addition to the usual instructions about fasting and so on, they were asked very clearly and explicitly to mark the side which was not to be operated on:

The secretary gave the patient a preoperative instruction sheet that provided him or her with several explicit instructions; one, which was stated in underlined, capitalized, bold-faced print, was to clearly mark the foot that was not to be operated on with the word 'NO' with a black indelible marker.

(DIGIOVANNI, KANG AND MANUEL, 2003)

Pretty clear instructions, you will probably agree. And a strong motivation, you would imagine, to avoid any chance of wrong site surgery. In spite of this, only 59 of 100 patients marked the site correctly, 37 made no mark and the others were partially compliant. Unfortunately, DiGiovanni did not interview the patients about their decisions, so can only speculate on the reasons for such low compliance. Some patients had obvious scarring and so might have presumed the operation site was clear. But most simply seemed to assume that the professionals would take care of everything and their input was unnecessary. Patients who had had surgery before were in fact less likely to mark the NO site, than those new to the procedure.

This study, admittedly a solitary example, at the very least shows that well intentioned efforts to engage patients need to be viewed with some caution and may also introduce new risks. Introducing an unreliable safety check is likely to be worse than having no check at all, potentially even increasing the chance of wrong site surgery because the absence of a NO mark could be a prompt to operate there, even though it is simply an omission by the patient.

Hand hygiene

Engaging patients is more straightforward when it is not actually imperative that every patient takes part or conforms to the procedure. This is the case with hand hygiene, in particular hand washing, where one just needs to engage as many people as possible, both patients and staff, in the general drive to improve hand washing and observation of other precautions. A series of small studies by Elizabeth McGuckin suggest that that this may well be a fruitful approach, though these studies have not been followed up in larger-scale trials. The programme trialled at the John Radcliffe hospital in Oxford, United Kingdom, provides an example. The main elements of the 'Partners in your care' programme were:

- Patients were visited by the infection control nurse within 24 hours of admission, to discuss the importance of hand washing by staff in preventing hospital acquired infections.
- Patients received an educational brochure, which provided information on hand hygiene.
- Patients were asked to become Partners in Your Care, by asking all healthcare workers who had direct contact with them, 'Did you wash your hands?'
- As a reminder to ask and for patients who said they might be too shy to ask, patients were given prompting aids that said, 'Did you wash your hands?'

Of the 98 patients approached, only 39 agreed to take part, though the reasons for this are not discussed. Nevertheless, compared with a baseline six-week monitoring period, hand washing, as reflected in use of soap and alcohol gel usage, increased by an average of 50% in the ward as a whole. Over 60% of patients felt comfortable asking staff if they washed their hands, few tackled the doctors and there was some unease (Box 15.6). These studies are promising pilots, but are small scale, lack direct observation of hand washing and without

BOX 15.6 Patients experience of challenging staff on hand hygiene

Surgical Patients

The nurses laughed when I asked them.

Didn't ask the doctors – didn't have much to do with them.

When I asked the doctor, he looked at me as if I had two heads. I thought I was going to have a heart attack but forced myself to ask.

The person who takes the blood didn't wash hands between three patients.

I asked them to, before taking my blood – didn't feel comfortable asking.

Some nurses washed their hands, but some said they'd put gloves on instead.

Didn't have to ask – because they saw the leaflet.

They saw the brochure. I think infections are mostly from long nails – it's important to keep nails short.

Got a positive response from most – not the doctor.

Doctor didn't wash his hands before taking blood. I asked two nurses – both said they'd already washed their hands.

Medical

Everyone wore gloves anyway!

Comfortable asking most.

One care assistant said she always wore gloves to protect herself – but didn't change them between patients – I explained to her why she should.

Very positive responses from nurses. I asked one doctor. Doctors and nurses responded well.

Was not comfortable asking doctors, as they were always in a group.

Nurses always washed their hands when prompted. Didn't ask doctors because I noticed doctors did wash hands.

(REPRINTED FROM *AMERICAN JOURNAL OF INFECTION CONTROL*, MARYANNE MCGUCKIN, ALEXIS TAYLOR, VERONICA MARTIN, LOIS PORTEN AND RICHARD SALCIDO. "EVALUATION OF A PATIENT EDUCATION MODEL FOR INCREASING HAND HYGIENE COMPLIANCE IN AN INPATIENT REHABILITATION UNIT". **32**, NO. 4, [235–238], 2004, WITH PERMISSION FROM ELSEVIER)

long-term follow-up. This approach does show some promise, and in any event, patients need to be active participants in maintaining a clean environment, but much more sustained trials and evaluation are needed if this is to be viewed as a routine part of hospital care.

Patients for patient safety

Our discussion of patient involvement has so far focused mostly on the role of individual patients and their families in their particular treatment. There are, however, many other ways in which patients or members of the public may fight for and contribute to safer care and more humane treatment of injured patients. 'Patients for patient safety' (PFPS) is a core programme of the World Alliance for Patient Safety which engages patients, many of whom have suffered serious harm themselves, in the quest for safer care. They have built up a truly global network of patients and consumers, whose purpose is to improve healthcare safety in all healthcare settings throughout the world by working as partners with healthcare professionals. These brave and thoughtful people often speak about their experiences at conferences on patient safety, which is a moving and sometimes painful experience for the audience and potentially distressing for the speakers too, even long after the original event. Although I believe it is critical to listen to these tragic stories in order to understand how best to help injured patients, as we discussed earlier, I remain uneasy that it seems to be necessary to use personal tragedy to motivate healthcare professionals. The equivalent in aviation, for instance, would be to begin a conference on safety with accounts from passengers who had survived a crash in order to motivate the audience to take the issue seriously. Surely we need to move beyond this, take the patient voice seriously and find ways of drawing on the unique perspective the patient (that is, any of us when we are patients) brings to patient safety. PFPS is very alive to all these issues, as the following excerpt from the World Alliance Web site shows:

When patients and families are included in gatherings of patient safety stakeholders, their primary contributions have been to share stories of preventable injury in healthcare and their impact on patients' lives. We are gratified to have made this contribution. The voice of patients and families who have suffered preventable medical injury is a powerful motivational force for healthcare providers across the globe who wish, first, to do no harm.

However, patients have much more to offer than visceral reminders to healthcare workers, administrators and policymakers that we are victims of tragic medical errors. Important as that perspective is, a victim orientation does not position us well as partners working with healthcare providers to prevent harm. Indeed, the perception that patients and their families are helpless or antagonistic victims has served to distance us from playing meaningful roles in the development and implementation of patient safety work in the past and generated fear among some clinicians who would have otherwise engaged with us. Patients and their families have needs and wants when things go wrong. We need to be told that something has gone wrong and we want healthcare service deliverers to be open and involve us in the investigation to find the root causes.

At the healthcare service delivery level, consumers who wish to contribute knowledge gained or lessons learned have often found few effective pathways for doing so. Particularly after healthcare accidents occur, a 'wall of silence' may descend and productive interaction may cease. When consumers register concerns, their actions often are perceived as adversarial threats or unscientific anecdotes that lack evidence, rather than potential knowledge contributions.

Although there are notable exceptions, at the policymaking level consumer participation tends to be marginalized, often by well meaning leaders who assume consumers to be unable to appreciate the complexity of healthcare. Such an approach fails to take into account that many consumers offer the richest resource of information related to medical errors, as many have witnessed every detail of systems failures from the beginning to end.

Establishing a proper and fruitful role for patients to play in patient safety is not straightforward and there are many issues to be resolved. There are, however, already some impressive examples of patients being actively involved in the management of a hospital, entirely changing the nature and tone of the usual patient clinician relationships. For example, by involving patients, the Dana Farber Cancer Centre in Boston learnt that patients with neutropenia (a reduction in white blood cells occurring in many diseases) often experienced long, wearying waits in emergency departments, seriously delaying the start of treatment. Telephone screening and direct admission to appropriate wards transformed this process and reduced the risk of infections and other complications. Patients are members of several important hospital committees and regarded as an essential voice in the redesign or improvement of services.

References

Berwick, D.M. (2003) *Escape Fire. Designs for the Future of Healthcare*, Jossey Bass, San Francisco CA.

Cleopas, A., Kolly, V., Bovier, P.A. *et al.* (2004) Acceptability of identification bracelets for hospital inpatients. *Quality and Safety in Health Care*, **13**(5), 344–348.

Coulter, A. (1999) Paternalism or partnership? Patients have grown up –and there's no going back. *British Medical Journal*, **319**(7212), 719–720.

Coulter, A. and Ellins, J. (2007) Effectiveness of strategies for informing, educating, and involving patients. *British Medical Journal*, **335**(7609), 24–27.

Davis, R.E., Koutantji, M. and Vincent, C.A. (2008) How willing are patients to question healthcare staff on issues related to the quality and safety of their healthcare? An exploratory study. *Quality and Safety in Health Care*, **17**(2), 90–96.

Davis, R.E. (2009) Patient involvement in patient safety, Imperial College, London.

DiGiovanni, C.W., Kang, L. and Manuel, J. (2003) Patient compliance in avoiding wrong-site surgery. *Journal of Bone and Joint Surgery of America*, **85-A**(5), 815–819.

Langewitz, W., Denz, M., Keller, A. *et al.* (2002) Spontaneous talking time at start of consultation in outpatient clinic: cohort study. *British Medical Journal*, **325**(7366), 682–683.

Marella, W., Finley, E., Thomas, A.D. and Clarke, J. (2009) Healthcare consumers' inclination to engage in selected patient safety practices: a survey of adults in Pennsylvania. *Journal of Patient Safety*, **3**(4), 184–189.

Marvel, M.K., Epstein, R.M., Flowers, K. and Beckman, H.B. (1999) Soliciting the patient's agenda: have we improved? *Journal of the American Medical Association*, **281**(3), 283–287.

McGuckin, M., Taylor, A., Martin, V. *et al.* (2004) Evaluation of a patient education model for increasing hand hygiene compliance in an inpatient rehabilitation unit. *American Journal of Infection Control,* **32**(4), 235–238.

Unruh, K.T. and Pratt, W. (2007) Patients as actors: the patient's role in detecting, preventing, and recovering from medical errors. *International Journal of Medical Informatics,* **76**(Suppl. 1), S236–S244.

Vincent, C.A. and Coulter, A. (2002) Patient safety: what about the patient? *Quality and Safety in Health Care,* **11**(1), 76–80.

Waterman, A.D., Gallagher, T.H., Garbutt, J. *et al.* (2006) Brief report: Hospitalized patients' attitudes about and participation in error prevention. *Journal of General Internal Medicine,* **21**(4), 367–370.

Weingart, S.S. (2005) What can hospitalized patients tell us about adverse events? Learning from patient-reported incidents. *Journal of General Internal Medicine,* **20**(9), 830.

Weissman, J.S., Schneider, E.C., Weingart, S.N. *et al.* (2008) Comparing patient-reported hospital adverse events with medical record review: do patients know something that hospitals do not? *Annals of Internal Medicine,* **149**(2), 100–108.

CHAPTER 16
Procedures, violations and migrations

The safety of healthcare is such a huge problem and the causes so diverse and complex that it may seem as if the individual clinician can do little to influence the overall safety of care. Safety is, as is often said, a property of the whole healthcare system. Making healthcare safer will require clinical innovation, process improvement, information technology and cultural change. However, the people who work in an organization are part of that system and each brings their own contribution to safe high-quality care. Clinical staff, in addition to simply doing their jobs well, actively create safety as they work. Atul Gawande expresses this eloquently when discussing the limits of a systems view:

It would be deadly for us, the individual actors, to give up our belief in human perfectibility. The statistics may say that some day I will sever someone's main bile duct, but each time I go into a gallbladder operation I believe that with enough will I can beat the odds. This isn't just professional vanity. It's a necessary part of good medicine, even in superbly 'optimized' systems. Operations like that lap chole have taught me how easily error can occur, but they've also showed me something else: effort does matter; diligence and attention to the minutest detail can save you.

(GAWANDE, A. COMPLICATIONS. PROFILE BOOKS LTD, HOLT METROPOLITAN, 2002 AND PICADOR USA, APRIL 2003. REPRODUCED WITH PERMISSION)

Although there is a certain amount of work in industry on safety behaviours and attitudes, comparatively little attention has been paid in the patient safety movement to the precise ways in which individuals, whether singly or in teams, can contribute to safer healthcare. People partly create safety by being conscientious, disciplined and following rules; however, they also create safety recognizing when one must think beyond standard procedures. Delivering safe, high-quality care is an interplay between disciplined, regulated behaviour and necessary adaptation and flexibility, considered in the following chapter. In this chapter, we consider the vexed issue of procedures in healthcare, why people often do not follow them and what might be done about it. The term 'procedures in healthcare' can encompass everything from giving an injection

---

Patient Safety, 2nd edition. By Charles Vincent. Published 2010 by Blackwell Publishing Ltd.

to complex surgery; in this chapter however, we are concerned with the basic rules, procedures and guidelines that govern clinical practice and behaviour.

Creating safety by following rules and procedures

Clinical work is founded on tried and tested ways of diagnosing and treating patients; being willing to follow procedures is fundamental to being a good clinician. Running an outpatient clinic for chronic asthmatics or diabetics, for instance, while still requiring much clinical acumen, requires good organization, good communication and reliable information technology delivering tried and tested, evidence based care. Much flexibility in healthcare stems not from necessary adaptation to changing circumstances, but from unnecessary, casual and inappropriate departure from good clinical practice. One way in which people create safety, therefore, is observing rules and by boring, conscientious following of standard procedures.

Protocols and guidelines for clinical care come in various forms. Most are disease centred and describe the procedures for the treatment of a particular condition in a particular context, such as the management of acute asthma in emergency departments or the management of diabetes in primary care. Clinical guidelines are 'systematically developed statements to assist practitioner and patient decisions about appropriate healthcare for specific circumstances' (Foy, Grimshaw and Eccles, 2001). Previously derided by some as 'cookbook medicine', they are increasingly both accepted and embedded in formal decision support systems, care pathways and in national frameworks and targets. In these situations the protocol provides guidance, but there is an expectation that the standard procedures may always be modified according to the judgement of the clinician and the preferences of the patient. There will always be occasions when guidelines cannot or should not be followed; for instance, patients with multiple conditions and problems cannot easily be treated according to strict guidelines or the patient themselves may simply decide against a particular course of action.

In this chapter however, we are mainly concerned with protocols that define a standard clinical procedure for a routine task which, broadly speaking, should be carried out in a standardized manner; some variation may be expected for skilled tasks when the patient is a child or requires special care of some kind. Protocols for routine tasks are standardized and specified precisely because variation is thought to be at the very least unnecessary and, on some occasions at least, positively dangerous. Protocols of this kind are equivalent to the safety rules of other industries, defined ways of behaving which are intended to either improve safety or achieve a required level of safety (Hale and Swuste, 1998). Examples in healthcare include: checking equipment; washing your hands; not prescribing dangerous drugs when you are not authorized to; following the procedures when giving intravenous drugs; and routinely checking the identity of a patient. Such standard routines and procedures are the bedrock of a safe organization.

Breaking the rules and bucking the system

Why don't people follow procedures? This was the despairing, indeed anguished, question put to me by a Director of Nursing after she had reviewed yet another case in which blatant disregard for the rules put a patient at serious risk. A review of the case showed marked lapses from basic procedures, seemingly for no good reason and the nurse in question was disciplined. Are these isolated incidents or are procedures often disregarded? Recall that James Reason speaks of 'routine' violations, implying that they are by no means uncommon. Routine and frequent violations? It seems incredible, until one begins to look more closely at the way human beings react and adapt to organizational policies and rules.

Fiona Moss is a chest physician and, for 10 years, editor of *Quality and Safety in Healthcare*. In her last editorial for the journal, she chose to focus on an intractable issue that she sees as fundamental to improving the safety of healthcare, which is the fact that clinicians, by which in this instance she meant doctors, routinely break rules and ignore basic and reasonable organizational procedures and practices. As Moss puts it, there is a 'chasm between organizational intention and individual action' (Moss, 2004). Recall the death of David James described in Chapter 8, in which several staff departed from standard procedures, and then consider this paragraph:

Learning to buck the system is a frequent early learning experience for many doctors. For example, hospitals in the UK do not allow house officers to prescribe or administer cytotoxic chemotherapy. Although this 'organizational rule' has been in force for several years, we sometimes find that it has been broken. This usually happens at night, when a patient has not been given chemotherapy; the person who should give it is no longer on duty and the 'covering' doctor is called. Although this very inexperienced doctor and the nurse may both be aware that the doctor should not give the chemotherapy, neither perceives any real danger as the action needed is simply to attach an infusion bag to an already sited drip; both are concerned that the patient get the treatment and so the treatment is given. An organizational rule is broken. Nothing happens, no one knows. A culture that ignores the system of the delivery of care is enforced and the system becomes a little more dangerous.
(REPRODUCED FROM *QUALITY & SAFETY IN HEALTH CARE*, FIONA MOSS. "THE CLINICIAN, THE PATIENT AND THE ORGANISATION: A CRUCIAL THREE SIDED RELATIONSHIP". **13**, NO. 6, [406–407], 2004, WITH PERMISSION FROM BMJ PUBLISHING GROUP LTD.)

Notice first that there are many plausible reasons for breaking this rule. The patient needs the treatment and it would probably be time consuming to call another doctor with the authority to administer the treatment. The other doctor may in any case be off site or dealing with an emergency elsewhere; there may be good reason for breaking the rule on at least some occasions. But, in healthcare, the fact that it is sometimes necessary to think beyond rules very easily shades, by sleight of hand, into simply ignoring rules, because it is inconvenient for some reason. Once ignoring rules is socially, if not organizationally, sanctioned, the system becomes a little more dangerous, then more dangerous still, and so on until there is a major disaster. Within healthcare organizations, there are some rules which are never broken, others more on the margins, and some which are routinely flouted. These shifts in what is acceptable are known as migrations, in the sense that an individual or a team steadily drifts from behaviour that is, if not optimal, at least reasonable in the circumstances towards serious violations of procedures and behaviour that are frankly dangerous (Polet, Vanderhaegen and Amalberti, 2003; Amalberti *et al.*, 2006).

Hand washing

Hand washing is an example of a rule that is routinely flouted; studies have found that average levels of compliance have varied from 16 to 81% (Pittet, 2001); compliance is probably higher in environments such as the operating theatre where the routine of getting scrubbed is solidly embedded. The causes of infection are undoubtedly complex and there are various routes of transmission. However, contamination through hand contact is a major source and hand hygiene a major weapon in the fight against infection (Burke, 2003). In spite of this, it has proved extraordinarily difficult to persuade healthcare workers to wash their hands.

The history of research into hand washing was for a long time a litany of failure, in the sense that most interventions had shown only small or transient effects; however, it was coupled with a steadily increasing sophistication in understanding the many factors that influence this behaviour and of the need for multifaceted interventions (Larson *et al.*, 1997). Previous interventions to change clinicians' behaviour had included education, feedback, financial rewards and penalties, and administrative changes. The lack of washing facilities at the patient's bedside, skin problems through frequent washing and shortage of time were major barriers to hand washing for busy clinicians. Didier Pittet and colleagues (2000) solved these latter problems by introducing a fast bedside procedure of hand disinfection with an alcohol based rub. In a four-year intervention in the University of Geneva hospitals, they improved compliance from 48 to 66%; in the same period the prevalence of nosocomial infection reduced from 16.9 to 9.8% and the transmission rates of MRSA halved. The intervention involved a massive and continuing educational campaign, regular surveys and observations and the backing and involvement of all professional groups at all levels of the hospital. Compliance increased most markedly for nurses and nursing assistants but they were at a loss to explain, or at least would not publicly state, why compliance remained poor amongst doctors. There is now considerable political and regulatory pressure in many countries for improvements in both rates of nosocomial infection and hand hygiene, and major campaigns to replicate the improvements demonstrated in Geneva across the world (Pittet *et al.*, 2005).

Understanding deviations from procedures

Are clinical staff particularly poor at following procedures compared with staff in other safety-critical industries? Healthcare is possibly more lax, but certainly not unique. Human beings never fully comply with rules and deviation from procedures occurs in all industrial systems, even those regarded as extremely safe. For instance, an extensive observational study of aircrews' deviations from procedures showed that 'intentional non-compliance' represented 45% of all errors and violations, but only 6% of these affected the flight in any adverse way (Helmreich, 2000). To understand why this is, we will examine studies of violations in two contrasting settings.

Rebecca Lawton (1998) is an enterprising researcher who qualified as a railway shunter while investigating safety on the railways. Being a shunter involves ensuring the safe movement of rolling stock in sidings, depots and stations and coupling and uncoupling of trucks and engines; if a shunter is trapped between two trucks or hit by a train, the chances of survival are slim. At the time of her study, the British railways network had 2000 shunters; an average of two shunters were killed each year, with investigations commonly revealing violations of basic safety procedures. Being a railway shunter is an extraordinarily dangerous occupation providing, you would have thought, every incentive for following safety procedures.

Interviews established that the shunters were well aware that safety procedures were often bypassed and could estimate frequencies for them. For instance:

- Even though he has lost sight of the shunter, the driver does not stop during a movement (High risk, high frequency).
- The shunter works without wearing the high visibility clothing provided (Low risk, high frequency).
- The shunter remains in between the trucks and asks the driver to ease up (High risk, low frequency).
- The shunter fails to look both ways before crossing the line and does not take extra care when stepping out from behind a truck (High risk, high frequency).

The main study asked shunters to endorse different reasons for the violations of safety rules, with revealing results. The reasons (Table 16.1) fall into three basic categories, reflecting the earlier discussion of the psychological classification of error and violation (Reason, 1990). Some are not strictly violations in the strict sense of the word, but arise more through lack of understanding or inexperience; in these circumstances, there is no sharp dividing line between errors and violations. A second group were labelled 'exceptional violations', when rules are bent in order to find a solution to an unusual situation. Finally, there are 'routine violations', which are frequent and considered low risk, often justified by the belief that the shunter is sufficiently experienced and skilful to cut corners. The same belief, or rather delusion, underlies a lot of dangerous driving (McKenna and Horswill, 2006).

Look again at Table 16.1 and substitute nurse, doctor, pharmacist or psychologist for shunter. Imagine your own working environment and the routine tasks you should carry out, but may not. Does this list of reasons seem familiar? A similar study of violations was carried out with anaesthetists using common scenarios, such as the ones below to elicit the reasons for potential violations:

Table 16.1 Railway shunters' reasons for violations

Reason for violation	%
This is a quicker way of working	39
Inexperienced shunter	38
Time pressure	37
High workload	30
The shunter is lazy	19
A skilled shunter can work safely this way	17
The rule can be impossible to work to	16
Design of the sidings makes the violation necessary	16
Management turns a blind eye	12
Physical exhaustion	7
No-one understands the rule	6
It is a more exciting way of working	6
It's a macho way to work	5
The rule is outdated	5

Reprinted from *Safety Science*, Rebecca Lawton. Not working to rule: "Understanding procedural violations at work". **28**, no. 2, [199-211], 2004, with permission from Elsevier.

You have an elective surgery list tomorrow morning. It is a routine list which you have done often before. Most patients on the list are ASA I–II. However, from time to time the list has thrown up unusually difficult cases where patients have been ASA III–IV. The list you have just completed has over run by an hour. You decide not to visit the patients but to speak to them the following morning in the operating theatre reception.

When you arrive at the list and enter the induction room there is no one about. The operating list is there and you note that a new case has been added to the end of the list. You cast a quick eye over the anaesthetic equipment in the operating theatre and everything appears to be normal. You decide not to do a 'cockpit' equipment check so that you may use the time to check up on the new patient.

(BEATTY AND BEATTY, 2004)

The researchers used a questionnaire examining anaesthetists' views of the factors that would influence the likelihood of following, or not following, these standard procedures. Three classes of belief were examined: beliefs about the consequences of the act; normative beliefs which are an assessment of the views and influence of other relevant people; and beliefs about control over the situation, factors such as time and resources which influence what is manageable in the circumstances (Table 16.2). Clinical reasons, such as preventing incidents, a vulnerable patient and ASA status were not surprisingly very important influences on behaviour. However, most striking was that equal importance was given to normative influences such as the views of colleagues, friends and teachers. From this pen and paper exercise, one cannot really say that these factors determine whether an anaesthetist checks their equipment or not, but it does suggest that the social environment and

Table 16.2 Influences on anaesthetists' willingness to violate safety rules

Scenario	Behavioural beliefs. What happens if?	Normative beliefs. Who influences me?	Control beliefs. What influences me?
Pre-operative visits	Decrease peri-operative risk Protect against litigation Help detect unusual patient conditions Decrease the anxiety of the patient	Competent anaesthetists Anaesthetic colleagues Non-anaesthetic colleagues Friends and family Patients Hospital managers My anaesthetic teachers	Patients with higher ASA grades Lack of time Patients in vulnerable groups
Pre-operative equipment checks	Equipment failure reduced Protects against litigation Helps detect faults	Competent anaesthetists Anaesthetic colleagues Non-anaesthetic colleagues Friends and family	Checking by the ODP or anaesthetic nurse Previous use of equipment Lack of time Patients in vulnerable groups
Alarm silencing on pulse oximeter	Hypoxia really present False alarms Okay if other monitors checked May lead to litigation	Competent anaesthetists Anaesthetic colleagues Non-anaesthetic colleagues Friends and family Hospital managers My anaesthetic teachers	Type of equipment Lower ASA grade False alarm rate Patients in vulnerable groups

Adapted from Beatty and Beatty (2004).

the cultural norms play an important role in understanding violations. The 'way we do things round here' includes basic clinical procedures, as well as less tangible attitudes and values.

A theory of migrations and violations

Violations can be understood from a number of different perspectives, which vary in the nature of the explanation advanced and the discipline from which they are derived. We will briefly sketch some of the principal theories and then discuss a framework developed by Rene Amalberti, which integrates the various approaches and which illuminates the whole problem of procedures and how people respond to them.

Previous writers on violations have put forward a number of explanations. Some have simply looked to individual characteristics, variously pointing to laziness, moral turpitude or personality. Certainly, some people are much more prone to ignore basic procedures and safety standards than others, whether these be anaesthetic checks, dangerous overtaking or drunk driving. Persistent and reckless behaviour can, and should, be understood in personal terms and disciplinary action and restraint may be necessary. But this hardly explains the frequency and widespread character of minor violations.

A second group have looked to organizational and cultural characteristics. A classic example of this approach is Diane Vaughan's analysis of the Challenger space shuttle explosion, when safety standards were progressively eased and finally ignored to the point of disaster. Her evocative phrase 'the normalization of deviance' perfectly captures the gradual erosion of standards, the tacit acceptance by the people concerned and the eventual loss of any sense of where the boundary of safety lies.

A third approach views violations as a necessary adaptation of professionals coping with the conflicting demands of complex work situations. From this perspective, violations are not a hazard or indeed necessarily a problem; they reflect the intelligence and flexibility of frontline workers. When people are short of time or the procedures are unworkable, people do whatever is needed to 'get the job done'; these are respectively the routine and necessary violations discussed earlier (Reason, 1990). This particular perspective was most powerfully developed and extended by Jens Rasmussen in his studies of nuclear power workers. You might think that maintenance in nuclear plants would be governed by the strictest rules and procedures, and so it is; the problem is that the demands of the work and the procedures do not always cohere. Rasmussen emphasized that front line workers do not follow procedures in a strict and logical manner, but try to follow the path that seems most useful and productive at the time. Workers operate within an envelope of possible actions, which is influenced all the time by wider organizational and social forces. Rasmussen also described the pressures on individuals and systems to move towards the boundaries of safe operation, as workers are constantly having to adapt and react to pressures for increased performance and productivity, which erode the margins of safety (Rasmussen, 2000).

Rene Amalberti used Rasmussen's framework to study violations of basic safety procedures in aviation, train driving and operating of rotary presses, finding that violations occurred in all settings in response to a range of pressures (Amalberti *et al.*, 2006). In his integrative model, he also considered how a system might evolve, or rather migrate, away from an initial sphere of safe

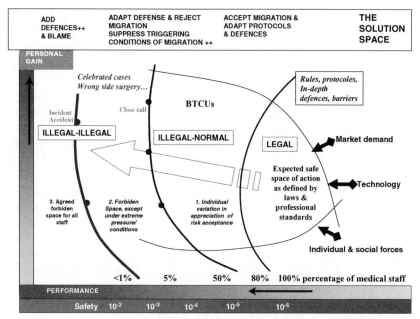

Figure 16.1 A framework for violations and migration (Reproduced from *Quality & Safety in Health Care*, R Amalberti, C Vincent, Y Auroy et al. "Violations and migrations in health care: a framework for understanding and management". **15**, no. suppl_1, [66–71], 2006, with permission from BMJ Publishing Group Ltd.).

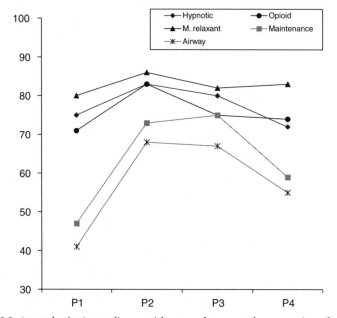

Figure 16.2 Anaesthetists' compliance with new safety procedure over time (from Saint Maurice *et al.*, 2010).

operations towards danger and then finally disaster. Amalberti's illustrative diagram is shown in Figure 16.1; many people, including me, find it baffling at first, but it really captures the fluid nature of procedures and violations. Think of it as an image that brings the concepts to life rather than as a formal quantitative graph.

On the right-hand side, there is a 'safe space' more or less corresponding to the way the system is designed to work according to specified standards and procedures. Imagine an operating theatre or outpatient clinic on a day when everything runs smoothly without too much hurry, there is time to reassure the patients, do all the checks and so forth. However, over time, pressures of various types accumulate to threaten this ideal world and push the system towards the boundary of what he calls the 'borderline tolerated conditions of use' which, just as it says, is the degree of deviation from procedure that is tolerated by those who work there, both front line staff and others. Typically, in a smooth running system, there will be pressures for greater productivity, less use of resources (does this sound familiar?) and occasions where missing or broken equipment forces adaptations and short cuts; add to this that we all, occasionally or frequently, are in a rush to get home, get on to the next case, tired or stressed and apt to stray over the edge. Crucially these occasional lapses become more tolerated over time and move, in Rene's wonderful phrase, to the 'illegal normal' phase of operations. This exactly captures the day-to-day running of many systems where, as we have seen, deviations from procedure are widespread but occasion no particular alarm. Recall, for example, the regular departures from procedure seen in the administration of intravenous medications discussed in Chapter 4 (Taxis and Barber, 2003). The concept routine violations is not part of the thinking of managers and regulators; in truth it is a very uncomfortable realization that much of the time systems, whether healthcare, transport or industry, operate in an 'illegal normal' zone. The system continues in this state however, because the violations have considerable benefits, both for the individuals concerned and for managers who may tolerate them, or even encourage them, in the drive to meet productivity standards.

Over time these violations can become more frequent and more severe, so that the whole system 'migrates' to the boundaries of safety. The same violations may be committed as in the second phase, but these are now routine and so common as to be almost invisible to both workers and managers. The organization becomes accustomed to operating at the margins of safety, echoing the normalization of deviance noted by Diane Vaughan. At this stage, any further deviance may easily result in patient harm, and is generally counted as negligent or reckless conduct. A limited number of individuals, in the absence of a tight social control, are willing to violate basic procedures to the point of recklessness and actual patient harm. Moreover, these individuals are not only a danger to themselves, but also may influence the other workers if no action is taken to control them. Eventually an accident or major incident occurs, forcing some reflection and a renewed emphasis on basic safety standards.

The natural lifespan of a safety rule

The framework presented above, when well explained, brings an immediate sense of recognition in clinical staff, that sense of having something described that you know implicitly but could not necessarily have articulated. However, while the existence of violations and some of the main reasons for them have been documented, there is relatively little empirical data linking violation frequency to the various factors that have been implicated. The idea that a system might migrate over time has been hardly explored, except in cases of extreme breakdown of all standards and procedures. Such cases tend to attract massive publicity but the route to disaster often remains obscure. What we need to understand though is how much deviation is usually tolerated and how systems drift towards disaster over time. One study, carried out by Guillaume St Maurice and colleagues, has explored this issue.

The chief of an anaesthesia unit in a major French hospital introduced a new safety rule stipulating that on the day before surgery anaesthetists had to record in the patient's file the drugs to be used for the induction and maintenance of anaesthesia and the method of upper airway control; this new rule was mandated by the French Society of Anaesthetists and was being introduced across France. These instructions had not previously been formalized as a rule; it was carefully explained and the anaesthetists signed a formal document to confirm their intention to adhere to the new standard. The researchers then assessed compliance with this rule for a year afterwards by checking the anaesthetic records; the anaesthetists involved did not know this but were later informed and interviewed about the rule. Compliance reached over 85% for some items after three months but never reached 100%; after six months it was dropping, but reasonably high. After a year though, compliance with the procedure had dropped to the informal level before the rule had been introduced; its lifespan as an 'effective intervention' was thus less than one year.

When interviewed, it was clear that most of the anaesthetists had intended to follow the rule but, for a number of reasons, gradually slipped back. The rule was not absolutely critical to safety, and there was little feedback or problems if it was not followed. Time pressure, weekend work and unscheduled cases produced lower adherence, while more complex cases led to higher adherence and greater attention to detail. There were also marked differences in individual compliance, with one anaesthetist conspicuously failing to adopt the new rule.

This study does not suggest that rules are not important; far from it. However, if confirmed, it would suggest that rules and procedures do, in a sense, have a natural life span in an organization. They are born, they have a vigorous youth where most people take note of them, they begin to get old and less notice is taken of them and finally they die. The lifespan of individual rules will vary considerably, with core safety standards being maintained, but more peripheral rules can just fade away unless reinforced or monitored. How can this be done?

Managing violations in the clinical team

The arguments set out above suggest that violations present considerable challenges for the management of safety. In most settings they are numerous, and yet comparatively few lead to harm or real danger. They are therefore tolerated and even viewed as normal occurrences in routine work. Furthermore, they are influenced by a range of personal, social and organizational factors and their occurrence may also have a distinct time course as a system migrates to the boundaries of safety or recalibrates following an adverse incident. As yet violations are incompletely understood and the research base remains extremely slender. However, even with this limited knowledge there are some important and immediate practical implications.

First, and most critically, many violations are in a sense invisible to those in the workplace. They know they happen, as we understood from interviews with railway shunters and anaesthetists, but on a daily basis they largely pass unnoticed so no one knows how often they occur. For these reasons, they do not feature in incident reporting systems, unless they have some serious consequence, which is very occasional.

The issue can nevertheless be addressed in meetings between staff, but only if they first accept the reality of constant migration and system drift. Violations are in part a socially determined phenomenon, relying on complicit acceptance by the group, so they can be reduced by a mutual decision that such behaviour will no longer be tolerated. Such discussions can take place in a meeting of clinical staff, provided the culture is open enough to allow such conversations to take place. For such a discussion to be productive, senior clinical staff, and ideally managers, also need to be involved to discuss the acceptability and elasticity of 'rule interpretation'. The very fact that such a discussion takes place is itself a safety measure, in that it makes violations more visible and allows the clinical team to reflect and to pull back from the dangerous edge. In passing, we might note that the frequency of violations is why cross monitoring is so important in high performance teams; team members watch and protect each other and strive to remain in the safety space.

The sheer number of guidelines and procedures in existence ensures that they cannot all be followed, or even remembered. Having a large number of rules that are only partially followed is a particularly dangerous situation, in that some will be really safety critical and others are desirable but not critical; a mixture of 'need to follow' and 'nice to follow' safety rules (Saint Maurice et al., 2010). In a hospital where I work, important anaesthesia guidelines such as 'How to manage anaphylaxis' are pasted on the wall of the anaesthesia room; however, mixed amongst these are relatively trivial matters such as the recent staff policy on clothing and footwear. This indiscriminate juxtaposition has the effect of trivializing all guidelines. When the inevitable deviations occur, compliance with the 'nice-to-follow' rules will be eroded first, but this increases the tolerance for deviation from procedure and so begins to affect compliance with more important rules. When introducing a new policy or procedure therefore, it is important to start by identifying potential barriers and having realistic expectations about compliance. On occasions one might decide against the introduction of a new policy with a limited, even if proven, capacity of safety improvement, particularly if the system was already under pressure.

Procedures are an ideal world

We can begin to see that many rules and procedures are designed without regard for the actual conditions of daily use, as if you designed a car which worked perfectly on a flat indoor surface but was never tested going up a hill in the wind and rain. Although most clinical procedures are written by clinicians who know full well what clinical life is like, the procedures themselves tend to be written as exemplars of a perfect anaesthesia, central line insertion or whatever. When thinking about safety we tend to think of an ideal world of clear rules and procedures, but actually these defences can be extremely fragile. The rules and procedures give a sense of reassurance, but we seldom test them in a different context, for example, during week-ends, or with poorly qualified staff (Amalberti *et al.*, 2006). We need first to understand the pattern of violations and system migration, while gradually changing the staff's behaviour within these systems. In other words, it is best to manage risk than to try to artificially eliminate it, because history shows that sooner or later, defences will be overturned.

References

Amalberti, R., Vincent, C., Auroy, Y. and Saint Maurice, G. (2006) Violations and migrations in health care: a framework for understanding and management. *Quality & Safety in Health Care*, **15**, I66–I7I.

Beatty, P.C. and Beatty, S.F. (2004) Anaesthetists' intentions to violate safety guidelines. *Anaesthesia*, **59**(6), 528–540.

Burke, J.P. (2003) Infection control – a problem for patient safety. *The New England Journal of Medicine*, **348**(7), 651.

Foy, R., Grimshaw, J. and Eccles, M. (2001) Guidelines and pathways, in *Clinical Risk Management*, 2nd edn (ed. C.A. Vincent), BMJ Publications, London.

Gawande, A. (2003) *Complications: A Surgeons Notes on an Imperfect Science*, Picador, New York.

Hale, A.R. and Swuste, P. (1998) Safety rules: procedural freedom or action constraint? *Safety Science*, **29**, 163–177.

Helmreich, R.L. (2000) On error management: lessons from aviation. *British Medical Journal*, **320**, 781–785.

Larson, E.L., Bryan, J.L., Adler, L.M. and Blane, C. (1997) A multifaceted approach to changing handwashing behavior. *American Journal of Infection Control*, **25**(1), 3–10.

Lawton, R. (1998) Not working to rule: Understanding procedural violations at work. *Safety Science*, **28**, 77–95.

McKenna, F.P. and Horswill, M.S. (2006) Risk taking from the participant's perspective: the case of driving and accident risk. *Health Psychology*, **25**(2), 163–170.

Moss, F. (2004) The clinician, the patient and the organisation: a crucial three sided relationship. *Quality and Safety in Health Care*, **13**(6), 406–407.

Pittet, D., Hugonnet, S., Harbarth, S., *et al.* (2000) Effectiveness of a hospital-wide programme to improve compliance with hand hygiene. Infection Control Programme. *Lancet*, **356** (9238),1307–1312.

Pittet, D. (2001) Compliance with hand disinfection and its impact on hospital-acquired infections. *Journal of Hospital Infection*, **48**(Suppl A), S40–S46.

Pittet, D., Allegranzi, B., Sax, H.,*et al.* (2005) Considerations for a WHO European strategy on healthcare-associated infection, surveillance, and control. *The Lancet Infectious Diseases*, **5**(4), 242–250.

Polet, P., Vanderhaegen, F. and Amalberti, R. (2003) Modelling border-line tolerated conditions of use (BTCU) and associated risks. *Safety Science*, **41**, 111–136.

Rasmussen, J. (2000) The concept of human error. Is it useful for the design of safe systems in healthcare, in *Safety in Medicine* (eds C.A. Vincent and B. de Mol), Elsevier, Oxford.

Reason, J.T. (1990) *Human Error*, Cambridge University Press, New York.

Saint Maurice, G., Auroy, Y., Vincent, C. and Amalberti, R. (2010) The natural lifespan of a safety policy: violations and system migration in anaesthesia. *Quality and Safety in Health Care*, vol. In press.

Taxis, K. and Barber, N. (2003) Ethnographic study of incidence and severity of intravenous drug errors. *British Medical Journal*, **326**(7391), 684–687.

CHAPTER 17
Safety skills

Clinical staff, in addition to simply doing their jobs well, actively create safety as they work. At the coal face, minute by minute, safety may either be eroded by the actions and omissions of individuals or, conversely, created by skilful, safety conscious professionals. As we discussed in the previous chapter, people partly create safety by being conscientious, disciplined and following rules. However, the treatment of complex, fluctuating conditions also requires thinking ahead and being prepared to adjust treatment as the patient's condition changes. When thinking about safety however, we are also calling on a broader vision in which the clinician is anticipating not only the disease, but the functioning of the organization in which they work, assessing the hazards emanating from both. Safety, from this broader perspective, requires anticipation, awareness of hazards, preparedness, resilience and flexibility, the qualities that those studying high reliability organizations have sought to capture and articulate.

In this chapter, we will examine some of the critical, but somewhat intangible personal skills and behaviours that are particularly relevant to safety. Anyone in healthcare will know nurses, doctors and others who have the qualities of anticipation, awareness of hazards, the calm and the confidence to navigate the dangers of clinical work, and indeed the dangers of healthcare organizations. Expert clinicians, indeed experts in many fields, have always developed such skills; we are not making new discoveries. However, these skills are seldom explicitly identified or formally trained, though there have been very important developments in the training of non-technical skills in the operating theatre. We will focus on hazard awareness, situation awareness, anticipation, foresight and decision making; leadership and other team orientated skills will be considered in the following chapter, which examines teamwork.

Safety skills, attitudes and behaviour in industry

The idea of teaching specific safety attitudes and behaviours is unusual in healthcare but deeply embedded in a number of hazardous industries. For instance, the Western Mining Corporation in Western Australia is an exemplar of creating 'error wisdom' within its organization and front line staff. Their motto is 'Take time, take charge', which aims to get workers to stop and think, to

Patient Safety, 2nd edition. By Charles Vincent. Published 2010 by Blackwell Publishing Ltd.

spend time assessing potential hazards before acting. Those training British Army officers at Sandhurst Military Academy have developed an approach called the Seven Questions to develop foresight skills. Trainee officers are taught to carry out mini-risk assessments of their environment, resources, terrain and contingencies by repeatedly cycling through a series of questions as they plan and implement a mission. The approach involves the use of the acronym DODAR: Decide, Overview, Diagnose, Act, Review, which provides a structured ways of analysing the environment. This is supported by realistic simulated training exercises to ensure that the skills become a fundamental component of an officer's way of working in the field (Taylor Adams *et al.*, 2008).

The oil industry has driven safety particularly strongly, with concern for people, pressure from regulators and business efficiency all being powerful drivers. Lost time, accidents and fatalities have a major impact on the people involved and can cost millions if a plant needs to be shut down. In the oil industry, ESSO has introduced a programme called 'step back by five'. The idea of this programme is that before starting a new job the employee should metaphorically take five steps back and take time to think about what might go wrong during a task and what action they would take if the risk became realized. British Petroleum has a set of 'Golden Rules' (Boxes 17.1 and 17.2) covering all the major hazards which are rigorously enforced; making an error is accepted, but recklessly ignoring safety standards is a sacking offence, whether or not one 'gets away with it'.

Healthcare also has some similar strongly reinforced rules through health and safety regulations; however, these are largely aimed at protecting the staff from injuring themselves. Curiously, the same standards are not applied to the delivery of clinical treatments, with some notable exceptions such as the delivery of radiotherapy which is heavily regulated. Just imagine if healthcare strictly applied BPs permit to work to every hazardous clinical activity; the system would grind to a halt within hours. In the longer term though, both staff and patients would probably be considerably safer.

BOX 17.1 BP's Golden rules of safety:

- Permit to Work
- Working at Heights
- Energy Isolation
- Vehicle Safety
- Ground Disturbance
- Confined Space Entry
- Lifting Operations
- Management of Change

(BRITISH PETROLEUM, HTTP://WWW.BP.COM)

BOX 17.2 Permit to work: an example of a golden rule

Before conducting work that involves confined space entry, work on energy systems, and ground disturbance in locations where buried hazards may exist, or hot work in potentially explosive environments, a permit must be obtained that:

- defines scope of work;
- identifies hazards and assesses risk;
- establishes control measures to eliminate or mitigate hazards;
- links the work to other associated work permits or simultaneous operations;
- is authorized by the responsible person(s);
- communicates above information to all involved in the work;
- ensures adequate control over the return to normal operations.
  Are you trained and competent to perform this work?
  You have an obligation to stop the work if it's unsafe.

(BRITISH PETROLEUM, HTTP://WWW.BP.COM)

An interesting and instructive aspect of the approach taken to safety in the oil industry is the way that safety thinking and action permeates all aspects of the work and workplace, even areas which are not generally thought of as hazardous. During a talk, an oil industry head of safety recalled reminding his chief executive not to tip his chair back during meetings and, more remarkably, was thanked rather than abused for this reminder (Motterhead, personal communication). Not tipping your chair back at a meeting? Surely this is petty in the extreme, health and safety taken to absurd lengths? Not necessarily. First, British Petroleum knows from the analysis of safety data that minor injuries in offices cost them a great deal of lost time and money. More important though, this approach inculcates a constant awareness of hazard and attention to safety issues, whether on an oil platform or in the board room. This extends to life outside work, as seen by the way oil industry people are more likely to check for fire exits in hotels, counting doors to the exit to know how many to pass if the corridor is full of smoke.

Safety skills in healthcare

In an earlier chapter, we examined the tragic case of David James as a means of showing that a full understanding of such events can only be achieved by considering the wider healthcare system, its structure, flaws and conflicts. However, taking a systems view of medical error in no way implies ignoring the contribution of the staff; the case can equally be used to examine the actions of individuals. Neale (2004) re-examined the case of David James, pointing out that, although it reveals many organizational problems, the death might have been avoided if individuals had been more safety aware and taken responsibility:

If the appropriate person in the Department of Health (who had known of the problems for many years) had taken real responsibility; if David and his family had accepted the need to adhere to appointments; if the consultant had provided a fail safe means of contact and insisted that he alone had the skills necessary to ensure safe administration of chemotherapy; if the pharmacy technician had been made to feel that he was more than a provider; if the unit managers had insisted that no one would be allowed on the unit without adequate induction; and if the SHO and registrar had striven to know how to safely administer chemotherapy, David would be alive today.

(*CLINICAL RISK*, NEALE, G. "SYSTEMS FAILURE". **10**, NO.5, 195–196, 2004. REPRODUCED WITH PERMISSION OF THE ROYAL SOCIETY OF MEDICINE PRESS)

The case, used to illustrate systems failure, equally illustrates the role of personal qualities and skills as a key factor in the erosion, or creation, of safety. Those involved failed to see the inherent hazards in the system.

In an effort to reflect on the key skills and attributes of safe, but effective, clinicians, Sonal Arora and Susy Long interviewed a number of clinical staff who identified dozens of relevant characteristics which were then grouped into several broad categories. This work is in an early stage of development but some of the initial skills and personal attributes identified are shown in Box 17.3. Reviewing the preliminary list of categories introduces us to the concept of safety skills and shows that clinical staff are very conscious of the importance of these attitudes, behaviours and skills. Note especially that people identified a large number of character traits such as humility, honesty and conscientiousness; we perhaps cannot train these attributes, but we can certainly foster them in the wider culture and ethos of the organization. Some of the skills however, are more tangible and we will examine some of the key ones: hazard awareness, situation awareness, anticipation, vigilance and decision making. Be aware though, that books have been written about these topics and we will only be able to highlight some key points of particular relevance to healthcare.

BOX 17.3 Safety skills, behaviours and personal attributes in healthcare

Conscientiousness

Being thorough and meticulous with administrative tasks, looking up results and so on.

Not always assuming that the information you have been provided with is correct and checking things yourself.

Humility

If I have a junior who is over confident, I actually see him as more dangerous than someone who's inexperienced.

Not being too proud or overly confident to ask for help. Will take advice from nurses and juniors.

Honesty

If you make a mistake, take it personally and do blame yourself for it, because then prevention will also become personal. Don't blame the system completely for everything.

Openly communicating mistakes, issues and areas of concern.

Self awareness

Be aware of your own abilities and state of mind at times when negative life events may affect your judgements and working ability.

If you are very tired, you have to take a break. You actually stop and . . . you say, I'm going out.

Confidence

To be able to question oneself and others without indicating that this is due to a lack of confidence.

Confidence to speak up if you notice any potential hazards.

Situation awareness

Being error-aware and recognize situations that may give rise to errors, such as stress or high workload.

Being aware of the situation in your immediate and somewhat less immediate work environment – for instance, difficult patients, or patients that have undergone major procedures, or patients who have been transferred to a remote ward and might fall off staff's radar, and so on.

Vigilance and open mindedness

Recognizing clinical patterns but not ignoring facts that don't fit. Vigilance for any deviation from the expected course of events.

Being mentally alert – a situation soon to get out of hand may or may not manifest itself in advance via warning signs. Think what you might be missing. What is the worst case scenario?

Anticipation and preparedness

Contingency planning – if patient fails to improve with a, we will try b and c. If x happens, we will escalate care to y. This instead of 'let's wait and see and we'll make up our minds if and when something goes wrong.'

One thing that I do on a daily basis is to think, what could go wrong today? And I try to cover for that; so the equipment that I need, the people that I need, the information that I think is critical, but could be missing.

Team working and communication

Communication with everybody, regardless of status. Sharing views and management plans. Staff should not assume that others will think similarly, or have the same perception of a situation.

If you initiate an action, make it absolutely clear who is to do what, when – and who is to be called if the patient goes 'off track'– and who will review progress when.

Leadership

Being available and ensure this is perceived by all colleagues: this allows people to approach, discuss issues, ask for help and facilitates learning and immersion into work environment.

Projecting a sense of calm, even when internally uncertain or stressed. Awareness of the need to provide effective leadership.

Putting on your second hat: awareness of fallibility and hazard

Mostly we do not have time to reflect or study our working environment because we have to just get on with the work. And yet, where safety is concerned, a reflective attitude and some anticipation of potential problems are essential. My surgical colleague Krishna Moorthy describes this as putting on his 'second hat'. His first hat is as a surgeon engaged in the daily routine, and occasional crises, of complex surgery. The second hat describes the mental stepping back to reflect and anticipate problems, to see the vulnerabilities of the system and to see the world through safety spectacles as replete with hazard and uncertainty. Let us think a little more about what this might mean in practice.

The first step towards safety for the individual healthcare professional is to appreciate the ubiquity and multiple sources of error and hazard and then consider how it applies in one's own environment. Which are the most dangerous processes on the ward? Which are most prone to error and failure? When is the system at its most vulnerable? When are errors most likely to occur? What are the principal forms of harm that may afflict patients in this environment? Really grappling with this requires openness about error and a willingness to discuss the hazards and dangers of the environment, as a team is much more likely to be able to monitor and prevent error than an individual. Anyone at any level can foster openness about error and hazard. A nurse running a ward can make it clear that it is acceptable to discuss the possibility of error; can constantly reinforce the possibilities for error, the need for anticipation and cross-checking. The most junior nurse can steer a new doctor away from a hazardous situation. All of this is critical safety conscious behaviour.

An understanding of error and its causes can help one become error aware, in the sense of heightening one's vigilance in error prone situations. James

Reason (2004) has suggested a simple, but memorable way of doing this: the three bucket model. This provides a simple way of assessing when alarm bells should be ringing in your head. The three buckets correspond to three factors that affect performance and the likelihood of error: yourself, the context and the task you are carrying out. If, for instance, you are carrying out a new procedure for the first time unsupervised, you are tired and hungry and the environment is noisy and distracting, then all three buckets are full and you should be very wary (you may decide for yourself what the buckets are full of, conjuring up your own particular image). When conditions are particular bad, particularly error prone as it were, it is best to step back if at all possible to see if the procedure can be delayed until conditions are more favourable, such as when you have had a chance to get some food, get some help or deal with some of the distractions. This is a much more skilful approach to hazardous environments than just ploughing on regardless with an impregnable belief in one's own abilities and a trusting assumption that things will turn out alright. Whether approaches of this kind can be learned and applied as a particular error skill remains to be seen.

Does reading about safety, researching safety and reflecting on the ways things can go wrong make any difference to clinical practice? Consider the findings summarized so far in this book. Patients are frequently harmed, often preventably; errors are common in every area of medicine yet examined; while people are resourceful, there are certain limitations to human cognition that markedly increase the chance of error; healthcare systems and processes have evolved, rather than been designed, and tend to be long, unnecessarily complex, unco-ordinated and prone to failure; the working conditions of many healthcare professionals are far from ideal, thus increasing the chances of error. Anecdotally, being involved in safety research and practice does seem to influence clinical work. When I asked some of my clinical colleagues if their engagement in safety research had influenced their practice, their response was that it certainly had (Box 17.4).

BOX 17.4 Safety in clinical practice

- Being more vigilant in terms of errors that occur in day-to-day practice, which I may have missed in the past. Being willing to address loose ends rather than say this is not part of my problem.
- Involving the patient in their care. For example, always asking the patient which side they thought they were having the operation.
- Being more explicit about my instructions, discussing everything I think or intend to do to with the patient and gaining opinions of other colleagues.
- At handover always summarizing the situation, outlining the plan and being absolutely clear about what to monitor and at what point I want to be called.

- Ensuring documentation of everything.
- I do not undertake any procedure unless I am sure I am competent in performing it or have adequate supervision.
- Senior clinicians say they want their juniors to err on the side of safety, yet many younger clinicians do not follow that principle for fear of seeming weak. I make a point of reminding myself day after day that I want to be safe first and brave afterwards.
- Spending longer with patients, explaining and discussing the risks and benefits of treatment.
- Being obsessive about hand washing. I am now very aware of why we are asked to do this and so less irritated about the time it takes.
- Having enough humility to recognize when you are stepping beyond your depth and willingness to ask for help.

(JACKLIN, OLSEN, SARKER, UNDRE, PERSONAL COMMUNICATION)

Safety and non-technical skills

In the rest of the chapter, we will draw heavily on the pioneering work of Rhona Flin and colleagues (Flin, O'Connor and Crichton, 2008), who have studied, analysed and been involved in developing training for non-technical skills in surgery, anaesthesia, aviation, oil and gas industry, nuclear power and the military. Non-technical skills are very similar to the safety skills attitudes and behaviours discussed above, but focused more on skills and behaviours that can be identified and trained. Flin, O'Connor and Crichton (2008) define non-technical skills as:

The cognitive, social and personal resource skills that complement technical skills and contribute to safe and efficient task performance. They are not new or mysterious skills but are essentially what the best practitioners do in order to achieve consistently high performance and what the rest of us do on a good day.
(FLIN, O'CONNOR AND CRICHTON, 2008)

The identification of non-technical skills rests partly on studies and direct observation of experts, but also on analyses of accidents in many different arenas where a lack of these skills has precipitated or failed to prevent disaster. As Flin, O'Connor and Crichton point out, these skills are essential for day-to-day work as well as in crises, but emerge as particularly critical at times of danger. Front line personnel are the last line of defence, whether in acting promptly to prevent an oil refinery fire or in controlling bleeding during an operation. These skills are not 'soft skills' but critical skills that are essential to safe and efficient technical operations; communication usually means communication about technical issues, decision making usually means decisions about technical issues and so on. Nor are these skills tied to particularly personalities. Perhaps some people are naturally better communicators or team players than others but, when the skills are clearly delineated, anyone can learn them. Rhona Flin quotes one airline telling its pilots 'you can have any personality you like, but this is the behaviour we expect on our flight decks.'

Situation awareness

Situation awareness conveys something more than just paying attention to what you are doing. As the term implies, in a hazardous environment, one needs to have a broader understanding of the task, the environment, and how events might unfold in the future. So, a nurse in intensive care might be recording observations, but also thinking about the coming shift change, the fact that the doctor is new to the unit and that the patient is not responding as rapidly as they should be to the treatment. These are the three core elements of situation awareness:

• Gathering information in the sense of ongoing monitoring of the situation;
• Interpretation of that information – why is the patient not responding?
• Anticipation – what is the critical information to hand over at the shift change?

The term originates in the military through the need to have a constant awareness of the enemy's movements and to interpret and anticipate their plans. Situation awareness emerged as a critical focus of safety training because of the numerous accidents in which a loss of awareness of the wider environment played a part. 'Controlled flight into terrain' is the classic example, where a pilot flies a well functioning plane into the ground because they have misinterpreted the height above ground. In accident enquiries, people report 'I hadn't noticed that ...', 'We were very surprised when ...' Loss of situation awareness is being 'out of the loop' (Flin, O'Connor and Crichton, 2008).

Gathering information involves scanning and monitoring the environment for relevant information and in particular for signs of change from the expected state. Rhona Flin provides an illuminating and memorable example of a fire fighter appraising the situation on arrival at the scene (Box 17.5). Anaesthetists watch the monitors to detect a fall in blood pressure or changes in oxygen saturation, but may also be alert for tensions in the surgical team, the fact that the surgeon has been distracted by a conversation about another patient and the tension in the team because the case is taking longer than expected and the next case is an emergency. The interpretation lies in assessing the clinical state of the patient or in realizing that the team is reacting to the inexperience of the surgeon and the wider organizational pressures to maintain productivity, potentially at the expense of safety.

BOX 17.5 A fire fighter assesses a fire

It is important for the firefighter to train his mind to 'tune in and observe' the essential features as he responds to every fire call.... Get an early glimpse of the structure from a distance where possible and scan all faces on the road for signs of fire. What is the roof access like? What type of structure is it? Is the construction likely to present unusual hazards? Is there a haze in the air that may suggest smoke is already in view? The more information you absorb at this stage, the more effective you will be when it comes to taking any necessary rapid action. All this should be taken in during the time it takes to walk off the pumper and into the building.

(ADAPTED FROM FLIN, O'CONNOR AND CRICHTON, 2008).

Anticipation and vigilance

Anticipation is a key component of expertise in many areas, and an essential component of full situation awareness. Essentially it involves thinking ahead and envisioning possible problems and hazards. If you drive a car in heavy rain you need to constantly think about what might happen. Suppose the types don't grip? Suppose the car in front brakes suddenly? Suppose a car pulls out in front, having failed to see my car? In a study of the control of fighter aircraft, Amalberti and Deblon (1992) found that in pre-mission planning, which often took longer than the mission itself, pilots spent a great deal of time analysing each part of the route for possible threats, whether from hostile aircraft, personal factors, weather or technical breakdown. During the flight itself, pilots devoted over 90% of the time when they were free to think to anticipation; typically they developed a 'tree' of events which might occur, which became more or less salient over the course of the flight.

Experts are constantly thinking ahead and looking to the future. For instance, Cynthia Dominguez showed surgeons a video of an operation involving an 80-year-old woman with an infected gallbladder that needed to be removed. She used the video as a prompt to ask the surgeons how they prepared for such an operation and what they would be thinking at each stage. She found that experienced surgeons made more predictions about likely problems than their junior colleagues. In particular, they predicted, and were thus prepared for, that they would have difficulty in dissecting and identifying the surrounding structures, because the gallbladder and surrounding areas would be swollen and inflamed. Second, they predicted a higher risk of complications such as an injury to nearby structures or tearing of the gall bladder itself, thus releasing bile and increasing the chance of abdominal infection (Dominguez *et al.*, 2004). With these predictions in mind, they were therefore mentally prepared for the hazards that lay ahead; like the fighter pilots, they mentally mapped the route and anticipated likely hazards along the way.

Having tried to anticipate all possible threats and hazards, the pilots in Amalberti and Deblon's study would then mentally simulate a response to see if it would resolve the problems; if not they would see if they could adjust the flight in some way so that they could deal with all contingencies. A key component of the pilots' expertise lay in predicting and avoiding dangerous situations. Expertise is not so much an ability to improvise and escape danger (their improvised solutions were often quite poor) but the ability to stay within an envelope of safe operation and to have prepared strategies to deal with problems. Similarly expert clinicians do not rely on their brilliance at escaping from dangerous situations but on trying to avoid them in the first place and having solid routines to fall back on when a crisis does emerge. Running through in your mind what you will do if some particular problem occurs, is a powerful way of preparing yourself for the eventuality (Box 17.6). Bob Wears, an emergency physician, reminded me that when a crisis occurs one does not so much rise to the occasion as fall back on one's preparation and training.

BOX 17.6 Anticipation and preparedness in surgery

You need to have a strategy ready when there is bleeding: cold, automatic responses to a hazardous situation ingrained in your mind so that it can be done without stress and strain. What to do if the groin starts to bleed is one of the worst situations. When teaching I give them a list of things they're going to do. I get them to repeat it to me over and over again so that when it does happen to them, and it will eventually, they don't need to think, they just go into autopilot.

The first thing is to put a pack in, which stops the bleeding. The second thing is to ask for some extra help; you need another person to use the sucker, because often you're on your own with the theatre sister. Third, you need to tell the anaesthetist you've got some bleeding. You then need to elevate the foot of the bed, which lessens the amount of bleeding and to extend the wound without moving the pack. Once you've got it controlled, you can get everything else you need sorted out. Make sure you've got the right instruments, the right support, the anaesthetist knows what's going on and you have everything ready, so when you take the pack out you have help and suction and view and all the things you need to deal with the situation. The sucker will show you where the bleeding's coming from and you deal with it. When they know all this by rote, then dealing with the problem becomes routine.

In healthcare, it is critical to anticipate problems that may arise in the clinical team or the wider organization. Anaesthesia is ideally a routine procedure but a life threatening emergency can occur at any time; anaesthetists are trained in numerous emergency routines and in maintaining a constant awareness of what might happen. Experienced anaesthetists ensure that they have a supply of equipment for emergencies and drugs that will, for instance, correct a rapidly falling heart rate. This kind of preparation sounds obvious and, in a sense it is, but it is difficult to constantly maintain this kind of 'emergency awareness' day after day, especially if few emergencies actually occur. Paradoxically, the safer a unit is, the harder it is to believe that disaster may strike at any time.

Vigilance means anticipating the disease but also the vagaries of the organization and the possibility that others may not check as assiduously as you would wish. My colleague Ros Jacklin expresses this clearly in an example that spans all the stages of situation awareness:

I feel that one of the keys to being a safe practitioner comes down to vigilance – looking for problems before they happen, when they still are in the brewing stage. For instance, if you are on call, find out who has been operated on that day, and have a brief look at them before you go to bed, whether or not anyone specifically asks you to. If the patient looks dry, you might check that there's nothing to suggest bleeding, and increase their fluids a little overnight. Otherwise, no one notices that they are dry until their urine output has dropped. If that were to happen, you can probably easily rectify the patient's fluid status with IV fluids at this stage, but if for any reason there is a delay, the patient may find themselves in established renal failure.
(JACKLIN, PERSONAL COMMUNICATION)

In addition to being vigilant oneself, the clinician looking ahead at potential problems will also be assessing how vigilant the staff on the next shift are likely to be.

Sometimes a clinician will end a shift knowing that they have left the patients in safe hands; at other times, with a less than conscientious person taking over, a nagging anxiety remains and they may consider that a few additional checks and enquiries are warranted.

Decision making

Decision making lies at the heart of all clinical practice, yet has attracted relatively little attention within either patient safety or in the broader quality improvement literature. The emphasis on systems and process improvement has deflected attention from human performance in general and decision making in particular. One reason for this is that decision making, and failures of decision making, fall into the 'too hard' category that have been set aside while we addressed more tangible process and system problems. Decisions making is also a sensitive issue, deeply bound up with professional identify and personal pride in professional work. To be challenged on the clinical decisions one has made, especially if they had adverse consequences, can be a wounding experience.

Decision making has been extensively studied and there is a vast psychological literature, and related work in economics, management, military and industrial settings. There is also an extensive and long established literature on medical decision making, but it has not had the impact on clinical practice and training that it deserves. All we can hope to do in a short section in the context of safety and quality is to highlight its importance and to suggest that developing methods of teaching and training clinical decision making are going to be a critically important to patient safety in the next few years. We will use decision making in surgery to illustrate the main approaches.

Clinical decisions: adapting strategies to context

Decision making is essentially the process of making a judgement or choosing an option in a condition of uncertainty. The extent of uncertainty will vary enormously, particularly within clinical work. A patient may arrive in the emergency room with an acute shortness of breath and a known history of asthma and the decision to give the standard treatment may be relatively clear cut; the next patient may present with a mystifying and atypical range of symptoms, which could stem from a dozen or more different conditions. The extent of uncertainty, and indeed the potential for use of decision support, depends very heavily on the extent to which a problem is already framed and structured.

In the context of clinical skills, Flin, O'Conner and Crichton present a useful classification of decision-making methods (Table 17.1). We will briefly consider three of the four approaches, setting aside the rarer need for completely improvisational, creative decision making:

Table 17.1 Senior surgeons' decision making

Decision making method	Surgeon's Statement
Recognition primed decisions	I am under extreme time pressure … the bleeding must be controlled rapidly and I have 20 min before the kidney dies. I tell the anaesthetists immediately as I find the source of the bleeding and arrange for it to be clamped. I need to keep the good kidney alive so get some cold saline into the kidney
Rule-based decision making	If damage is occurring then you want to stop, especially according to clinical governance guidelines. Part of the clinical expertise lies in doing but the other part is in recognizing when you are struggling and knowing that 'first do no harm', so I decided to stop and get a second opinion
Choosing between options	There were three options to consider and at this point we had to balance the potential risk of problems in the post-operative period with the risks of doing something intra-operatively
Creative decision making	None of the usual joints would work so we had to adapt a different one in order to make it fit

Adapted from Flin, O'Connor and Crichton, 2008: p. 56.

Intuitive recognition primed decision making

Classical decision theory espouses an orderly vision of rational actors weighing and balancing choices. It is grounded in a strong tradition of ingenious, laboratory based experiments generally using well structured problems and volunteer subjects, who are often undergraduates. Sophisticated experimental methods have emerged from this, some of which have proved applicable to surgery (Jacklin *et al.*, 2008a). However, these approaches have seldom used expert decision makers and the structured, formal approaches have not proved to be easily translatable into contexts where decisions must be made rapidly and without obvious deliberation.

Naturalistic decision making (NDM) emerged in the late 1980s, partly in response to the realization that poor decisions had led to major accidents in a variety of settings. NDM researchers aimed to study experts making decisions in their own working environments, usually in conditions of high uncertainty, time pressure, shifting goals and often inadequate resources for the task. Firefighters, military personnel and acute medicine all require this kind of decision making. Work pioneered by Gary Klein (1998) and others suggested that decision making in these contexts was characterized, not by a formal weighing up of options, but by an immediate recognition of the nature of the challenge being faced. Experts in these contexts recognized a roof that was about to collapse or a patient who might arrest and reacted immediately, basing their response on memories of previous similar emergencies and drawing on a repertoire of previously used strategies. Typically, the situation evolves rapidly, depending on whether the roof does or does not fall, requiring a sequence of decisions on a moment-by-moment basis. The emphasis in on immediate workable decisions and solutions that are good enough, rather than a perfectly calculated choice.

Rule-based decision making

With rule-based decision making, the clinician, pilot or operator has to identify the situation they are facing, but is then able to identify a learned set of rules or procedures that should be adopted. Pilots, for instance, are trained in a wide variety of both routine and emergency procedures that, once initiated, follow a standard pattern. Pilots of commercial airliners are expected to have memorized all standard emergency procedures, for which they will have rehearsed mentally and trained in practice in simulators; where time allows, they are also expected to actually check the flight manual to ensure they follow the procedure to the letter.

Medicine too has an extensive set of rule-based procedures, such as giving drugs or setting up intravenous lines, and emergencies, such as a failed intubation or resuscitation after a cardiac arrest. Such routines are much better developed in some specialties than others, depending on the precision with which they can be identified and the taste of the practitioners for living dangerously and relying on an intuitive response. Anaesthesia is particularly rich in standardized emergency routines, particularly appropriate and necessary for a speciality which involves long periods of vigilance, monitoring and adjustment interspersed with periodic life threatening emergencies (Williamson and Runciman, 2009). The use of such procedures is critical for both novices, as a guide as to what action to take, and for experts who, while they may understand what action to take, can react much more quickly if they have acquired a repertory of established routines. Such routines will never, of course, encompass all possible crises and there is always the danger of choosing the wrong procedure and then struggling to regain control. As one expert expressed it, 'true decision making starts when procedures run out, and they will in my experience' (Flin, O'Connor and Crichton, 2008).

Clinical judgement and choices

Choosing one of several options is a much more analytical process than either intuitive or rule-based procedures, involving assessing the information available, assessing the support it lends to the options available, then weighing up and comparing the options before making a choice. This may be done very rapidly, as an emergency physician diagnoses a myocardial infarction within a couple of minutes, or slowly, as the possibility of lung cancer or pneumonia are assessed in a series of investigations. These diagnostic choices are the most immediate examples and it is tempting to think that the initial diagnosis is the primary focus of such choices. In fact such 'choice points' occur throughout the patient journey and the decisions made are variously governed by recognition, rules and analytic choice and weighing of options. This is well illustrated in a study carried out by Ros Jacklin and Nick Sevdalis, in which they interviewed expert surgeons to identify the decisions they made while assessing and treating symptomatic gallstones; these can be summarized in a single diagram illustrating the complexity of the process and the considerable number of critical decisions. Curiously, this decision chain is not usually mapped out and seems never to be explicitly taught.

Some of these decisions are rule-based, though interestingly many of the 'rules' are personal ones which may or may not be more widely accepted by the surgical community or backed by any available evidence. An initial decision is whether to do an open (Hasson) port insertion or use a Verres needle. This decision relates to the technique used to gain access to the abdominal cavity in order to inflate it with carbon dioxide, thereby creating a working space within which to insert the instruments via ports through the abdominal wall.

Which technique to use remains a matter for individual preference, with surgeons expressing their own personal rules, ranging from always using the open method through to always using a Verres needle, with an intermediate category in which some surgeons use the Verres needle unless there is abdominal scarring with associated risk of adhesions. This was illustrated by the following excerpts:

I always use an open technique to do this, sometimes it can be a time-consuming part of the operation, particularly in a fat person.

Even though the recommendation is of an open pneumoperitoneum, if it's a virgin abdomen, I would probably still use the Verres. However, if there's any scars or any history to suggest intra-abdominal adhesions, then an open Hasson technique.
(JACKLIN *ET AL.*, 2008A, 2008B)

Other choices, however, are much more solidly based on risk estimation and a more formal judgement process, involving weighing the evidence and choosing the best course of action. For instance, patients have to be warned that there is a risk of conversion from a closed (laparoscopic) procedure to an open (traditional) operation:

I would give them a 2% conversion risk and tell them about risks of bleeding and biliary tree damage.

There is about a 4% risk they might be converted to open and obviously we could not wake them up to ask them, so we consent them for both.
(JACKLIN *ET AL.*, 2008A, 2008AB)

In practice, clinicians, and other experts, do not of course carefully weigh up each choice – this would take too much time; instead they rely on rules of thumb based on experience, reading and observation of colleagues' practice. These heuristics are essentially simple, but approximate rules, which aid decision making by simplifying the situation and decision to be made. 'Common diseases occur commonly' is an example, simply reminding the clinician of the base probability of a particular disease; a myocardial infarction is, statistically speaking, a more likely explanation of symptoms than an obscure myopathy seen only once or twice a year. However, these heuristics can also lead one astray, hence the frequent use of the term 'heuristics and biases'. In extensive combing of the psychological and medical literature, Pat Croskerry, an emergency physician with a background in psychology, has identified almost 30 of these heuristics, which have implications for clinical medicine (Table 17.2). Croskerry (2009a) uses the term 'cognitive dispositions to respond' (CDRs) as a neutral descriptive term, which captures the sense that these dispositions can both help us (when they are described as heuristics) or lead us astray (when they are described as biases).

Training in decision making

Doctors, nurses and other healthcare staff receive almost no training in decision making. This statement is at first glance transparently false; surely medical and nursing students are endlessly drilled in the signs and symptoms of disease and in recognizing particular constellations. A distinction has to be made though between the content of decision making and the process; students and trainees receive plenty of training in the signs and symptoms of disease. However, few of us in any field are ever given any guidance in how best to make decisions. Can we improve the accuracy of clinical decision making?

As Pat Croskerry notes, most researchers have taken a very pessimistic view of the possibility of influencing apparently hard wired cognitive dispositions; the experimental literature has apparently not encouraged a more positive view (Croskerry, 2009b). The reality, however, is that there are quite a number of potentially useful strategies and at the moment we just do not know which of them, if any, might have positive effects. Training in decision making, as opposed to describing the signs to look for, barely exists in medicine. Somehow

Table 17.2 Examples of cognitive dispositions to respond

Diagnostic biases	
Availability	Overestimating probability of a diagnosis when instances are relatively easy to recall
Confirmation	Selectively gathering and interpreting evidence that confirms a diagnosis and ignoring evidence that might disconfirm it
Hindsight bias	Overestimating probability of a diagnosis when the correct diagnosis is already known
Regret	Overestimating probability of a diagnosis with severe possible consequences because of anticipated regret if diagnosis were missed
Representativeness	Overemphasising evidence that resembles a class of events. Can lead to undervaluing of relevant base rates, ignoring regression to the mean and gambler's fallacy
Treatment biases	
Regret/outcome	Feeling worse about adverse outcomes due to active treatment than to inaction, and taking more credit for treatment decisions that lead to positive outcomes than those that lead to adverse outcomes
Framing	Choosing riskier treatments when they are described in negative (e.g. mortality) terms rather than positive (e.g. survival terms)
Number of alternatives	Choosing a treatment option more often when there are additional alternatives

From Jacklin (2008)

though clinicians do appear to become more expert over time, at least within a narrow range, so it is at least plausible that we might speed this process up and possible that we might improve decision making at every level of experience. Croskerry's suggestions (Table 17.3) are wide ranging, encompassing innovative types of training in which multiple clinical scenarios are presented, essentially mimicking and accelerating the conditions of acquiring expertise, but combined with specific training and feedback of cognitive patterns and the development of the habit of always seeking alternatives, no matter how clear cut the diagnosis seems. Even in this most private and interior process however, the system plays a part. Fatigue, stress and time pressure will impair the most expert diagnostician and attempting to plan work schedules efficiently will also enhance decision making accuracy.

The influence of working conditions

I have been awake for 30 hours and still have at least 5 more hours of work, not to mention 3 procedures. Every time I sit down to try and figure out why Mrs Long's kidney is deteriorating, I fall asleep.
(VOLPP AND GRANDE, 2003)

Table 17.3 Strategies to improve clinical reasoning

Strategy	Mechanism or Action
Improve critical thinking component of clinical reasoning	Establish formal training for critical thinking in medical curricula
Develop insight and awareness	Provide detailed description of known CDRs together with multiple clinical examples illustrating their effects
Consider alternatives	Establish forced consideration of alternative possibilities. The routine generation and consideration of alternative diagnoses. 'What else might this be?'
Decrease reliance on memory	Improve the accuracy of judgements through cognitive aids: mnemonics, clinical practice guidelines, algorithms, handheld computers
Simulation	Develop mental rehearsal, cognitive walk-through strategies or specific clinical scenarios to allow cognitive biases to be made and their consequences observed
Optimise working conditions	Ensure adequate provision of resources and optimize work schedules to reduce fatigue, sleep deprivation and sleep debt
Minimize time pressure	Provide adequate time for quality decision making
Provide feedback	Provide feedback to decision makers that is as rapid and reliable as possible so that errors are immediately appreciated, understood and corrected, which will provide better calibration of decision makers

Adapted from Croskerry (2009b)

Anticipation, preparedness, the ability to think straight, personal drive and personal responsibility are all vulnerable to fatigue. Any clinician is hugely affected by their working environment and the demands, not only of the immediate task, but of the wider organization. Absurdly long hours, with consequent fatigue and stress, are one of the principal factors contributing to errors. The impact of a night's sleep deprivation on hand-eye co-ordination is comparable to that induced by a blood alcohol concentration of 0.10% (Dawson and Reid, 1997). Being cared for by a doctor exhausted by the loss of a night's sleep is, at least in respect of hand-eye co-ordination, equivalent to being cared for by someone who is moderately drunk.

Reviews of the effects of sleep deprivation in other domains show substantial effects on a variety of mental tasks, sustained vigilance and motor skills. Studies in clinical settings have demonstrated a decrement in surgical skills after a night on call (Taffinder *et al.*, 1998), reduced ability to interpret electrocardiograms and slower responses in anaesthetic simulations with some sleep deprived clinicians actually falling asleep during the anaesthetic simulations (Veasey *et al.*, 2002; Weinger and Ancoli-Israel, 2002). Most of these studies have addressed simulated clinical tasks not involving actual patients. However, two substantial recent studies (Lockley *et al.*, 2004; Landrigan *et al.*, 2004) examined the sleep schedules of doctors on different shift systems using continuous recording of eye movements while concurrently assessing the rate of serious clinical errors. The rate of serious clinical errors, monitored by methods that included direct observation, was 22% higher on critical care units during the traditional shift schedule (extended shifts of 24 hours or more) compared with a revised schedule which eliminated long shifts and reduced the number of hours worked each week. Thankfully, several countries are now beginning to take action to reduce doctors' hours, although progress is slow and there are many issues, such as loss of clinical experience during training, to be addressed. In many places however, we still suffer the ludicrous situation in which it is illegal to drive a coach, lorry or train while exhausted, but perfectly acceptable to look after an intensive care unit.

The purpose of raising this issue here, at the end of a chapter on personal contributions to safety, is to stress once again the limits and constraints on human performance. Fatigue and excessive working hours provide us with a particularly powerful example of the way in which individual capacity is constrained and influenced by the working environment and the wider organizational context. The system view neglects the individual, but the individual perspective must always be set in the wider organizational context and address the interplay between the many factors that ultimately determine the care that is delivered to the patient.

References

Amalberti, R. and Deblon, F.(1992) Cognito modelling of fighter aircraft process control: a step towards an intelligent on-board assistance system. *International Journal of Man Machine Studies*, **36**, 639–671.

Croskerry, P. (2009) A universal model of diagnostic reasoning. *Academic Medicine*, **84**(8), 1022–1028.

Croskerry, P. (2009) Critical thinking and reasoning in emergency medicine, *Patient Safety in Emergency Medicine* (eds P. Croskerry *et al.*.), Lippincott Williams & Wilkins, Philadephia, pp. 213–218.

Dawson, D. and Reid, K. (1997) Fatigue, alcohol and performance impairment. *Nature*, **388**(6639), 235.

Dominguez, C., Flach, J.M., McDermott, P.C. *et al.* (2004) The conversion decision in laparoscopic surgery: Knowing your limits and limiting your risks, *Psychological Investigations of Competence in Decision Making* (eds K. Smith, J. Shanteauand P. Johnson), Cambridge University Press, Cambridge, pp. 7–39.

Flin, R., O'Connor, P. and Crichton, M. (2008) *Safety at the Sharp End. A Guide to Non-Technical Skills*, Ashgate, Guildford.

Jacklin, R., Sevdalis, N., Darzi, A. and Vincent, C. (2008a) Mapping surgical practice decision making: an interview study to evaluate decisions in surgical care. *American Journal of Surgery*, **195**(5), 689–696.

Jacklin, R., Sevdalis, N., Harries, C. *et al.* (2008b) Judgment analysis: a method for quantitative evaluation of trainee surgeons' judgments of surgical risk. *American Journal of Surgery*, **195**(2), 183–188.

Klein, G. (1998) *Sources of Power. How People Make Decision*, MIT Press, Boston.

Landrigan, C.P., Rothschild, J.M., Cronin, J.W. *et al.* (2004) Effect of reducing interns' work hours on serious medical errors in intensive care units. *New England Journal of Medicine*, **351**(18), 1838–1848.

Lockley, S.W., Cronin, J.W., Evans, E.E. *et al.* (2004) Effect of reducing interns' weekly work hours on sleep and attentional failures. *New England Journal of Medicine*, **351**(18), 1829–1837.

Neale, G. (2004) Systems failure. *Clinical Risk*, **10**(5), 195–196.

Reason, J. (2004) Beyond the organisational accident: the need for 'error wisdom' on the front line. *Quality and Safety in Health Care*, **13**(suppl_2), ii28–ii33.

Taffinder, N.J., McManus, I.C., Gul, Y. *et al.* (1998) Effect of sleep deprivation on surgeons' dexterity on laparoscopy simulator. *Lancet*, **352**(9135), 1191.

Taylor Adams, S., Brodie, A. and Vincent, C.A. (2008) Safety skills for clinicians: an essential component of patient safety. *Journal of Patient Safety*, **4**(3), 141–147.

Veasey, S., Rosen, R., Barzansky, B. *et al.* (2002) Sleep loss and fatigue in residency training: a reappraisal. *Journal of the American Medical Association*, **288**(9), 1116–1124.

Volpp, K.G. and Grande, D. (2003) Residents' suggestions for reducing errors in teaching hospitals. *New England Journal of Medicine*, **348**(9), 851–855.

Weinger, M.B. and Ancoli-Israel, S. (2002) Sleep deprivation and clinical performance. *Journal of the American Medical Association*, **287**(8), 955–957.

Williamson, J. and Runciman, W.B. (2009) Thinking in a crisis: use of algorithms, *Patient Safety in Emergency Medicine* (eds P. Croskerry *et al.*), Lippincott Williams & Wilkins, Philadephia, pp. 228–234.

CHAPTER 18
Teams create safety

Healthcare is delivered by teams of people rather than by individuals. Even when a patient has a particular relationship with their family doctor, surgeon or nurse, that person is supported by a network of people who are essential for the delivery of safe, effective care. Understanding the variety of healthcare teams, the way they work, the factors that promote or impede teamwork, is critical to the achievement of safe high quality care. As so often in patient safety, we are looking at a small corner of a vast area. There is a substantial literature on teams in many different kinds of organization, and research from a variety of psychological, sociological and management perspectives (Paris, Salas and Cannon-Bowers, 2000). We will briefly introduce some of the principal ideas and findings from this wider literature, but will concentrate on what is known about teamwork in healthcare and its role in improving safety and quality, using examples from obstetrics, intensive care, surgery and anaesthesia.

What is a team?

A team in a formal sense is a group of individuals with a shared, common goal who, while they each have defined individual tasks, achieve their goal by working interdependently and cooperatively. Teams are sometimes little more than a group of individuals brought together by chance, haphazardly struggling to work together; alternatively they may work seamlessly, fluidly and, with few words, communicate, anticipate and respond to each other and to the ebb and flow of the work. Healthcare teams vary hugely in size, complexity, the mix of skills, professions involved and seniority of members. They include, for instance, surgical teams, nurses running a ward, management teams, primary care groups and mental health rapid response teams who deal with acute psychosis across wide geographical areas. Furthermore, each staff member, and in a sense each patient, is a member of a number of different teams.

If you work in a team, as we almost all do, you may not think much about how it functions and what factors make a team work well. Some days, everything just seems to go smoothly and it's a joy to work with your colleagues; on another day, the team is fragmented, every communication seems to be misunderstood, the work takes twice as long as usual and you go

Patient Safety, 2nd edition. By Charles Vincent. Published 2010 by Blackwell Publishing Ltd.

home stressed and exhausted. It's easy to blame others for being difficult or obstructive, which people sometimes are. However, in healthcare, if we look a little deeper, we see that there is a fundamental underlying problem; teams are not designed, teamwork processes are not specified and the whole system relies on goodwill and the native resilience and adaptability of healthcare staff.

Healthcare has much to learn here from teamwork in military and industrial settings. While we try out checklists and other quick interventions, they begin from trying to understand the team. While checklists are valid and useful, we need in the longer term to think more in terms of designing teamwork in the same way as we design equipment. Designing teams, or even thinking about them seriously, means that we have to examine the components and processes and how these fit together to produce a functioning team.

Lemieux-Charles and McGuire (2006) identify three different broad types of healthcare team: teams that deliver care, teams that engage in specific projects such as quality improvement, and management teams. The first two have featured prominently in patient safety initiatives but, as yet, we have less understanding of how boards of hospitals, for instance, approach patient safety. Lemieux Charles and McGuire set out an integrated model of healthcare team effectiveness, which melds organizational and healthcare team models to provide an overview of factors that influence team performance and outcome. I have combined some aspects of this model with our own framework for surgical teams (Healey *et al.*, 2004) to describe the main influences and determinants of clinical team performance (Figure 18.1).

The model first describes the team tasks and formation, sometimes referred to as 'Input factors'. This refers to the basic team set-up – who is in the team, what it is meant to be doing, how much autonomy it has and the rules and standards by which it operates. Team processes describe the actual day-to-day operation of communication between members, the co-ordination of work and so on. The model also points to more subtle group processes, such as how cohesive the team is as a group. The accepted norms and standards are also critical and, as we saw when discussing both procedures and culture, may vary widely. Cutting corners in, for instance, the identification of a patient, might be shrugged off on one ward but attract widespread disapproval on another. The outputs and effectiveness of the team are the quality and safety of care delivered to the patient, but note that they also include the experience of the team members and their reflections on team performance. Finally, the model includes team interventions and a feedback loop in which team training, clinical outcomes and experiences within the team can all influence subsequent team performance.

Underlying a number of specific team skills, such as prioritizing tasks, monitoring each other's work and communicating effectively, is the idea that the team has a common understanding of the task in question and the nature of team work. This is sometimes referred to as a 'shared mental model', analogous to the mental models of the world that each of us has as individuals. One tends to assume that everyone else in the team has the same understanding as you do

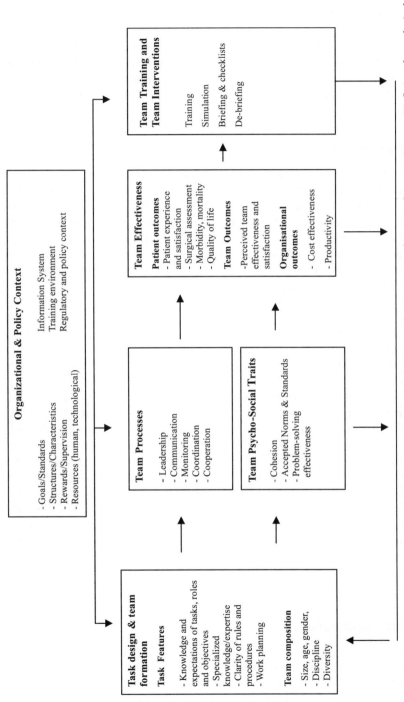

Figure 18.1 Team effectiveness model (Reproduced from *Quality & Safety in Health Care*, A N Healey, S Undre, C A Vincent. "Defining the technical skills of teamwork in surgery". **15**, no. 4, [231–234], 2006, with permission from BMJ Publishing Group Ltd.).

about what is happening, but this may be far from the case. Think back again to the catastrophic role played by assumptions about competence and supervision in the death of David James. Effective, safe teams continually check each other's assumptions so that they never drift too far from a common understanding of the task in hand and their own role in it. This is the reason, in highly skilled and effective teams, for constant team briefing and exchange of information.

Why work in teams?

There is extensive evidence from many different settings, including healthcare, that effective teamwork improves organizational performance in terms both of efficiency and of quality. Reviews of literally hundreds of studies in industry and financial services for instance, have concluded that improved team working can lead to increases in productivity, quality and financial performance (Paris, Salas and Cannon-Bowers, 2000). We know there are many differences between healthcare and other settings, but at the very least this should make us think there may be more to good teamwork than a sense of camaraderie, shared grievances about working life and occasional, though welcome, alcohol-induced team bonding. As we will see, many quite simple team interventions have as their primary goal the re-introduction of these basic team processes.

In their comprehensive review of team effectiveness in healthcare, Lemieux-Charles and McGuire (2006) found some evidence that structuring work in healthcare teams improved quality. For instance, team interventions in the Veterans Administration geriatric service, improved functional status, mental health and even reduced mortality (Caplan *et al.*, 2004). West and colleagues (2002) found an association between management practices in hospitals and patient mortality; in hospitals where more than 60% of staff worked in formal teams, mortality was around 5% lower than would have been expected (West *et al.*, 2002). In a major study of 44 sites and over 6000 people, Daniel Davenport and colleagues (2007) found that reported levels of communication and collaboration in surgical teams, though not team climate or working conditions, were associated with risk adjusted morbidity and mortality in the Veterans Health System. These are important findings but there is still much to learn both about the nature of team performance in healthcare and where our priorities should be for strengthening teamwork.

Teams and safety

Teams, like individuals, may erode or create safety. For instance, in their study of communication in the operating theatre, Lorelei Lingard and colleagues (2004) classified about a quarter of operation relevant communications they observed as communication failures. Events were classified as failures because they were made too late or too early, because essential content was missing, they were addressed to the wrong person or the purpose was simply unclear. The nurses and anaesthetist, for instance, discussed the positioning of the patient for surgery without consulting the surgeon, resulting in wasted time and interpersonal friction later in the case. A team that is not working effectively multiplies the possibility of error. Conversely teams, when working well, have the possibility of being safer than any one individual, because a team can create additional defences against error, by monitoring, double checking and backing each other up; when one is struggling, another assists; when one makes an error, another picks it up.

Patient safety has been particularly influenced by aviation teams and the use of simulation in pilot training; this approach has been particularly important in anaesthesia, and latterly in surgery and emergency medicine (Cooper and Taqueti, 2004). Crew resource management (CRM) is the term commonly used to describe the training of cockpit teams and other aviation teams; the detection and management of error has always been a central component of the more successful training programmes (Helmreich and Merrit, 1998). The CRM training includes instruction in human vulnerability to stressors, the nature of human error and error counter-measures. The objective of the training is to reduce the risk that crews will make a series of important errors, because they failed to foster teamwork, solve problems, communicate and manage their workload effectively (Risser *et al.*, 1999). Notwithstanding the importance of CRM, it is important to realize first that aviation will only be a good parallel for some healthcare teams and second that, as patient safety matures as a discipline, we should be drawing on a wider range of models, research literature and methods of training.

Watching what goes on: observing teamwork

Most teams believe their teamwork is pretty good. But, what do you see when you actually watch a team work? We will look at two examples from surgery, and one from emergency medicine. In the first, my colleagues Shabnam Undre, Andrew Healey and Nick Sevdalis (2007) and others developed a method of assessing the performance of surgical teams, Observational Team Assessment in Surgery (OTAS), in which two observers, usually one clinician and one psychologist, observe team tasks and team behaviours, respectively. For the moment we will just review the team tasks which were divided into three categories:
- *Patient tasks* – related to actions or information associated directly with the patient;
- *Equipment and provisions tasks* – included items such as checking and counting surgical instruments;
- *Communication tasks* – included confirming consent, patient details and operative site.

In an initial study of general surgery, we found that up to a third of standard team tasks were not completed. In a second study of urology surgery teams, we found that the average level of task completion across the three categories of tasks that we observed was higher, in that 83% of the tasks were completed; 93% of patient tasks, 80% for equipment/provisions tasks and 71% for communication tasks. Many fewer equipment/provisions tasks were completed during the preoperative phase (61%) than during the intraoperative phase (91%) or the postoperative phase; the opposite was found for communication tasks (Box 18.1).

BOX 18.1 Examples of team communication tasks

Observational Team Assessment in Surgery (OTAS)

Pre-operative	Surgeon informs of any co-morbidity
	Anaesthetist informs team of special patient needs
	Surgeon briefs team on the surgical procedure
	Scrub-nurse and circulating nurse confirm instruments check
	Correct patient is confirmed verbally by team
Intra-operative	Surgeon asks team whether they are ready to start
	Okay to start acknowledged by team members
	Surgeon provides clear instrument requests to scrub nurse
	Nurses confirm final counts on swabs and instruments
	Anaesthetist instructs assistant on reversal of anaesthesia
Post-operative	Anaesthetist instructs team to move patient
	Anaesthetist informs recovery of operation
	Anaesthetist informs recovery of patient condition
	Anaesthetist informs recovery of drugs used
	Recovery staff acknowledge information about patient

In a second example, Elaine Hart and Harry Owen observed 20 anaesthetists carrying out the difficult, and increasingly uncommon, procedure of general anaesthesia for Caesarean section in a simulated environment. They had first prepared a checklist of 40 items all viewed as important procedural checks by an expert panel. They found that on average the anaesthetists failed to carry out about a third of the recommended checks:

Some items were omitted because staff assumed they had been checked by others. Such assumptions can have disastrous consequences. . . Most participants admitted that they did forget to check an item that they would deem as important and would routinely want to check.
(HART AND OWEN, 2005)

In spite of these findings, only 40% of participants felt that a checklist would be useful in a clinical situation. Many expressed concerns about increased anxiety in the patient associated with its use, in that hearing the list being read out loud might be disconcerting to an awake patient in what is often an already stressful situation for them. But, if you were a patient, what would you think? Hart and Owen appositely remark that airline passengers are reassured by visible routines and checklists as being evidence that everything has been checked and nothing ignored or overlooked by the flight crew; the same may well be true of patients.

The third observational study concerns the critical team handover within emergency medicine. Accurate communication of information at shift change is one of the primary functions of handover to ensure safe transition of shift responsibility from the outgoing to the incoming teams in a healthcare setting. The shift leader is required to have knowledge of the all patients in the department, in order to prioritize them and organize investigations necessary to make decisions. This requires knowing how many patients are in the emergency department, what beds are available and whether side rooms are needed because of infection control. They also need to be able to anticipate problems in the forthcoming shift due to staffing problems and have identified the senior doctors on call for the various specialties. They would expect to know about serious incidents and patients who had died in the department, as well as equipment problems and any other problems or special circumstances (Farhan, personal communication).

When Maisse Farhan began her observations, the need for this information to be transferred was well understood by senior staff, but the handover was informal. Although having worked in the department for some years she was surprised to find, when she actually watched, just how little information was actually transferred. Only about a third of the deaths and serious incidents were discussed, the hospital bed situation was hardly ever mentioned, equipment problems although quite frequent were never mentioned and seriously ill patients often not discussed. In these circumstances, the incoming shift leader has, in effect, to go round and find out everything for themselves; the handover, being inaccurate, serves little purpose and conveys false and dangerous reassurance.

Direct observation of clinical care has not been used to a great extent in studies of safety and quality, but deserves a much higher profile. Compared, for example, to the laborious and expensive analysis of hundreds of incidents, invaluable information can be extracted relatively quickly. This is just a small selection of studies, but fairly typical of those I have reviewed; always, the care actually provided falls far short of what the staff concerned imagine is happening (and indeed the patients). The most remarkable feature of these studies is that the clinical observers themselves, although they know these environments intimately, can still be surprised by what they see. As human beings, we quickly become accustomed to our working environments and in a very real sense fail to actually see the many inefficiencies and lapses. This is perhaps less surprising than it first seems. Clinicians are almost always busy and do not have time to stand about watching. Once you do stand back though and watch attentively, a whole new landscape emerges. Suddenly one is simultaneously deeply impressed by how everyone copes with the rapidly changing and sometimes chaotic environment, while being simultaneously appalled by how far teamwork in practice diverges from the tidy guidelines and protocols mandated by professional organizations. Teamwork can, however, be improved by effective leadership and by a variety of interventions.

Team leadership

Team leadership in all its forms is particularly critical in high risk activities. For example, team leaders influence safety attitudes and behaviour in the workplace, such as compliance with safety related rules and procedures and are key to the effective management of emergencies (Flin and Yule, 2004). Rigid hierarchies in healthcare teams may not be conducive to high quality care; however, leadership, clarity of purpose and roles remain critical.

I once attended a talk on surgical leadership in which Ernest Shackleton, the Antarctic explorer, was held up as a model for surgeons to emulate. The talk was very inspiring, thoughtful and reflective. However, I remember thinking that healthcare was in serious trouble if all leaders were expected to develop the same qualities as Shackleton. This story directs us to one particular vision of leadership, prominent in early research, in which leadership is founded in character and associated with charisma, drive, intelligence and endurance; one might call it the heroic model. Latterly, however, writers on leadership began to see that effective leaders adapt their style and behaviour to the context and demands of the task. For instance, a completely autocratic string of commands might be absolutely appropriate during an emergency; the same leader would be ill advised to adopt the same approach when trying to engage ward staff in an improvement programme.

Consider the range of leadership responsibilities in a maternity unit. Maternity services are organized in different ways in different countries. In Britain, Canada and other countries, normal births are managed by midwives with obstetricians managing complex births and associated medical problems. The leadership roles in this context include:

- The individual midwife leads the team caring for the woman and her baby, which may include a midwifery student and a maternity support worker. In an emergency, leadership passes to an obstetrician, co-ordinating a larger team, including paediatricians, midwives, anaesthetists and more junior obstetricians.
- The senior obstetrician on call needs to provide similar leadership to the team of obstetricians on duty and is ultimately responsible for all the care provided on an obstetrician-led labour ward.
- Midwifery co-ordinators are the leaders of a labour ward midwifery shift, providing support to all midwives on duty, taking decisions about staff deployment and reviewing professional decisions where appropriate.
- Other clinical areas also have their own leaders: antenatal and postnatal wards have a midwifery shift leader; operating theatres have separate

structures of leadership, involving anaesthetists, scrub nurses, and recovery nurses.

- Specific leadership and support on safety issues may be provided by a dedicated unit safety lead or risk manager.
- At a higher level, the unit's head of midwifery, clinical director or service lead, and general manager lead the entire maternity unit team.

Clearly leadership is very widely distributed in organizations, and not just confined to those in senior positions. Almost everyone in healthcare has some leadership responsibilities.

Leadership skills

Leadership requires specific skills, in addition to clinical ability but these skills are often lacking:

Our experience on the ground is that there are a lot of core management skills that people in very key roles are lacking, and that's to do with managing conflict, getting teams to work effectively together, being able to analyse incidents and drawing out learning from that. When we do development work with people, some of the basic management skills appear to be a revelation.

We had people telling us either that they didn't know who was in charge or that those in charge never seemed to be around unless there's a crisis.

(SAFE BIRTHS: EVERYBODY'S BUSINESS, 2008. REPRODUCED BY PERMISSION OF THE KING'S FUND, LONDON)

Leaders must manage not only their own work but also those of the team. They need therefore to be knowledgeable not only about their own speciality, but to also appreciate the work and challenges faced by other members of the team. Ideally they are respected by other team members for their experience in their own field, but also for their willingness to appreciate the skills of others (Flin, Crichton and O'Connor, 2008). Team leaders have three main tasks (Zaccaro, Rittman and Marks, 2009), which are to:

- Create the conditions that enable the team to do its job. This means making sure the team has clear objectives and that the necessary resources are available.
- Build and maintain the team as a performing unit. This includes making sure the team includes members with the necessary skills and abilities. The leader must also develop processes that help the team to perform effectively by nurturing good decision making, problem solving and conflict management.
- Coach and support the team. The team leader has to be sensitive to the mood of the team and to note how well members are interacting and communicating. A key task is to ensure that everyone is on 'the same page' while training and working together, which is why the best teams engage in constant team briefing and exchange of information.

Team leadership is different from traditional hierarchical leadership. Traditional leaders tend to direct rather than facilitate and support, to give rather than seek advice and to determine rather than integrate views. Effective team leaders, on the other hand, encourage members to offer solutions when things are not going well and do not insist on having the final say when decisions need to be made. Team leaders differ most clearly from traditional leaders in focusing on the team as a whole rather than on its individual members and in sharing responsibility with the team (West, 2004). Leaders must be easily available and visible to junior staff and have a crucial role to play in supporting more junior staff to be confident about asking for help.

Team interventions: briefing, checklisting and daily goals

Watching teams and teamwork quickly reveals that a group of well intentioned individuals does not make a team and furthermore, that teamwork has to be planned and organized. In this section we will review some apparently simple interventions, which turn out to have quite profound effects. Daily goals, pre-operative and post-operative checklists seem mundane, and this partly accounts for clinicians' resistance to their use. However, a checklist is not a piece of paper or even a list; it is a team intervention which, used well, can affect the wider team functioning, the relationships across professions and hierarchies and even the values and safety culture of the team. To my mind, the impact of these simple tools on clinical processes and patient outcome suggests that their effect can only be fully understood by appreciating their wider impact on team performance.

Clarity and communication: the adoption of daily goals

Recall the case of David James, who died from a spinal injection of Vincristine. One of the features of this case was that almost everyone involved made assumptions about the knowledge and abilities of those around them. We assume, by default, that other people have the same understanding of a situation as we do and, even worse, that we have correctly communicated our intentions and wishes. Many instructions for patient care are given rapidly, in a hurry, often in a kind of clinical shorthand and with many assumptions about the kind of basic care that will be provided. In a fixed team that works together day in and day out, this generally works pretty well. However, few teams, especially ward teams, are like that; it's a shifting population of people on a variety of shift patterns, supported to varying degrees by temporary staff.

Pronovost *et al.* (2003) posed two simple but critical questions to intensive care doctors and nurses after the daily rounds: (1) How well do you understand the goals of care for this patient today? and (2) How well do you understand what work needs to be accomplished to get this patient to the next level of care? These questions seem unnecessary, almost insulting.

BOX 18.2 Daily goals in intensive care

Room No	Date Initial as goals are reviewed		
	07.00–15.00	**15.00–23.00**	**23.00–07.00**
What needs to be done for the patient to be discharged from the ICU?			
What is the patient's greatest safety risk? How can we reduce that risk?			
Pain management/ sedation			
Cardiac volume status Pulmonary/ventilator (PP, elevate HOB)			
Mobilization			
ID, cultures, drug levels			
GI/Nutrition			
Medication changes (can any be discontinued?)			
Tests/procedures Review scheduled labs; morning labs and CXR			
Consultations			
Communication with primary service			
Family communication			
Can catheters/tubes be removed?			

Is this patient receiving DVT/PUD prophylaxis
Mgt. management; PP, plateau pressure; HOB, head of bed; ID, infectious disease; GI, gastrointestinal; labs, laboratory tests; CXR, chest radiograph; DVT, deep vein thrombosis; PUD, peptic ulcer disease

(REPRINTED FROM JOURNAL OF CRITICAL CARE, PETER PRONOVOST, SEAN BEREN-HOLTZ, TODD DORMAN, PAM A. LIPSETT, TERRI SIMMONDS AND CAROL HARADEN. "IMPROVING COMMUNICATION IN THE ICU USING DAILY GOALS". 18, NO. 2, [71–75], 2003, WITH PERMISSION FROM ELSEVIER)

These people are caring for very sick patients; surely they know what they are meant to be doing? A formal survey revealed however, that only 10% of nurses and doctors surveyed understood the goals of care for specific patients.

Following some interviews and exploration, the team introduced a daily goals sheet that asked staff to state the tasks to be completed, care plan and communication plan (discussions with patient and family or with other caregivers). This sheet went through many iterations and refinements before reaching its final form. The sheet is basically a checklist and plan, but like many such apparently simple interventions, its impact is more wide ranging than one might think. The daily goals sheet first forces explicit objectives to be stipulated for each patient, which can be reviewed and monitored. Second, it ensures that everyone works from the same set of assumptions and to the same plan. Third, it was designed to facilitate communication between team members both in the sense of communication of the goals themselves and, necessarily, by making sure that all members of the team are engaged in the care of each patient. All providers, doctors, nurses, respiratory therapists and pharmacists review the goals for the day and initial the form three times a day. Care is thus structured, systematic and forward-looking plans are integral to the daily work.

The impact of this simple intervention was remarkable. Within eight weeks, the proportion of nurses and doctors who clearly understood the daily goals for the patient increased from 10 to 95%. Staff found the short-term goals sheet to be a simple tool for setting priorities and guiding the daily work. Nurses felt that they were an active part of the team working in partnership with physicians, so this basic change to the clinical process also impacted on relationships within the team.

Remarkably, following the introduction of the daily goals sheet, ICU length of stay reduced from 2.2 days to 1.1 days, allowing an additional 670 patients each year to receive intensive care. The research team did not set out to assess impact on length of stay and are cautious about attributing the improvements to the daily goals approach. Nevertheless, it is plausible as the impact on clinical practice seemed to be immediate and profound. Before this approach was introduced, the team might discuss each patient for 20 or 25 minutes, but the discussion would centre on pathology and the clinical literature; staff could leave the discussion after 20 minutes, still not clear about what they should actually be doing. After an explicit discussion of goals and tasks, care was sharper, better co-ordinated and patient specific. In a word, reliable.

Briefing and checklisting in surgery

At Orange County Hospital in the United States, theatre teams have used a routine pre-operative briefing for many years (Leonard, Graham and Bonacum, 2004). Their peri-operative briefing checklist highlights a number of the key themes we have discussed: the team first sets out exactly what will be happening, prioritizes tasks as either standard or non-standard procedure, considers whether this procedure presents any particular threats (long operation, hypothermia, other potential problems), looks ahead to the possible need for other services and inputs, and allows each member of the team to review the information given by the other. Most importantly, the very fact of a briefing in which all team members take part embeds the idea of open communication from the beginning of the operation, whether or not the team has worked together before. Implicit in the fact of the briefing is the idea that everyone in the team has a right, in fact a responsibility, to communicate and to speak up if they foresee or notice any errors or problems. Such briefings, whether formal or informal, are certainly not confined to surgery. Wards, for instance, which have a regular daily meeting at which all patients are reviewed with both nurses and doctors present, are building in checks against false assumptions, miscommunication and errors of all kinds, as well as anticipation of potential problems.

A number of studies have now been carried out, which demonstrate the value of checklisting and briefing which, although sometimes described separately, in practice usually occur together. For instance, Lorelei Lingard and colleagues (2008) demonstrated a substantial reduction in communication failures after training the entire division of general surgery in a Canadian tertiary referral hospital in the use of briefing and checklisting. However, the most influential study of surgical checklists has undoubtedly been that led by Atul Gawande, as part of the World Health Organization (Figure 18.2) (WHO) World Alliance for Patient Safety 'Safe Surgery Saves Lives' campaign (Haynes *et al.*, 2009).

The WHO surgical safety checklist ensures that the entire operating theatre team understands the patient, the surgical procedure, the equipment needed and that evidence based interventions such as antibiotic prophylaxis or deep vein thrombosis prophylaxis are reliably given. The 19-item checklist is completed in three stages – before induction of anaesthesia (sign in), just before skin incision (time out) and before the patient leaves the operating theatre (sign out). Items on the checklist must be verbally confirmed with the patient and other team members (Soar *et al.*, 2009). The WHO Safe Surgery Saves Lives Study Group introduced the checklist in eight countries worldwide, studying 3733 patients before and 3955 patients after the implementation of the checklist. After implementation, deaths were reduced by 47% (from 1.5–0.8%), and in-hospital complications by 36% (from 11–7.0%). In some sites, the checklist prompted the introduction of techniques that are now standard in developed countries; for instance, use of a pulse oximeter rose from 60 to over 90% in one study site over the course of the study.

Briefings and checklists are, however, not a panacea and, according to how they are used, can be either a positive or negative influence on team performance. This is well illustrated in a study on the paradoxical effects of team briefings by Sarah Whyte, Lorelei Lingard and colleagues. They

Surgical Safety Checklist

World Health Organization | Patient Safety
A World Alliance for Safer Health Care

Before induction of anaesthesia

(with at least nurse and anaesthetist)

Has the patient confirmed his/her identity, site, procedure, and consent?
☐ Yes

Is the site marked?
☐ Yes
☐ Not applicable

Is the anaesthesia machine and medication check complete?
☐ Yes

Is the pulse oximeter on the patient and functioning?
☐ Yes

Does the patient have a:

Known allergy?
☐ No
☐ Yes

Difficult airway or aspiration risk?
☐ No
☐ Yes, and equipment/assistance available

Risk of >500ml blood loss (7ml/kg in children)?
☐ No
☐ Yes, and two IVs/central access and fluids planned

Before skin incision

(with nurse, anaesthetist and surgeon)

Confirm all team members have introduced themselves by name and role.

Confirm the patient's name, procedure, and where the incision will be made.

Has antibiotic prophylaxis been given within the last 60 minutes?
☐ Yes
☐ Not applicable

Anticipated Critical Events

To Surgeon:
☐ What are the critical or non-routine steps?
☐ How long will the case take?
☐ What is the anticipated blood loss?

To Anaesthetist:
☐ Are there any patient-specific concerns?

To Nursing Team:
☐ Has sterility (including indicator results) been confirmed?
☐ Are there equipment issues or any concerns?

Is essential imaging displayed?
☐ Yes
☐ Not applicable

Before patient leaves operating room

(with nurse, anaesthetist and surgeon)

Nurse Verbally Confirms:
☐ The name of the procedure
☐ Completion of instrument, sponge and needle counts
☐ Specimen labelling (read specimen labels aloud, including patient name)
☐ Whether there are any equipment problems to be addressed

To Surgeon, Anaesthetist and Nurse:
☐ What are the key concerns for recovery and management of this patient?

© WHO, 2009

This checklist is not intended to be comprehensive. Additions and modifications to fit local practice are encouraged. Revised 1 / 2009

Figure 18.2 Surgical Safety Checklist (from WHO, 2009) Reproduced with permission by WHO, © World Health Organization 2009, WHO Surgical Safety Checklist.

identify five types of negative events (Box 18.3), which can occur from failing to use the briefings in the way it is intended:

- Team briefings can mask knowledge gaps.
- Team briefings can disrupt positive communication.
- Team briefings can reinforce professional divisions.
- Team briefings can create tension.
- Team briefings can perpetuate a problematic culture.

BOX 18.3 Misuse of checklists and briefing

Masking knowledge gaps

At the 'operative medications' prompt, the staff anaesthesiologist confirmed that he would give the antibiotics (no specific antibiotic mentioned) and then took over from the surgeon in leading the briefing. He read the list of prompts followed simply by 'yep' ('anaesthesia, yep; blood products, yep; positioning, yep')... When he finished, I [the observer] commented that I had never seen a briefing that involved so few words. The anaesthesiologist responded, 'Was that not good?'

Closing down communications

This was a very poor checklist. The surgical fellow led as though he were speed reading, focusing his eyes only on the checklist, including no prompts for participation, and continuing to prep the surgical area at the same time. The circulating nurse also continued with tucking in the patient's arm.

Reinforcing professional boundaries

This briefing covered significant details about the patient's history and the operative plan. However, staff surgeon gave something of a monologue and didn't invite questions or contributions from others. The circulating nurse and staff anaesthesiologist each interjected at particular points in the briefing, but the scrub nurse (a novice nurse) stood at the scrub table with her back to the group as she listened. After the briefing, she told me (the observer) that the staff surgeon 'hadn't really included' her, so she didn't want to appear to be intruding on the exchange.

At the 'team' prompt, the staff surgeon looked up at the surgical fellow and [the observer] and said, 'We've done a few of these before.' He proceeded to the next prompt. There was no mention or introduction of the student scrub nurse.

(WITH KIND PERMISSION FROM SPRINGER SCIENCE + BUSINESS MEDIA: COGNITION, TECHNOLOGY & WORK, PARADOXICAL EFFECTS OF INTERPROFESSIONAL BRIEFINGS ON OR TEAM PERFORMANCE, **10**, NO.4, © 2008, [287–294], SARAH WHYTE)

As the examples show, it is not really that the briefing or checklist causes negative events, rather that they can be used in a way that simply reinforces patterns of interaction that are already there. So a surgeon, for instance, can ostensibly take part in the briefing but express their superiority and detachment by not really listening and carrying out other tasks at the same time. A checklist can be read in a clipped and dismissive way, which closes down all possibility of discussion within the team.

Formula 1 and post-operative handover

The handover of infants after complex congenital heart surgery from the theatre team to the intensive care team is a critical phase in the care of these vulnerable patients. During this period, all the technology and support (ventilation, monitoring lines, multiple inotropes and vasodilators) is transferred twice, from theatre systems to portable equipment, then to the intensive care systems, within 15 minutes. At the same time, knowledge of the patient gained by the surgical team in the four to eight hour procedure is conveyed to the intensive care unit staff. This handover is carried out by people who are tired after a very long and difficult operation and is extremely vulnerable to error (Catchpole *et al.*, 2007).

A team from Great Ormond Street Hospital London found inspiration in Formula 1 motor racing, where the pit stop is a supreme example of a highly co-ordinated, multi-professional team performing a complex activity under huge time pressure; four tyres are changed and the car is fuelled in under seven seconds (I can't believe this either). The association with Formula 1 has endeared the study to many, but to my mind the beauty of the approach lies in the analysis and appreciation of the teamwork. In effect, the surgical team looked at the Formula 1 team and asked themselves 'How do they do that?' The answer was a combination of factors: clear leadership, task allocation, task sequence, checklists coupled with a highly disciplined, composed approach to the task underpinned by training, rehearsal and review meetings (Box 18.4). In contrast, the surgical team were serious and disciplined, but the handover process was informal, unstructured and somewhat haphazard in comparison.

The surgical team explicitly and carefully redesigned the handover, as shown in the table and the handover summary. The results were clear; after the intervention, there were fewer technical errors in the handover, fewer instances of lost information and the revised, more formal handover was actually slightly quicker than the previous informal one. Better still, the new, explicit process was simple to understand, and training of new staff could be carried out within 30 minutes.

Redesigning the wider team

The team interventions we have reviewed so far have focused mainly on specific parts of the team process, whether during surgery or ward care. Friedman and Berger (2004) restructured the operation of an entire general surgical unit in order to produce more reliable and efficient care for patients.

BOX 18.4 Redesigning post-operative handover

Process	Old approach	New approach
Leadership	Unclear who was in charge	Anaesthetist was given overall responsibility for co-ordinating the team, which was transferred to the intensivist at the end of the handover
Task sequence	Inconsistent and nonsequential	Three phases defined: 1. equipment and technology handover; 2. information handover; 3. discussion and plan
Task allocation	Informal and erratic	People allocated to tasks: ventilation – anaesthetist; monitoring – ODA; drains – nurses. The anaesthetist identified and handed information over to the key receiving people
Predicting and planning	Risks identified informally and often not acted upon	A modified FMEA was conducted and senior representatives commented on highest areas of risk. Safety checks were introduced, and the need for a ventilation transfer sheet was identified
Discipline and composure	Ad hoc and unstructured, with several simultaneous discussions in different areas of the ICU and theatres	Communication limited to the essential during equipment handover. During information handover the anaesthetist, then the surgeon, speak alone and uninterrupted, followed by discussion and agreement of the recovery plan
Checklists	None.	A checklist was defined and used as the admission note by the receiving team
Involvement	Communications primarily within levels (e.g. consultant to consultant or junior to junior).	All team members and grades encouraged to speak up. Built into discussions in phase 3

Briefing	A process was already in place, where planning begins in a regular multidisciplinary meeting, and is reconfirmed the week before surgery problems highlighted on the day	
Situation awareness	Not previously identified as being important.	The consultant anaesthetist and intensivist have responsibility for situation awareness at handover, and regularly stand back to make safety checks
Training	No training existed	Formal training was introduced, and laminated training sheets detailing the process are provided at each bedside. The protocol could be learnt in 30 min
Review meetings	A weekly clinical governance meeting, attended 50 + people, was already in place where problems and solutions could be openly discussed	

(PEDIATRIC ANESTHESIA, KEN CATCHPOLE ET AL. "LEADERSHIP FOR SAFETY: INDUSTRIAL EXPERIENCE". **34**, NO.3. 470–478. 2007. REPRODUCED BY PERMISSION OF BLACKWELL PUBLISHING LTD.)

They took the same basic principles of clear leadership, task allocation, task sequencing and so on and simply applied them on a wider scale:

The general surgery team was previously an informal... lacking structured collabora-tion between physicians, nurses, and managers. Meetings were unscheduled and often did not include all necessary team members. This disorganized system led to poor communication... Duplication of roles... frustrated team members and compounded problems.
(FRIEDMAN AND BERGER, 2004)

Following a thoroughgoing review and restructuring, a new system was introduced, which was carefully evaluated over a two-year baseline, followed by a three-year follow-up after the intervention. Length of stay was reduced by one day for all patients, from an average stay of about a week. As they comment, in a year when 4400 patients were admitted to their hospital, this represents an additional 4400 bed days to reduce the strain on services or use to treat additional patients. As well as benefits for the patients, there were considerable benefits for the staff. They reported a much stronger sense of collaboration between team members and a sense of working towards a common goal. Although there was still a formal hierarchy, every member of the team had the opportunity to make a contribution to a patient's care plan and, with the reduction in overlapping responsibilities, the unique contribu-tion of each team member became apparent (Friedman and Berger, 2004).

Team training for safety

Enormous resources are rightly devoted to the training of healthcare profes-sionals but almost all training takes place within disciplines. This is, to put it mildly, completely crazy, given that almost all the work happens in teams. There are, of course, many historical, social and political pressures for training within disciplines and it is organizationally complicated to bring different professions together. However, the nearer training comes to clinical practice, the more important joint training becomes. The increasing attention paid to patient safety, the appreciation of the role of teamwork in both the occurrence and prevention of error and the influence of other safety critical industries, have given an increased impetus to team training. We will examine two examples of safety orientated team training, one more technically orientated using simulation and the other, in emergency medicine, with a stronger focus on communication and team relationships. Before we turn to interventions to improve teamwork however, we must briefly consider a critical prerequisite of training.

Assessing teamwork

An absolute requirement of any serious training is to have a means of assessing teams and of feeding back performance to the team members. We feel we know what good teamwork is (primarily from experiencing bad teamwork), but identifying it formally requires a proper assessment instrument. This in turn means having a clear conception of what good teamwork actually looks like. When constructing such a measure, a researcher immediately faces a number of problems. Do you assess the whole team together or do you rate individual members? Do you assess communication globally or examine particular communication tasks? What are the core dimensions of teamwork and how many are there? And finally, what do we mean by 'good' teamwork? None of these questions is simple to answer and the answers in any case vary with context. Assessment of a hospital board will require a very different approach to the assessment of a surgical team. We cannot review even a fraction of the substantial literature on team assessment, but we can illustrate the approaches by considering some instruments that assess surgical teamwork.

The assessment of non-technical skills was discussed in the previous chapter. Systems have been developed for anaesthetists (ANTS) and surgeons (NOTS), which can be used to give feedback to individuals in simulation and other settings on such skills as leadership, communication and decision making. Each of these was carefully developed and tested to ensure that the assessment instruments really did reflect core professional skills and that they could be reliably assessed by senior anaesthetists and surgeons. My colleagues and I have developed an observational instrument (OTAS) to assess an entire surgical team; the focus was different because the purpose was different. We were primarily interested in the overall functioning of a team in real operations and simulations, because we considered that the performance of the team as a whole was most critical to good patient outcomes. In contrast, the purpose of ANTS and NOTS is to assess individuals during training. OTAS has two elements: broad behaviours and specific task performance. Five broad dimensions of team performance are assessed: leadership, communication, co-ordination, cooperation and monitoring. Note that these dimensions primarily assess interactions and reflect what is happening between people, rather than the behaviours of individuals. The tasks are highly specific, pointing, as we saw earlier in the chapter, to very specific points of process that are often neglected. The neglect of individual items may have little effect but, cumulatively, they can erode team performance and the migration to the edges of safety begins (Chapter 16).

Simulation

Anaesthesia was the first speciality to develop simulation scenarios (Gaba, 2000). Anaesthetists' emulated crisis management training that was developed in the context of commercial aviation in the late 1970s and has become known as Crew Resource Management (CRM). This work led to the development of Anaesthetic CRM training (ACRM) modules, usually known in this context as Crisis Resource Management. Surgical training has followed – with studies in real operating theatres (Undre et al., 2007a, 2007ab; Moorthy et al., 2006), furnishing relevant evidence to be fed into simulation and, critically, challenging tasks for the entire team (Box 18.5).

BOX 18.5 Simulation in surgery

The scenario consisted of a day surgery unit patient for a routine high-tie ligation of a saphenofemoral junction for varicose veins. The simulated patient had been marked and had given consent prior to entering the operating theatre, and his notes and investigations were available. A full set of notes was prepared and included the patient's history of well-controlled angina, a recent ECG report, blood investigations and a drug chart. The anaesthesia trainee and ODP commenced set-up of anaesthesia, while the scrub nurse set up the surgical trolley. During the anaesthesia phase, the anaesthesia team were presented with a crisis that was tailored according to the level of experience of the trainee. These included rapid sequence anaesthesia and difficult intubation. Once the patient had been stabilized, surgery commenced. The surgical crisis consisted of bleeding from the femoral vein. The team crises consisted of haemorrhage or cardiac changes leading to cardiac arrest. Throughout the routine and the crisis phases, the assessors rated online the technical and non-technical skills of their trainees

(UNDRE *ET AL.*, 2007A, 2007B).

Simulations can take a variety of forms. They can be focused on individual trainees or teams; they can be static or interactive; they can be more or less technology driven. Some simulations replicate the 'real thing' (e.g. procedure, clinical environment) and require complex and expensive equipment, such as mannequins that 'breathe' and display vital signs; others however may be simple, inexpensive mock-ups that are nevertheless quite adequate for the skills being trained (Arora and Sevdalis, 2008). Kneebone and Aggarwal (2009), for instance, have achieved excellent simulation of both the technical and interpersonal elements of minor surgical procedures, using an actor, basic kit and an inexpensive backdrop; seeing this makes one realize what can be achieved by skilled actors working with minimal props.

The major goal of this type of simulation-based team-training is to improve the safety and quality of care that is provided to patients, because many key failures in patient care are not attributable to lack of individual technical skill, but rather to lack of accurate and timely communication amongst members of clinical teams, lack of leadership when required, and compromised crisis management. Crises can be simulated, managed and failure can be experienced and recovery can be practised, without risk to patients. Initial evidence suggests that simulations offer effective learning environments and are very much appreciated by those given the opportunity for this kind of training (Arora and Sevdalis, 2008).

Emergency medicine: team training to reduce error

In Emergency Medicine, the MedTeams Consortium has drawn heavily on CRM but has also founded their training on the findings of research on emergency medicine teamwork failures. These problems are well illustrated in a case described by Risser and colleagues (1999) (Box 18.6).

BOX 18.6 Failures in teamwork and the death of a patient

A 39-year-old woman with a history of documented coronary artery disease came to the emergency department complaining of increased frequency of anginal chest pains over the past two weeks. She was triaged as 'urgent', the second highest triage category in a 4-tier triage system, even though she had abnormal vital signs and a history that should have placed her in the highest category. The emergency department was extremely busy, and almost one hour elapsed before she was evaluated by a medical student. At that time she complained of chest pain and was found to have weak-to-absent peripheral pulses.

Ninety minutes after she arrived, a reassessment of her vital signs showed her blood pressure to be 61/32, but this was not communicated to the medical student or the physician. To relieve the patient's chest pain, the physician ordered sublingual nitroglycerin. Later, the nurse reported on a written statement that she was uncomfortable giving nitroglycerin, a drug she knew could lower blood pressure, to a hypotensive patient but assumed that the physician 'knew what he was doing'. The patient continued to complain of chest pain and shortness of breath; morphine sulfate was given and a nitroglycerin drip was started. Finally, almost half an hour after the initial hypotensive episode, her low blood pressure was noted by the physician, the nitroglycerin infusion was discontinued and an internal medicine specialist was called who arrived a further half hour later. The patient remained hypotensive, short of breath and continued to have chest pain. Finally, she became extremely bradycardic, lost her blood pressure, and a 'code' was called. Advanced cardiac resuscitation was carried out, including epinephrine, atropine, defibrillation, external pacing and pericardiocentesis. However, this was unsuccessful and the patient was pronounced dead, 3 hours and 10 minutes after entering the department.

This case demonstrates a chain of errors in which poor organizational climate, lack of team structure, poor task prioritization, poor communication, lack of cross-monitoring (team members checking each other's actions) and lack of assertiveness within the emergency department contributed to a catastrophic patient outcome. The consequences of this team failure were dramatic: the patient died, the family was devastated, the staff were distressed and demoralized and the hospital's reputation was harmed.

(REPRINTED FROM ANNALS OF EMERGENCY MEDICINE, DANIEL T RISSER, MATTHEW M RICE, MARY L SALISBURY, ROBERT SIMON, GREGORY D JAY AND SCOTT D BERNS. "THE POTENTIAL FOR IMPROVED TEAMWORK TO REDUCE MEDICAL ERRORS IN THE EMERGENCY DEPARTMENT,". **34**, NO. 3, [373–383], 1999, WITH PERMISSION FROM ELSEVIER)

Risser and colleagues identified key team behaviours which would protect and defend against errors, drawing on team enhancement strategies fostered in other high risk environments, such as navy teams (Box 18.7). Implicit in these strategies is an acceptance that errors will always occur, that no one can function effectively all the time and that the environment will always present unexpected threats. Individuals can respond to these threats and challenges to some extent, but a team has a better chance of bringing a patient through a critical phase if they constantly watch each other, communicate openly and effectively and back each other up when necessary.

BOX 18.7 Team behaviours to prevent, detect and recover from errors

Identify the protocol to be used or develop a plan. It must be clear to everyone on the team what protocol or plan is being used.

Prioritize tasks for a patient. Team members must understand the plan and how their individual tasks fit into the overall task.

Speaking up. The healthcare professional must speak up when a patient is at risk; team leaders must foster a climate in which this can occur.

Cross monitoring within the team. Team members should watch each other for errors and problems; this needs to be seen not as criticism but as a support to other team members and additional defence for the patient.

Giving and accepting feedback. Feedback is not restricted to team leaders; any member of the team can provide feedback to any other. Implicit in this is that team members understand each other's roles.

Closed loop communications. Messages and communications are acknowledged and repeated by those who receive them; often the senders of these messages will again repeat them. This is seen as an additional check and defence.

Backing up other team members. Team members are aware of other's actions and are ready to step in to support and assist.

(FROM RISSER *ET AL.*, 1999; ILGEN, 1999)

The Medteams training programme (Morey *et al.*, 2002) is focused on teaching core team skills underpinned by an understanding of the nature of team work and how it impacts on clinical practice. Led by a doctor and a nurse, the teamwork training entails groups of about 16 clinical staff completing 8 hours of formal instruction on the fundamentals of team training and on specific behaviours with direct clinical application. The team training is then taken into clinical settings in the deliberate formation of specific teams at the start of each shift, additional instruction in specific team behaviours for each member of staff and coaching and mentoring of teamwork behaviours by staff during normal working hours.

Team training produced significant improvements on standardized team measures, as assessed by observers in nine emergency departments. These observers also monitored a sample of cases in each department, recording overall teamwork and any specific errors. For instance, in one case a technician did an electrocardiograph on a patient with chest pain; he prepared the patient but neglected to tell anyone and the patient was left unobserved for 25 minutes. Following team training, there was a substantial reduction of errors of this kind. Clearly there are many questions to be asked about the impact of such training on a wider scale, the extent to which enhanced team performance would be maintained and so on. Nevertheless the overall programme, specifically targeted at clinical practice and clinical errors, produced impressive benefits.

Leadership and learning: how do teams train themselves?

The Medteams project was based on an initial formal training programme, but clearly relies for its eventual success on the adoption of these practices and the fact that members of each team then foster and develop them. A few hours of training by itself would have little direct impact; rather it acts as a catalyst for the team to develop itself. So how can we foster this kind of continuous team learning?

In an intriguing study, Amy Edmondson and colleagues (2001) examined 16 cardiac surgery teams who were learning a new procedure. The basic coronary bypass operation is well established, but teams were learning to carry out these procedures endoscopically via small incisions in the chest wall. There are technical challenges for the surgeon in the use of endoscopic techniques in any area of surgery but these surgeons were already fairly skilled in the new techniques; the real challenge was that the new technology required much greater co-ordination and communication between team members. Initially, operations using the new technique took two to three times as long as conventional open procedures.

Edmondson and colleagues examined how long teams took to develop these new skills, assessing progress by the length of the operation and other measures. Interestingly, many conventional assumptions about organizational and team change were not upheld. The support of senior management, which varied considerably from place to place, did not have much effect; nor did the status or seniority of the surgeon. Having regular briefings and debriefings was also not critical, although most teams did examine performance data retrospectively. Rather, the learning took place as the process unfolded in real time; the more effective teams were able to take full advantage of the operation itself as a place of learning and training. How did they achieve this? There were three key factors. First, considerable thought was given to choosing the right people to take on this new challenge; people were chosen not just for their seniority or technical skills but ability to work in a team. Second, and particularly important, was the way the team approached the task. In some institutions, the surgeons viewed the challenge as simply one of instructing the team what to do; these teams learned slowly. In others, the surgeon emphasized the challenge, the requirement of each person to contribute and the need for ongoing learning and communication throughout the process; these were the teams who progressed most rapidly (Box 18.8). Finally, in the rapidly learning teams, the leaders and team members created an atmosphere of what Edmondson and colleagues call psychological safety. In these teams, members were able to make suggestions, point out potential problems, and admit mistakes when they occurred. By contrast, when people felt uneasy about acting in this way, the learning process was stifled (Edmondson, Bohner and Pisano, 2001).

BOX 18.8 A tale of two cardiac surgery teams

New technology as a plug-in component

The surgeon, senior and well established in a major hospital, played no role in choosing the team, which was assembled according to seniority. He also didn't participate in the team's dry run prior to the first case. He later explained that he did not see the new technique as particularly challenging technically. Consequently, he explained, 'it was not a matter of training myself but of training the team.' Such training would not require any change in his style of communicating with the team. 'Once I get the team set up, I never look up. It's they who have to make sure that everything is flowing.' Mastering the new technology proved slow and difficult for this team, with operations times remaining long, even after 50 cases.

New technology as a team innovation project

Although this cardiac surgery department had no history of undertaking major research or innovation, it had recently hired a young surgeon who took an interest in the new approach. This surgeon realized, more than any other surgeon, that implementing the new technology would require the team to adopt a very different style. 'The ability of the surgeon to become a partner, not a dictator, is critical. You really do have to change what you're doing during an operation based on a suggestion from someone else in the team.' Team members noted that the hierarchy had changed, creating a free and open environment with input from everybody. This group was one of the two who learned the new technique most quickly, with operation times over an hour below the average after 20 procedures.

(REPRODUCED FROM *HARVARD BUSINESS REVIEW*, EDMONDSON, A., BOHNER, R., & PISANO, G. "SPEEDING UP TEAM LEARNING", VOL. **79**, 125–132, 2001, WITH PERMISSION FROM HARVARD BUSINESS PUBLISHING SCHOOL)

References

Arora, S. and Sevdalis, N. (2008) HOSPEX and concepts of simulation. *Journal of the Royal Army Medical Corps*, **154**(3), 202–205.

Caplan, G.A., Williams, A.J., Daly, B. and Abraham, K. (2004) A randomized, controlled trial of comprehensive geriatric assessment and multidisciplinary intervention after discharge of elderly from the emergency department – the DEED II study. *Journal of the American Geriatric Society*, **52**(9), 1417–1423.

Catchpole, K.R., de Leval, M.R., McEwan, A. *et al.* (2007) Patient handover from surgery to intensive care: using Formula 1 pit-stop and aviation models to improve safety and quality. *Paediatric Anaesthesia*, **17**(5), 470–478.

Cooper, J.B. and Taqueti, V.R. (2004) A brief history of the development of mannequin simulators for clinical education and training. *Quality and Safety in Health Care*, **13** (suppl_1), i11–i18.

Davenport, D.L., Henderson, W.G., Mosca, C.L. *et al.* (2007) Risk-adjusted morbidity in teaching hospitals correlates with reported levels of communication and collaboration on surgical teams but not with scale measures of teamwork climate, safety climate, or working conditions. *Journal of the American College of Surgeons*, **205**(6), 778–784.

Edmondson, A., Bohner, R. and Pisano, G. (2001) Speeding up team learning. *Harvard Business Review*, **79**, 125–132.

Flin, R. and Yule, S. (2004) Leadership for safety: industrial experience. *Quality and Safety in Health Care*, **13**(suppl_2), ii45–ii51.

Flin, R., O'Connor, P. and Crichton, M. (2008) *Safety at the Sharp End. A Guide to Non-technical Skills*, Ashgate, Guildford UK.

Friedman, D.M. and Berger, D.L. (2004) Improving team structure and communication: a key to hospital efficiency. *Archives of Surgery (Chicago, Ill: 1960)*, **139**(11), 1194–1198.

Gaba, D.M. (2000) Anaesthesiology as a model for patient safety. *British Medical Journal*, **320**, 785–788.

Hart, E.M. and Owen, H. (2005) Errors and omissions in anesthesia: a pilot study using a pilot's checklist. *Anesthia and Analgesia*, **101**(1),246–250, table.

Haynes, A.B., Weiser, T.G., Berry, W.R. *et al.* (2009) A surgical safety checklist to reduce morbidity and mortality in a global population. *The New England Journal of Medicine*, **360**(5), 491–499.

Healey, A., Undre, S. and Vincent, C.A. (2004) Developing observational measures of performance in surgical teams. *Quality and Safety in Health Care*, **13**, 33–40.

Helmreich, R.L. and Merrit, A.C. (1998) *Culture at Work in Aviation and Medicine: National, Organisational and Professional Influences*, Ashgate, Aldershot UK.

Ilgen, D.R. (1999) Teams embedded in organizations: some implications. *American Psychologist*, **54**(2), 129–139.

Kings Fund (2008) *Safe Births. Everybody's Business*, Kings Fund, London.

Kneebone, R. and Aggarwal, R. (2009) Surgical training using simulation. *British Medical Journal*, **338**, b1001.

Lemieux-Charles, L. and McGuire, W.L. (2006) What do we know about health care team effectiveness? A review of the literature. *Medical Care Research and Review*, **63**(3), 263–300.

Leonard, M., Graham, S. and Bonacum, D. (2004) The human factor: the critical importance of effective teamwork and communication in providing safe care. *Quality and Safety in Health Care*, **13**(suppl_1), i85–i90.

Lingard, L., Espin, S., Whyte, S. *et al.* (2004) Communication failures in the operating room: an observational classification of recurrent types and effects. *Quality and Safety in Health Care*, **13**(5), 330–334.

Lingard, L., Regehr, G., Orser, B. *et al.* (2008) Evaluation of a preoperative checklist and team briefing among surgeons, nurses, and anesthesiologists to reduce failures in communication. *Archives of Surgery (Chicago, Ill: 1960)*, **143**(1), 12–17.

Moorthy, K., Munz, Y., Forrest, D. *et al.* (2006) Surgical crisis management skills training and assessment: a simulation[corrected]-based approach to enhancing operating room performance. *Annals of Surgery*, **244**(1), 139–147.

Morey, J.C., Simon, R., Jay, G.D. *et al.* (2002) Error reduction and performance improvement in the emergency department through formal teamwork training: evaluation results of the MedTeams project. *Health Services Research*, **37**(6), 1553–1581.

Paris, C.R., Salas, E. and Cannon-Bowers, J.A. (2000) Teamwork in multi-person systems: A review and analysis. *Ergonomics*, **43**(8), 1052–1075.

Pronovost, P., Berenholtz, S., Dorman, T. *et al.* (2003) Improving communication in the ICU using daily goals. *Journal of Critical Care*, **18**(2), 71–75.

Risser, D.T., Rice, M.M., Salisbury, M.L. *et al.* (1999) The potential for improved teamwork to reduce medical errors in the emergency department. The MedTeams Research Consortium. *Annals of Emergency Medicine*, **34**(3), 373–383.

Soar, J., Peyton, J., Leonard, M. and Pullyblank, A.M. (2009) Surgical safety checklists. *British Medical Journal*, **338**, 220.

Undre, S., Healey, A.N., Darzi, A. and Vincent, C.A. (2006) Observational assessment of surgical teamwork: a feasibility study. *World Journal of Surgery*, **30**(10), 1774–1783.

Undre, S., Sevdalis, N., Healey, A.N. *et al.* (2007a) Observational teamwork assessment for surgery (OTAS): refinement and application in urological surgery. *World Journal of Surgery*, **31**(7), 1373–1381.

Undre, S., Koutantji, M., Sevdalis, N. *et al.* (2007b) Multidisciplinary crisis simulations: the way forward for training surgical teams. *World Journal of Surgery*, **31**(9), 1843–1853.

West, M.A., Borrill, C., Dawson, J. *et al.* (2002) The link between the management of employees and patient mortality in acute hospitals. *International Journal of Human Resource Management*, **13**(8), 1299–1310.

West, M.A. (2004) Twelve steps to heaven: successfully managing change through developing innovative teams. *European Journal of Work and Organizational Psychology*, **13**(2), 269.

Whyte, S., Lingard, L., Espin, S. *et al.* (2007) Paradoxical effects of interprofessional briefings on OR team performance. *Cognition Technology & Work*, **10**(4), 287–294.

Zaccaro, S.J., Rittman, A.L. and Marks, M.A. (2009) Team leadership. *The Leadership Quarterly*, **12**, 451–483.

The Journey to Safety

CHAPTER 19
Safe organizations: bringing it all together

In the previous seven chapters we have reviewed a number of strategies for improving the safety and quality of care, some concerned with changing the way people work and others with technological change and process improvement. The multifaceted, systemic nature of safety problems suggests that sustained improvement will only be achieved by integrating these various components within a comprehensive strategy for safer care. In this and the following chapter we will review some ambitious and potentially transformative approaches that hold out the promise of safer, high-quality healthcare. In this chapter we review the work of Peter Pronovost and colleagues in intensive care and the British Safer Patients Initiative, followed by a short review of campaigns targeting specific safety issues within organizations. In the following chapter we consider the even more challenging problem of improving entire systems of healthcare. The approaches described in this chapter are based primarily at the level of the clinical microsystem, which some have argued should be the primary target of safety and quality improvement programmes.

Clinical microsystems

A clinical microsystem is a group of clinicians and staff working together with a shared clinical purpose to provide care for a defined population of patients (Mohr, Batalden and Barach, 2004). The system includes the clinicians, support staff, the equipment and technology, the care processes and everything that needs to be done to provide care to the patients – essentially the structure and process in Donabedian's terms, but on the smaller scale of an extended clinical team. Examples of clinical microsystems include a cardiovascular surgical care team, a community based mental health centre, or a neonatal intensive care unit. Each example has in common core elements: a focused type of care; clinicians and staff with the skills and training needed to engage in the required care processes; a defined patient population; and a certain level of information and technology to support the work. Each hospital or healthcare economy will

Patient Safety, 2nd edition. By Charles Vincent. Published 2010 by Blackwell Publishing Ltd.

have a large number of these microsystems, each delivering a different type of care but interacting with each other and the larger organization.

Mohr, Batalden and others have argued that the clinical microsystem is a particularly critical target for safety and quality improvement. The microsystem concept stems from earlier studies of service organizations outside healthcare, which achieved particularly high quality; each of these organizations created small units, which could be replicated across the organization, organized and engineered to provide a high quality service to the customer. Clinical microsystems tend to be larger and more complicated, but the essential idea is similar. They are recognizable sub-systems within the larger organization, which have their own purpose, organization and delivery processes; they are small enough to permit defined improvement programmes to take hold relatively quickly but large enough to influence the care of considerable numbers of patients. In a series of studies in the 1990s and beyond, Mohr and Donaldson (Nelson, Batalden and Godfrey, 2007) defined the qualities of high performing microsystems:

- Constancy of purpose over time;
- Investment in improvement in terms of both time and resource;
- Alignment of role and training for efficiency and staff needs;
- Interdependence of the care team in meeting patient needs;
- Integration of information and technology into work flows;
- Ongoing measurement of outcomes;
- Support from the wider organization;
- Connection to the community to enhance care and extend influence.

Improvement then requires a simultaneous focus on processes, organization, supervision, training and teamwork, underpinned by leadership, constancy of purpose and support from senior leaders. In this chapter we will see how these ideas have been put into practice, but first we need to briefly consider the difficult topic of the evaluation of safety and quality improvement.

The evaluation of complex interventions

A clinical trial is conceptually similar but very different in practice from the comparatively tidy, isolated laboratory experiment on which a clinical trial is modelled. The concept is simple – comparing the response in two or more groups – but this can be challenging in practice, both methodologically and practically. A drug trial, for instance, has to separate the action of the drug from everything else that affects the course of a disease and must also encompass the variability in patients' lives, disease course and other illnesses. Now consider a surgical trial comparing, for instance, open and laparoscopic procedures. This is more complicated still because of the variations in the intervention as well as the patient: surgeons, facilities and post-operative care may all differ making it even more difficult to identify any advantages of the new surgical technique; the noise can drown out the signal. Now consider a still more complex problem, that of evaluating a safety and quality intervention within an organization; a number of methodological issues particularly stand out.

A hospital is a complex adaptive system

The structure of most healthcare organizations is a fairly rigid hierarchy, complicated by the inclusion of a number of distinct professional hierarchies. It can be very frustrating, and puzzling, to plan and set out a clear programme of organizational change and then find that in practice it doesn't proceed as expected. Organizations, in fact, change all the time, in response to both internal and external influences, and their dynamic quality is just one of the features that makes organizational change complex; one is constantly working with a moving target. Clinical microsystems, and indeed healthcare organizations, are complex adaptive systems (CAS), constantly evolving and changing. CASs are networks of many agents, which may be people, cells, species, companies or countries, in which all the agents constantly act and react to each other. The control of these systems tends to be highly dispersed and decentralized, in fact there may be no clear locus of control. Coherent and predictable behaviour in such systems arises from both competition and cooperation amongst the agents. The overall behaviour is the result of a huge number of decisions made every moment by many individual agents (Waldrop, 1992).

This definition of a CAS was coined by John Holland, Murray Gell Mann and others, at the Santa Fe Institute. Examples of CASs include the stock market, social insect colonies, the ecosystem, the brain and the immune system, the cell and the developing embryo, manufacturing businesses and any human social systems such as political parties or communities. The language of the definition is rather alarming and the extent to which analogies can really be drawn between the behaviour of the immune system and the functioning of a hospital is obviously not a simple question. Fortunately though, we do not have to worry about that at the moment. The essential point to grasp for our purposes is that hospitals are not just complicated, which they are, but complex in the sense that the coherence of the system can only be achieved by the many independent individual people acting and responding independently (Plesk and Greenhalgh, 2001). This is in a sense obvious, but in practice not how the organizations are necessarily run; the crisp diagrams of organizational structure and clear hierarchies suggest that orders proceed from the top and actions are taken. The complex view is that a hospital is more like a biological system with multiple interacting components. To clinicians who constantly struggle with the complexity and unpredictability of biological systems, the images are familiar, though few probably apply biological thinking to running their units. If one thinks in terms of trying to change a biological system, then the difficulties and the fluid, dynamic nature of change becomes less puzzling.

The intervention evolves over time

Assessing the impact of safety and quality interventions is difficult, partly because hospitals are complex, but also because the intervention itself may be complex, ranging over many different clinical areas and across different levels of the organization; front line staff, middle management and the executives are all involved. In a randomized trial, one endeavours to specify the treatment as

closely as possible; this is relatively straightforward for drugs, somewhat more difficult for surgery but both can be specified with reasonable clarity. For an organizational intervention over two years say, there is absolutely no way of knowing in practice how events will unfold or how it will be taken up. This is not necessarily a failure of specification, in that it may actually be counterproductive to try to specify and standardize all aspects of the intervention, leaving no room for local innovation. Plesk and Greenhalgh (2001) point out that the CAS perspective suggests that when planning interventions, one should specifically plan and allow for an evolving intervention by:
- Using biological metaphors to guide thinking;
- Creating conditions in which the system can naturally evolve over time;
- Providing simple rules and minimum specifications;
- Setting forth a good enough vision and creating a wide space for natural creativity to emerge from local actions within the system.

Each organization reacts to and embraces (or rejects) the intervention and so, in a very real sense, each organization actually gets a different intervention – even if all organizations went to the same learning sessions and had the same materials and information. To make matters worse, for those attempting to understand the impact of any intervention, the effects of such programmes evolve over a long time period and the effects continue after the formal programme has ended. Finally, there is an additional complication which is that organizations do not always start in the same place and are not equally ready for such interventions; this issue is discussed further below.

We might add to this that it is also not clear to what extent there is a 'right' way to do things. In practice, organizations approach improvement in very different ways, even when they are allegedly following the same programme (see below). We might see this as simply reflecting our ignorance. For instance, before antibiotics were discovered, there were dozens of different remedies and tests of treatments for tuberculosis, which all vanished like smoke once a true treatment emerged. However, although we may be able to isolate some fundamentals, it is unlikely that a 'one size fits all' model will ever emerge. Organizations always have to start from where they are, which varies considerably, and adapt their efforts to local conditions and the changing external environment.

Measurement of impact

We must return again to measurement. With some notable exceptions, not nearly enough attention as been paid to measurement in most quality and safety improvement programmes. Usually some indices are monitored, but not nearly enough to reflect the breadth of the actual change programme; the need to 'get on and change things' often seems to take precedence over the need to find out later whether all one's efforts were worthwhile. It is also tricky to predict all the potential variables of interest. Supposing, for instance, one aims to improve the reliability of antibiotic use on surgical wards; the surgical wards fail to make use of it and no improvement is seen but two of the medical wards hear about it, successfully adapt it and show major change. Is this a failure of the intervention or an unexpected success? Both, really.

Reviews and comparisons of different quality and safety improvement plans have generally found evidence for modest improvements (Schouten, Hulscher and Everdingen, 2008) but none of the various, and numerous, broad strategies and approaches really stands out as 'the way forward'. The situation was well summarized by Richard Grol and colleagues in 2002, and still applies today:

From what we know, no quality improvement programme is superior and real sustainable improvement might require implementation of some aspects of several approaches – perhaps together, perhaps consecutively. We just do not know which to use, when to use them, or what to expect.

(REPRODUCED FROM *QUALITY & SAFETY IN HEALTH CARE*, R GROL, R BAKER, F MOSS. "QUALITY IMPROVEMENT RESEARCH: UNDERSTANDING THE SCIENCE OF CHANGE IN HEALTH CARE". **11**, NO. 2, [110–111], 2002, WITH PERMISSION FROM BMJ PUBLISHING GROUP LTD.)

In reflecting on the programmes to be discussed in the remaining chapter, we need to be cognisant of both the methodological and practical difficulties. Certainly it is right that we should require evaluation of such programmes, but we should also be cognisant of the difficulties of defining the intervention, or predicting the course it might take as it evolves within the organization. Much more attention needs to be given to measurement and evaluation but we need to understand the difficulties and challenges.

Improving the safety of intensive care

Our first example of long-term, sustained change is the work of Peter Pronovost, Albert Wu and their colleagues in critical care medicine at Johns Hopkins Hospital. This work is remarkable on several counts. First, the leaders all have a serious and longstanding commitment to patient safety. Second, the work has been sustained over a decade now, with continuous evolution and refinement. Third, they have combined a desire for improvement with an equal passion for science and measurement and fourth, they have documented both the journey and the outcomes (Box 19.1). Many other leaders have a similarly longstanding commitment but the evaluation and publication of the Johns Hopkins team have made their work particularly influential. We cannot do justice to the entire programme, but we will review some of the salient features.

BOX 19.1 Safety, quality and science

When we started this work, the safety and delivery of care were often not viewed as science. Science seemed to include understanding disease biology and identifying effective interventions but not ensuring patients received those interventions; this work was viewed as the art of medicine. What I tried to do was to highlight to our hospital and medical school leadership that there *is* science in the delivery and that we often do this science poorly. As a result, patients suffer harm. By exposing that, we revealed the dissonance between our pride and our belief that we are a great institution and the reality that some people were being hurt by adverse events, or were not having the best outcomes or receiving evidence-based therapies. Through what admittedly was a bit of a risky strategy – discussing sentinel events with our CEO, department chairs, and board – and making the dissonance real to them – the institution was galvanized into realizing the need to apply science to the delivery of care, just as we apply it to everything else. The delivery of care is really a learning lab for safety and quality. We continually try to evaluate, in a rigorous way, how we are doing things and how we can do them better.

PETER PRONOVOST IN CONVERSATION WITH BOB WACHTER; ACCESSED WWW. AHRQ.ORG

Foundations of improvement

The Hopkins team assumed from the outset that safety interventions could only take root if the front line staff were aware of the hazards patients faced and a need for change. A positive safety culture was regarded as essential, by no means sufficient to produce change but a necessary foundation. The safety critical attitudes, beliefs and behaviours need to be embedded at all levels of the organization, so that as far as possible everyone begins with a shared set of assumptions.

They administered a safety climate survey to 395 nurses, doctors and managers, including all 8 of the ICU physicians. A safety leadership survey was carried out in parallel, which assessed the priority given to safety by leaders at various levels of the organization and also the perceived priority; leaders might believe they were prioritizing safety, but those on the ground might see things very differently (Pronovost, Weast and Holzmueller, 2003). Taken together, these surveys suggested that:

- A proactive strategic planning process was needed.
- Senior leaders needed to become much more visible to front line staff in their efforts to improve patient safety.
- Greater efforts were needed to involve and educate physicians about patient safety.

The ICU reporting system discussed earlier also provided an important window onto the systemic issues the team faced. The reports were used to surface safety problems and to make an initial assessment of their causes and contributory factors, such as the need for training and inadequate staffing. Note that the reporting system is simply analytical and diagnostic, not viewed as a solution or as a safety intervention in itself.

Translating evidence into practice

The safety interventions are grounded in clinical practice and evidence based medicine. The goals are to deliver evidence based practice reliably and without harming patients. That is, of course, every clinician's goal; however, as we have seen, the tricky part is making that happen. The approach has five key components (Pronovost, Berenholtz and Needham, 2008):

- A focus on systems (how work is organized) rather than care of individual patients;
- Engagement of local interdisciplinary teams to assume ownership of the improvement project;
- Creation of centralized support for the technical work;
- Encouraging local adaptation of the intervention;
- Creating a collaborative culture within the local unit and larger system.

This approach has evolved and matured into the Johns Hopkins Quality and Safety Research Group translating evidence into practice model (Figure 19.1). Considerable attention is paid to established clear objectives and the associated measures, such as infection rates from central lines. The evidence and the objectives form the core, but it is also necessary to understand the realities of the work process and its context, and the barriers to doing the job well. Some of this understanding comes from formal analytic methods, such as incident analysis, but much comes from simply watching and talking:

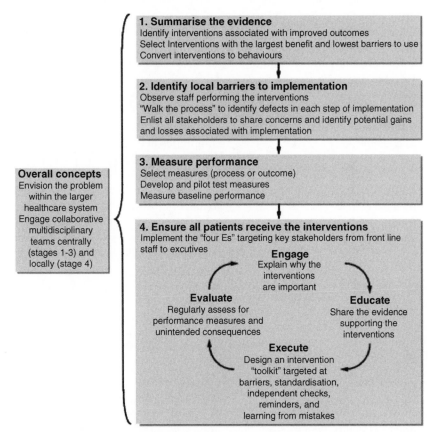

Figure 19.1 Strategy for translating evidence into practice (Reproduced from *British Medical Journal*, Peter J Pronovost, Sean M Berenholtz, Dale M Needham et al. "Translating evidence into practice: a model for large scale knowledge translation". **337**, no. 1, [1714], 2008, with permission from BMJ Publishing Group Ltd.).

Specifically, it helps to physically walk through the steps with clinicians to observe what is required to administer the intervention to patients. This helps identify where defects occur, or where the intervention is not implemented as intended. For example, while observing insertion of central lines, we watched clinicians gather equipment essential for complying with recommended practice (sterile gloves, full sterile drape, etc.) from up to eight different locations. To make compliance easier for clinicians we introduced a central line cart storing all the necessary supplies.
(PRONOVOST ET AL., 2008)

BOX 19.2 Patient safety initiatives at Johns Hopkins following the culture and leadership survey

Initiative	Status and progress
Write safety mission	Developed by the Ethics and Patient Safety Committees
Create non-punitive medical error reporting policy	Policy passed October 2001
Create education sheet for families regarding how to help ensure their safety in the hospital	Brochure available to patients June 2002
Develop and pilot comprehensive safety plan	Started in September 2001, this programme has evolved and currently includes five ICUs
Educate staff at all levels on the science of safety	This briefing, a component of the comprehensive patient safety programme, is being given throughout the health system
Educate staff on how to disclose medical errors	A medical error disclosure policy was passed
Initiate senior executive staff adopting a unit	Another component of the comprehensive patient safety programme has been initiated in four ICU units; adopters (current and pending) include the President of the Johns Hopkins University, President of the Johns Hopkins Health System, Chief Operating Officer of the JHH and the Vice President for Human Resources at the JHH
Develop an intranet site for patient safety efforts	This site has provided the organization with a means of disseminating project information and sharing ideas
Create the Centre for Innovations in Quality Patient Care	This centre reports to the CEO and university president and provides support for quality and safety improvement initiatives

Participate in the IHIs "Quantum Leaps in Patient Safety"	This initiative is scheduled to end in June 2002 but the efforts will be adopted by the 'safety team' created under the auspices of Innovations in Patient Care and Safety
Medication safety initiative	This initiative created a web based system to report medication incidents
Develop strategic plan for patient safety	In the process of development

(REPRODUCED FROM *QUALITY & SAFETY IN HEALTH CARE*, P J PRONOVOST, B WEAST, C G HOLZMUELLER ET AL. "EVALUATION OF THE CULTURE OF SAFETY: SURVEY OF CLIN-ICIANS AND MANAGERS IN AN ACADEMIC MEDICAL CENTER". **12**, NO. 6, [405–410], 2003, WITH PERMISSION FROM BMJ PUBLISHING GROUP LTD.)

The greatest change was the shift from treating safety as primarily a matter of reacting to and managing crises, to a proactive approach to reducing errors and addressing system problems. This group has engaged people at all levels and fostered a collaborative ethic in which safety is prioritized. This in turn led to unit based safety programmes across many areas of the hospital, modelled on the ICU approach, in which staff collaboratively work to address safety issues in their own environment. A fundamental component of this was the senior executive 'adopt a work unit' scheme (Box 19.3), which brought much closer links between senior executives and the front line and ensured that leaders could resolve blocks and barriers to the improvement process rapidly.

BOX 19.3 Senior executive adopt a work unit

A senior leader from hospital management is assigned to a programme or unit. In an orientation, he or she meets with the unit safety committee and programme leaders to discuss unit demographics, safety cultures cores, and answer questions and concerns of the executive. An orientation handbook outlines each step of CUSP, staff roles and responsibilities, and helpful hints when rounding and interacting with unit staff. The executive is responsible for meeting with the unit's safety committee periodically, monitoring the unit's safety efforts, meeting with unit staff monthly, and holding staff accountable for continued performance improvement.

Executives use the information in the shared stories during future monthly rounds as a shared learning tool with staff and to close the loop on completed projects. The executive plays an integral role in stimulating discussions about safety concerns and providing support, including making resources available and dealing with issues beyond a staff's reach (e.g. crossing departmental political barriers). In addition, executives are encouraged and reminded as needed to show their commitment by interacting with front line staff during their monthly safety rounds. This method of active leadership has proven effective in improving staff attitudes about management and their sense of commitment and accountability to the organization.

(FROM PRONOVOST, WEAST AND BISHOP, 2004)

The keystone project: state wide harm reduction

As the success of this and related programmes became apparent, a much wider intervention was launched led by the Michigan Health and Hospital Keystone Association for Patient Safety and Quality. 108 Michigan ICUs took part in an 18-month intervention programme aimed particularly at decreasing catheter related bloodstream infections, a common, costly and potentially lethal complication of ICU care. In the United States, 80 000 patients each year were affected, with up to 28 000 deaths in intensive care units from this cause.

Five clinical strategies were highlighted:
- hand washing;
- full barrier precautions during the insertion of central venous catheters;
- cleaning the skin with chlorhexidine;
- avoiding the femoral site if possible;
- removing unnecessary catheters.

All this was standard clinical practice, yet infection rates remained stable and were probably viewed by many as largely inevitable consequences of ICU care. As at Johns Hopkins, the clinical practices were the core of the programme, but were supported by a variety of other interventions: these included a central cart to bring all necessary supplies together, checklist of infection practices, the regular discussion of catheter removal at daily rounds, and measurement and continual feedback of catheter rates.

During the project, median rates of central line associated infections per 1000 catheter days were reported quarterly to each unit and compared with past performance using simple run charts. Within three months, the median infection rate per 1000 catheter days decreased from 2.7 (interquartile range 0.6–4.8) in the baseline period to 0 (0–2.4) in the 18 months after the intervention. Over the 18-month observation period, more than half of the units reduced their infection rate to zero, and the overall mean rate was reduced by 66% (Pronovost, Needham and Berenholtz, 2006).

This programme has improved safety dramatically for patients and saved a great deal of money in reducing length of stay in intensive care. However, achieving change on this scale requires investment:

The resources required to develop, implement, and evaluate programmes using this model are substantial. Thus, the model is intended for large-scale collaborative projects, in which centralised researchers support the technical development (e.g. summarise the research evidence and develop measures) and local teams throughout a hospital perform the adaptive work (engage staff in the project, tailor interventions to fit the local work processes, and identify how to modify work so that all patients can receive the intervention).
(PRONOVOST ET AL., 2008)

In many healthcare systems, improvement work is fitted in between other commitments, not properly resourced and usually continually under threat from recurrent crises and central demands for compliance to standards. In these circumstances, it is not surprising that progress is slow. Most organizations have yet to learn to invest in safety and quality improvement in the same way as they invest in buildings and equipment.

The Safer Patients Initiative

The Safer Patients' Initiative (SPI) is one of the most ambitious programmes of safety and quality improvement yet attempted. It was ambitious partly in scale, in that 24 hospitals were involved in total, but more in the speed of implementation and the bravura of the objectives. Studies in many countries have shown that about 10% of patients are harmed in hospitals and that there is little sign of any change over time. Yet the SPI programme boldly set out to achieve a 50% reduction in adverse events in two years, as well as a range of other changes. No one knew whether this was achievable or simply naïve; SPI was, in the best sense, a gigantic experiment.

The safer patients programme

The SPI is a long-term collaborative programme developed by the Health Foundation in partnership with the US Institute for Healthcare Improvement (IHI) and 24 participating UK NHS Trust sites. In structure and content, the programme followed IHI's Breakthrough Collaborative model, with a focus upon reliability and safety of care through application of continuous quality improvement (CQI) techniques adapted from process industries and manufacturing (Langley, Nolan and Nolan, 1996). Most collaboratives focus on a specific clinical area and a fairly narrow set of problems; SPI took aim at the entire hospital, albeit focusing on some specific clinical programmes. IHI essentially took all they knew and melded it into a single programme (Haraden, personal communication).

Following an initial two-year pilot programme initiated at four sites in 2004, the main programme began in 2006 focusing upon 20 participating acute care organizations across the United Kingdom in the period until the end of 2008. They aimed to improve safety culture, reduce overall mortality, adverse event rates and hospital acquired infection rates. Four hospital work areas were targeted: critical care, medicines management, general ward care and perioperative care. The programme additionally worked with senior leadership, including leadership walkrounds designed to facilitate senior level support for front line quality and safety issues (Benn, Burnett and Parand, 2009b).

The programme was driven by a series of four collaborative learning sessions led by an expert faculty team. These events were attended by multi-disciplinary teams from each participating site, representing all clinical work areas and all levels of the local organization from front line to executive. Participating sites were networked with each other and programme leaders by e-mail to promote inter-site learning and dissemination of emergent best practice in the improvement work. Support from programme leaders was provided through e-mail, conference calls and site visits.

Local process improvement efforts were supported by tools and techniques developed in industry for CQI. These included use of process measurement and statistical process control principles, including use of run charts to monitor process variability (Langley *et al.*, 1996; Grol, Baker and Moss, 2002). The data was used locally to guide improvement efforts but also reported monthly for review by programme leaders who then provided feedback on progress and performance to individual sites. A Plan-Do-Study-Act (PDSA) approach to the quality improvement activities of front line teams was promoted, involving rapid-cycle development and testing of small-scale local process changes. Once process monitoring indicated that a specific change had proven to be effectively and reliably implemented in an initial pilot area (Speroff, James and Nelson, 2004), the team then disseminated and spread the methods to other parts of the organization.

Ready for improvement?

Studies of organizational change have suggested that if improvement pro-grammes are to succeed, organizations have to be 'ready' in the sense of having the necessary conditions and capability to start with (Burnett, Benn and Pinto, 2010). For instance, research has identified senior management com-mitment, physician involvement and training as factors for a programme's success, along with provision of sufficient resources, careful programme management and the presence of the necessary culture. Management reorga-nizations and mergers tend to impede progress, with mergers producing periods of 'intensive introspection' that set organizations back. Being ready for change then seems essential if a programme on the scale of SPI is to be successful.

In our studies of SPI, we examined a number of dimensions of organiza-tional readiness, using surveys and interviews with staff involved in the programme. We found that an essential prerequisite for engaging in SPI was that the organization was financially stable and had broadly met all regula-tory and government targets; only then could they engage in their own improvement work. We found that these organizations all had the necessary culture, attitudes and values, as well as having suitably motivated people to lead the changes, probably because they had been chosen in open competi-tion as being suitable for the SPI programme. A history of being involved with previous safety and quality improvement initiatives seemed to confer an advantage, but with the proviso that the SPI programme needed to be well aligned with other improvement efforts. In the British NHS, with an endless series of directives and targets descending from above, a programme can fail simply because other imperatives consume everyone's time and attention.

The findings from this and other studies show that if organization-wide patient safety improvement programmes are to be successful, all aspects of an organizations infrastructure, processes and culture should be considered in advance. From a practical viewpoint, there are two major implications. First, before embarking on any kind of change programme, organizations need to assess their capacity and ability to take part; they may quite simply not be ready and an ambitious programme would be destabilizing.

Second, a better understanding of the preconditions that mark an organization as ready for improvement work, would allow the programme design to be tailored to the requirements of specific organizations, which may vary in terms of their initial status.

The impact of SPI

Well, did it work, you may reasonably ask? This sounds like a simple question, but in fact needs to be opened out. Remember that this is a complex, unfolding intervention that relies on engaging large numbers of people. It has to work in many different ways, which each build on each other. Such an intervention has to enthuse and engage people, has to raise awareness of safety issues, has to impact on clinical practice and, through that, make patients safer. So, we need to think about these issues in turn.

Engagement and motivation

Our research first showed clearly that the people involved in SPI valued highly the contribution of the IHI team and the methodologies they brought. They specifically praised the SPI programme leads, citing their extensive healthcare experience; experience with improvement work and good communication and training skills, all of which contributed to the credibility of the advice. Interviewees also reported that IHI learning sessions were essential in motivating local improvement teams, as well as providing a forum at which different sites could compare progress. Both surveys and interviews suggested that people believed that the SPI programme had markedly raised awareness of safety issues, engaged people in improvement and brought about a variety of positive changes in attitude and culture, such as a more thoughtful approach to error and blame. To a lesser extent they believed that the programme had a positive impact on clinical practice and important safety issues, such as infection control (Benn, Burnett and Parand, 2009a).

Process improvement

SPI placed a strong and very welcome emphasis on measurement, with a Web based data collection system to monitor all manner of clinical indices. These mostly concerned clinical processes, such as the treatment of pneumonia, but also staff behaviours such as hand washing. Some were derived from observation, others from case note review; adverse event rates were monitored using the IHI trigger tool. This data was rightly and properly classed as improvement data, meaning that it is good enough for local purposes and for guiding the improvement programme. However, it is difficult to go beyond this and draw firm conclusions about improvements in the overall safety of care. In interviews, we found that definitions and sampling approaches often changed midway through a programme, which was quite reasonable in the context of an improvement programme but disastrous for assessing interventions. Organizations monitored different indices, data was often missing and, when approached, there was almost no pre-intervention baseline data.

There were, however, some convincing examples of major improvements within the run chart data collected locally; some of the data capture was clearly both sustained and controlled (Box 19.4). For instance, patients received correctly timed antibiotics before surgery and the introduction of a care bundle in one site significantly reduced the incidence of ventilator associated pneumonia. In patients on mechanical ventilation, the cumulative risk of pneumonia increases with the duration of ventilation. This infection has serious potential complications and a high mortality rate, so improvement in the reliability of the care delivered has important implications.

BOX 19.4 Care bundles in intensive care

A 'care bundle' is the term used for a group of evidence based clinical practices that, when used on their own, are shown to improve care, but when applied together they result in substantially greater improvements. The challenge for healthcare is to apply these best practices reliably on every patient who needs them, every day, measuring compliance and monitoring the outcome.

The bundle drives people to examine their practice – arguably the discussion and examination of practice this generates is more important than the bundle itself. Though the ventilator bundle provides you with standardized care for a ventilated patient, it doesn't necessarily reduce VAP rates. What reduces your VAP is the whole culture created by being able to implement bundles reliably. Daily goals, teamwork, reliability and so on, have an effect on all infection control issues within a unit. That in itself reduces infection rates, whether it's VAP or central line infections. The ICU team built redundancy into the system by getting a nurse on each shift to check the bundle elements, so if something was missed, it would be picked up in the next 12 hours. This also created peer pressure within the nursing teams for others to complete their share of duty. The 95% target of complete compliance was achieved within 6 weeks; compliance with the necessary procedures was quite poor before SPI.

(ADAPTED FROM BENN *ET AL.*, 2009A)

Patient outcomes and system change

At the time of writing the impact of SPI on patient outcomes is not clear. There has been some evaluation of the clinical indices on the first four sites, but conflicting views on the effectiveness of the programme. Some have claimed that the adverse event rate, as measured by the global trigger tool, has reduced by 50% as promised but given little information as to how and where the trigger tool was used. These claims have not, however, been backed up by an external evaluation, which found some evidence of changes in clinical processes but little effect on clinical outcomes. There are, however, concerns that the focal external evaluation, which provided a close examination of critical care, did not adequately capture the broader programme.

Although results are still emerging, first impressions are that SPI has been a success, although it has almost certainly not achieved, never mind sustained, the rather fantastic aims that were set. SPI had a hugely energizing effect on the staff involved with the programme, although it remains to be seen how deep the effects reached in the wider organization. While, to my mind, some of the claims of reductions in adverse event rates are exaggerated, there do seem to have been substantial changes in certain clinical areas. The impact, spread and longer-term impact of the programme however, are probably much more variable than originally anticipated which, with the benefit of hindsight, is probably not surprising. A repeated observation in these final chapters is that safety and quality improvement tends to be much harder than people originally thought. Finally, SPI has certainly galvanized further action, being one of the main drivers of the Scottish Patient Safety Programme, which aims to take patient safety to an entire nation. These national campaigns are a relatively recent development, which we will briefly consider.

On the campaign trail

Campaigns have been a part of public health for decades, as governments have sought to tackle alcohol consumption, smoking and the wearing of seat belts. The first patient safety campaign was launched in later 2004 when Don Berwick, frustrated at the slow progress on safety, announced a campaign to save 100 000 American lives in 18 months. Learning from the political machines, they sought to engage both front line staff and senior executives in a massive sign-up to key objectives, accompanied by as much media attention as possible. It was certainly a different approach!

The Institute for Healthcare Improvement (IHI) chose six practices, which they had worked with in the past and which, for the most part, had a strong evidence base behind them:

- Preventing central line infections
- Preventing surgical site infections
- Preventing ventilator associated pneumonia
- Provision of evidence based care for myocardial infarction
- Medicines reconciliation
- Rapid response teams.

The first four practices are backed by strong evidence; in all four it is clear what should be done but in practice, as we have so often seen, it does not happen. The programme introduced care bundles and other tools to increase reliability in these areas. Medicines reconciliation essentially means making sure that the patient's drugs are correctly adjusted or maintained at points of transfer; far too often people are discharged from hospital without essential medication or remain on a drug which should have been stopped when they returned home. Rapid response teams aim to lower the threshold for calling for help when patients are deteriorating, by having a special team on call, which are constantly available; hopefully this encourages earlier action. These are certainly important issues, but there is less agreement on the strategies needed to deal with them.

Saving 100 000 lives was quite an ambition and, not surprisingly, aroused some scepticism. These practices had evidence behind them, so were in themselves completely justified, but the approach to implementation was radically different and without precedent. In terms of raising both public and professional awareness of patient safety, and galvanizing and engaging people, the campaign was an extraordinary success. Should other countries emulate this approach? It depends in large part on how you assess the impact and also, much more difficult to assess, what else hospitals might have been doing if they had not absorbed their energies in the campaign.

In June 2006, IHI announced that the campaign had saved 122 000 lives across America. An incredible claim. Should we believe it? Wachter and Pronovost (2006) address this question in a brave and thoughtful article: brave because it is hard to raise doubts in the face of such enthusiasm and thoughtful because they balance admiration for what has been achieved with careful analysis of the underlying claims. Following their argument, we need to examine two questions: can we believe the numbers and, if we can, then was the reduced mortality due to the campaign? We will take these in turn.

IHI based the claim of reduced mortality on risk adjusted comparisons of actual and expected mortality on a monthly basis using a base year of 2004. Two external organizations examined the data and made independent assessments of the effect of adjusting for case mix, essentially adjusting the estimates to allow for the underlying disease and other factors which made death more or less likely. The initial estimate of reduced death rates was 33 000; the additional 89 000 came from the case mix adjustment! Remember this is a comparison across years in the same hospitals; why were the patients so different from one year to the next? As there are no details of the case mix adjustment, all one can say is that it is hard to know what to make of this.

A second major query concerns the reliability of the information reported. All the data were supplied by the hospitals themselves; this is understandable, as the cost of collecting it would otherwise have been prohibitive. However, there was no external checking at all; IHI simply expressed confidence that hospitals would report accurately. The first problem is that 14% of hospitals did not submit any data at all and yet were included in the analysis on the basis that they would have been the same as the ones that did. But supposing the ones who did not report were ones where the death rate had gone up; this would be quite plausible in a high profile campaign, even if hospitals were not individually identified. At the very least we would expect to also examine the data with the assumption that nothing changed in the 14% who did not report. Similarly, where data was reported, there would undoubtedly be strong expectations internally to show change; after all, you would not want to report to your Chief Executive, who had just signed up publicly to this high profile campaign that, no, actually our hospital had not shown any change, in fact possibly more people had died. These problems exist in all forms of data collection, so we must not overstate this. However, the circumstances of the campaign, the pressure to perform, the voluntary submission of selected data and the absence of any other checks, make the campaign especially vulnerable to the biases that plague all forms of clinical research.

If we accept that mortality did reduce in this period to some degree, what role was played by the campaign? The principal issue here is that in-hospital mortality rates have been declining anyway, and there are a host of factors that might account for this, including specialist treatment for stroke, ongoing improvements in medical records, changes in patterns of admission and discharge and so on. It is genuinely very difficult to separate out the effects of any particular initiative, no matter how substantial. Wachter and Pronovost conclude:

Overall, we end our analysis of the science, unable to fully understand what actually happened at the organizational and patient levels as a result of the campaign ... and concerned about what appears, to us, to be substantial bias in the methodology behind the reported 'lives saved' numbers.
(WACHTER AND PRONOVOST, 2006)

Robert Wachter and Peter Pronovost are not condemning the campaign, or narrowly carping about methodology. Given the limited resources available, it was probably not feasible for the campaign to carry out a full evaluation. They state that they have nothing but admiration for IHIs courage in initiating the campaign and indeed for its wider role in improving care. They argue that the campaign effect may be there, but that it has probably been considerably exaggerated and that the findings have been presented without the caveats and caution that the data demands. Many of the internal documents from IHI express caution about interpretation, but almost none of this appeared in the media or the public presentations. Wachter and Pronovost also recognized that campaigns need to energize people, indeed that is their main purpose. IHI were astonishingly effective in achieving this and their energy and challenge to make fundamental change was inspiring. Too much statistical introspection could well have slowed things down. Yet a more thorough and thoughtful evaluation might have allowed us to answer a key question: What precisely was accomplished? (Wachter and Pronovost, 2006).

Does this matter? Wachter and Pronovost accept, as I would, that to the individual patient whose life may have been saved, none of this matters. The primary reason that these assessments matter is that we need to decide whether this is indeed a good way to drive patient safety; it is certainly good at raising the profile of patient safety, but is this short-term gain matched by clinical improvements? The 100 000 lives campaign has now been followed by the 5 million lives campaign and by parallel campaigns in England, Wales and Scotland variously based on 100 000 lives, the Safer Patients Initiative and various local admixtures. These campaigns are more than welcome; after decades of neglect, patient safety is a priority issue for health systems and their governments. But, few of these campaigns have seriously tried to assess their impact and after all the razzamatazz one question may still remain: what exactly was accomplished?

References

Benn, J., Burnett, S., Parand, A. *et al.* (2009a) Perceptions of the impact of a large-scale collaborative improvement programme: experience in the UK Safer Patients Initiative. *Journal of the Evaluation of Clinical Practice*, **15**(3), 524–540.

Benn, J., Burnett, S., Parand, A. *et al.* (2009b) Studying large-scale programmes to improve patient safety in whole care systems: challenges for research. *Social Science & Medicine*, **69**, 1767–1776.

Burnett, S., Benn, J., Pinto, A. *et al.* (2010) Organisational readiness: exploring the preconditions for success in organisation-wide patient safety improvement programmes. *Quality and Safety in Health Care* (in press).

Grol, R., Baker, R. and Moss, F. (2002) Quality improvement research: understanding the science of change in health care. *Quality and Safety in Health Care*, **11**(2), 110–111.

Langley, G.J., Nolan, K.M., Nolan, T.W. et al. (1996) *The Improvement Guide: A Practical Approach to Enhancing Organizational Performance*, Jossey-Bass Publishers, San Francisco CA.

Mohr, J., Batalden, P. and Barach, P. (2004) Integrating patient safety into the clinical microsystem. *Quality and Safety in Health Care*, **13**(Suppl. 2), ii34–ii38.

Nelson, E.C., Batalden, P. and Godfrey, M.M. (2007) *Quality by Design. A Clinical Microsystems Approach*, Jossey Bass, San Francisco CA.

Plesk, P.E. and Greenhalgh, T. (2001) Complexity science – the challenge of complexity in health care. *British Medical Journal*, **323**(7313), 625–628.

Pronovost, P.J., Weast, B., Holzmueller, C.G. *et al.* (2003) Evaluation of the culture of safety: survey of clinicians and managers in an academic medical center. *Quality & Safety in Health Care*, **12**(6), 405–410.

Pronovost, P.J., Weast, B., Bishop, K. *et al.* (2004) Senior executive adopt-a-work unit: a model for safety improvement. *Joint Commission Journal on Quality and Safety*, **30**(2), 59–68.

Pronovost, P., Needham, D., Berenholtz, S. *et al.* (2006) An intervention to decrease catheter-related bloodstream infections in the ICU. *The New England Journal of Medicine*, **355**(26), 2725–2732.

Pronovost, P.J., Berenholtz, S.M. and Needham, D.M. (2008) Translating evidence into practice: a model for large-scale knowledge translation. *British Medical Journal*, **337**, 963–965.

Schouten, L.M.T., Hulscher, M.E.J.L., Everdingen, J.J.E. *et al.* (2008) Evidence for the impact of quality improvement collaboratives: a systematic review. *British Medical Journal*, **336**(7659), 1491–1494.

Speroff, T., James, B.C., Nelson, E.C. *et al.* (2004) Guidelines for appraisal and publication of PDSA quality improvement. *Quality Management in Health Care*, **13**(1), 33–39.

Wachter, R.M. and Pronovost, P.J. (2006) The 100 000 lives campaign: a scientific and policy review. *Joint Commission Journal on Quality and Patient Safety*, **32**(11), 621–627.

Waldrop, M.M. (1992) *Complexity: The Emerging Science at the Edge of Order and Chaos*, Cardinal, London.

CHAPTER 20

High performing healthcare systems

Healthcare systems are huge, complex networks of numerous smaller micro-systems, each with their own people, processes and cultures. These systems also exist within a complex and changing regulatory, social, cultural and policy environment, which both support and constrain their efforts to deliver safe, effective care and to improve that care. So far we have examined change within processes, within teams and across clinical networks, but we now turn to the even greater challenge of bringing about sustained change across entire systems. In a very large system, no leader, however powerful, can hope to control or even fully understand an improvement process that embraces the whole system. The task is not just complicated, but complex in the sense that it cannot be completely planned or predicted. As many have pointed out, quality improvement is more like steering a ship than building a car; you plan, you have a goal and you steer a course, but you constantly have to react, make small adjustments, deal with crises and adapt to circumstances and the wider environment.

How can safety and quality in these huge systems be improved? This is the million dollar question or if you prefer, in these turbulent financial times, the million euro question. One of the principal strategies for understanding the nature of the process is to study high performing organizations that seem to have progressed faster than others towards the safe, high-quality care that as patients we wish to receive. In this last chapter we will review some of the factors that have been identified, consider the nature of the process and contrast two healthcare systems, the Veterans Affairs (VA) health system and the Jonkoping Health economy, that have been particularly admired for their success; others could have been chosen, but this pairing is particularly useful for illustrating different routes that have been taken. We will draw on the work of a number of researchers, but particularly on the study of high performing healthcare systems by Ross Baker and colleagues (Baker *et al.*, 2008).

Patient Safety, 2nd edition. By Charles Vincent. Published 2010 by Blackwell Publishing Ltd.

Conditions and drivers of change

We have already reviewed the conditions that provide the necessary foundations for change in clinical microsystems. The transformation of an entire health economy requires that all these basic conditions are in place but across a network of microsystems. Leaders of change on this scale cannot direct improvement at the front line; their task is to develop strategy and create the conditions in which change can occur. On this scale, different authors have identified and prioritized slightly different sets of factors. For instance, Ferlie and Shortell (2001) identify:

- leadership at all levels;
- a culture that supports learning;
- the development of effective teams;
- effective use of information and information technologies.

Other authors supplement these factors with the need for clear roles and responsibilities, specific structures and resources, education and training and so on. Ross Baker and his colleagues, following a literature review, have drawn these various studies together into a table of commonly identified factors (Table 20.1). In previous chapters we have already seen the importance placed on culture, information, measurement communication and teamwork, so it is no surprise that these are included. Before we turn to the case studies however, we need to address the critical role of leadership.

Leading system change

Leadership comes in many forms and is demonstrated at all levels of the organization. Senior leaders influence safety directly by setting up safety related committees and initiatives and allowing staff time to engage in fundamental safety issues, such as the redesign of systems. Leaders also influence safety indirectly by talking about safety, showing they value it and being willing to discuss errors and safety issues in a constructive way. Safety is also strongly influenced by people in supervisory roles, such as a nurse in charge of a ward, both in the efficient management of processes and in the attitudes and values they foster in the people they manage. In turn, an individual nurse demonstrates her personal commitment to safety to trainees by attention to detail, by performing checks and by rigorous adherence to basic standards of care.

In this chapter we are primarily concerned with senior leadership, with the style, behaviours and actions of those with executive responsibilities. The transformational leadership theory of Bass and Avolio (1991) distinguishes two types of leadership, both of which are important for safety. Transactional leadership is, broadly speaking, an effective and efficient management style: set objectives, get agreement on what needs to be done, monitor performance and reward or sanction as appropriate. A theatre nurse, for instance, may set clear guidelines for behaviour and the standard of care they expect from the staff reporting to her. Transformational leadership in contrast, which Bass and Avolio suggest is characteristic of high performing teams, is more concerned with conveying a sense of purpose and vision, with empowering people in the

Table 20.1 Attributes of successful improvement

Attribute	Elements
Culture	Organization/leaders support and expect learning and innovation Organization/leaders value staff and empower all members to participate Organization/leaders focus on customers/patients Organization/leaders value collaboration and teamwork Organization/leaders are flexible
Leadership	Strong administrative leadership that provides role models for organizational values Leadership celebrates and even participates in improvement initiatives Emphasis on developing, fostering and inclusion in decision-making for clinical leadership and champions Board support: Board sets expectations by asking for reports on improvement initiatives and results Board provides continuity of expectations if administrative leadership changes
Strategy and policy	Leaders set clear priorities for improvement Improvement plans are integrated in the overall strategic plan as the means to achieve key strategic goals Leaders demonstrate both constancy of purpose and flexibility Operational policies and procedures, including human resources policies, provide incentives, rewards and recognition Incentives, rewards and recognition are aligned to support improvement work
Structure	Roles and responsibilities for improvement are clearly articulated Steering/oversight committees provide direction Teams and teamwork are part of structure
Resources	Organization provides time for staff members to learn skills and participate in improvement work Financial and material resources and human resources are available for improvement Quality improvement support/expertise: a core group of improvement experts is available to help teams and individuals Quality improvement department coordinates and support initiatives
Information	Needed clinical and administrative information are readily available Information is available to support improvement
Communication channels	Organization has vehicles to communicate with stakeholders regarding priorities, initiatives, results and learning Ample forms of communication, including newsletters, forums, meetings and intranet sites
Skills training	Includes training in improvement methods, team and group work, project and meeting management, and epidemiology

Table 20.1 (*Continued*)

Attribute	Elements
Physician involvement	Physicians are involved in planning improvement initiatives and participate as team members
	Opportunities for physician and clinical leadership of improvement
	Clinicians 'own' improvement

(Reproduced from *High performing healthcare systems. Delivering quality by design* , Baker, G. R., Macintosh-Murray, A., Porcellato, C., Dionne, L., Stelmacovich, K., & Born, K. p.84, 2008, with permission from Longwoods Publishing Corporation, Toronto)

team and treating people as unique individuals. A growing literature suggests that transformational leadership is significantly related to safety climate, staff compliance with rules and procedures, reduced accident rates and higher levels of performance, commitment and employee satisfaction (Barling, Loughlin and Kelloway, 2002; Flin and Yule, 2004). Key behaviours are: articulating an attainable vision of safety; demonstrating personal commitment to safety; engaging everyone with relevant experience; and being clear and transparent when dealing with safety issues (Box 20.1).

BOX 20.1 Leadership behaviours for safety

	Transactional behaviours	Transformational behaviours
Supervisors	Monitoring and reinforcing workers' safe behaviours	Being supportive of safety initiatives
	Participating in workforce safety activities (*can also be transformational*)	Encouraging employee involvement in safety initiatives
Middle managers	Becoming involved in safety initiatives (*can also be transformational*)	Emphasizing safety over productivity
		Adopting a decentralized style
		Relaying the corporate vision for safety to supervisors
Senior managers	Ensuring compliance with regulatory requirements	Demonstrating visible and consistent commitment to safety
	Providing resources for a comprehensive safety programme	Showing concern for people
		Encouraging participatory styles in middle managers and supervisors
		Giving time for safety

(REPRODUCED FROM *QUALITY & SAFETY IN HEALTH CARE*, R FLIN, S YULE. "LEADERSHIP FOR SAFETY: INDUSTRIAL EXPERIENCE". **13**, NO. SUPPL_2, [45–51], 2004, WITH PERMISSION FROM BMJ PUBLISHING GROUP LTD.)

Safety and quality in high performing firms need not be seen as separate from financial and other matters, but an integral part of productivity and profitability. When Paul O'Neill, later US Treasury Secretary, was Chief Executive of Alcoa, he made safety his 'signature issue', starting all board meetings with that issue, always linking it to whatever was being discussed. Other people quickly learnt that paying attention to safety always engaged his attention, and the over riding importance of safety permeated the culture of the company (Berwick, 1999). As an example of someone who put safety at the very forefront of his tenure as Chief Executive, we consider Jim Conway at the Dana-Farber Cancer Institute in Boston, who led a root and branch reform after a high-profile patient death in 1994. Jim Conway's reflections on the crucial elements of leadership for safety (Box 20.2) summarize and give life to the more academic treatment earlier in this section.

BOX 20.2 Patient safety leadership in practice

The leader's role is part strategic, part organizational and part cultural. First and foremost, leaders must: 'Provide focus, make patient safety not just another "program de jour" but a priority corporate objective. You must make everyone in the institution understand that safety is part of his or her job description.' This is more than a general pronouncement; executive leaders need to provide the human and financial resources to safety teams necessary for them to design and implement an integrated programme for identifying risks and reducing errors.

Along with the required technology and systems investment, an effective safety programme entails a leadership-driven cultural shift. 'You have to set the tone, provide a supportive, non-punitive environment for your staff. The goal is transparency – an atmosphere of open communication about safety concerns and incidents.' In more specific terms, this means leaders have to learn how to listen and start talking about safety concerns continually – with front line staff and at the highest levels of the organization. 'If you're not hearing about errors, don't assume they're not happening.' He urges leaders to 'Go looking for trouble, probe your staff, ask people "What feels unsafe?" Your staff is incredibly worried about safety. You must provide opportunities for conversations.' At the other end of the spectrum, leaders must involve the board, trustees and executive committee in safety discussions. This can take a variety of forms: sharing adverse event reports; being included in root-cause analysis meetings; and hearing patients' stories.

Patients are very much at the centre of the safety mission. Conway speaks passionately about the rewards of forming partnerships with patients in the safety drive. 'Patients and their families can make unbelievable contributions,' he says. 'That errors happen and patients are at some risk when they come to your institution for treatment is no secret to them,' he adds, and the atmosphere of silence is outdated and counterproductive. Hearing their experiences is 'sobering but incredibly useful. Again and again I hear from patients and families that they want to find leaders in the hospital who will talk to them about safety. They want opportunities for conversations.'

(ADAPTED FROM AN INTERVIEW WITH JIM CONWAY WWW.IHI.ORG)

Leadership in complex organizational settings, such as a hospital, requires other characteristics which are closely associated with the transformational leadership style. Westrum (1997) calls such leaders 'maestros'. This wonderful image suggests that presiding over a large, complex organization, which marries people and technology, is akin to being the conductor of a great orchestra. This notion of leadership may be far from the common image of great military or political leaders, but may be closer to the style required to promote and maintain safe, high-quality care. When thinking of the wider organization, be it a clinical unit or an entire health system, the struggle for the aspiring maestro is to have the wider vision and to discern, predict and articulate the safety problems before they arise. The maestro should constantly watch for the weaknesses in the system and the conditions that may eventually combine to produce a catastrophe. Equally they try to create the conditions in which musicians can aspire to performances and achievements they think are beyond them – like safe healthcare.

High performing healthcare systems

Ross Baker and colleagues identified a number of healthcare systems which, by reputation, had achieved major gains in safety and quality. We do not have sufficient information, either across systems or for the most part within these systems, to really identify the high performers from data, so these choices were essentially made on reputation. Nevertheless, the systems they chose have all undoubtedly placed safety and quality at the heart of their endeavours and there is much to learn. Baker and colleagues reviewed documents, carried out interviews with a wide range of people and, in the context of a broader understanding of the nature of system change, reflected on the journeys that these organizations had made. We cannot attempt to show the full richness of the study, just point to some of the most important observations in order to illustrate that there are different routes to high performance.

Veterans Affairs, New England

The VA system in the United States provides healthcare for Americans who have served their country in the military and, unusually in the United States, is under government control. The VA, like other systems, must respond to many external pressures and is particularly susceptible to political and government initiatives. Almost all VA physicians are salaried employees, again unusual in the United States. The service is imbued with a military ethos and staff regard caring for veterans as a particular privilege. The system is divided into 21 Veterans Integrated Service Networks (VISNs), which emphasize integrated treatment across a whole geographical region, encompassing all aspects of community and hospital based medicine; the 1990s saw a massive transformation from a primarily hospital based service to one that provided healthcare across an entire area. Many factors contribute to the high standards of care delivered but, in comparing the descriptions of different systems, the VA places a strong emphasis on structure, standardization and measurement.

Standardization and systematization

The VA operates with a clear structure of national regulations, standards and practice guidelines. Care delivery is organized into five broad services, which are the same in each region: primary care, speciality and acute care, mental health, spinal cord injury and geriatrics. Standardization pervades every area of work, which brings a number of benefits. For instance, infusion pumps are standardized across the entire network, so training is simpler, mistakes are fewer and staff can easily move between units and regions. Summarized here in a few lines, this sounds simple enough; to achieve it was no doubt a monumental effort.

Performance measurement and accountability

From the 1990s onwards, the VA has set clear goals and performance targets which track the care delivered across the entire network, enabling comparison of units and regions within the VA and over time. Each network monitors a basic set of indicators, which now run into the hundreds. These are derived from their own information, but also by data collected from record review by the VA External Peer Review Programme. The external review ensures that the data collected is rigorous, independent and hard to argue with. As one of the staff commented when discussing trying to persuade a department that improvement was needed, 'the data speaks volumes' (Baker et al., 2008).

Electronic medical records and decision support

The VA has invested heavily in electronic medical records and information technology of all kinds and keeping records in electronic form is now mandatory in almost all circumstances. The electronic medical record is critical to several other features; without it the measurement, the monitoring of workload and clinical work and the accountability for performance would simply not be feasible.

Systems for implementing change

While the system is constantly monitored, it nevertheless also needs to evolve and change. Within the VA, the targets and goals are constantly stretched, though, ideally, not to the point of destabilizing the current system. Considerable thought has been given to how change is actually achieved, in contrast to many systems where improvement initiatives are run in spare time or treated as secondary activities. In VA Boston, improvement work is clear and organized, and much thought is given to the proper resources and clinical leadership:

The big change in approach that allowed improvements in the performance measures was assigning teams and supporting and encouraging them. . . We are very thoughtful about who we select for physician leaders and participants and we are very clear about endpoints and expectations. We are very clear about who we want, why we want them and what we want them to do (Quality manager).
(BAKER *ET AL.*, 2008)

While this selection of a few key features has emphasized internal structures, standardization and accountability, it would be quite wrong to see the VA simply in those terms. The VA also has a long history of external involvement with IHI improvement collaboratives and with engaging in new learning; their patient safety programme for instance, was one of the first to take learning from incidents seriously. We have not even touched on culture, leadership or the timescale of change. Nevertheless, the VA approach to improvement is undoubtedly grounded in an overall structure of performance measurement and accountability and, in a sense, driven from the top while accepting that the improvements themselves must be generated on the ground. This contrasts quite strongly with our next example, where the style of leadership and change is very different.

Jonkoping County

Jonkoping County is a regional health economy southwest of Stockholm in Sweden. Sweden's healthcare system is publicly funded, and at the local level controlled by 21 elected county councils. Jonkoping has 3 hospitals, 34 care centres and a staff of about 10 000, looking after the health needs of about 340 000 people. It is therefore a whole health economy, but on a relatively small scale. Jonkoping regularly tops the league of Swedish County Councils when ranked on the six goals of quality, efficiency, safety, patient centredness, equity and effectiveness. Their approach to high performance is distinctive in a number of ways, and we will select some of the most important.

Sustained leadership and commitment

Jonkoping Healthcare System has been led for almost 20 years by its Chief Executive, Sven Olof Karlsson, supported by Mats Boestig, medical director and Goran Henriks, who leads on learning and innovation. These three people and their enduring commitment have been hugely important in providing both the leadership and the stability necessary for serious, purposeful healthcare improvement. This has been achieved in spite of the fact that county councils are elected for four-year terms, and each new regime reviews the leadership of their healthcare. Jonkoping's healthcare leadership are fully aware of the necessity for structures and the usual organizational processes and their achievements rest on a bedrock of strong financial discipline. However, they also believe that there are limits to this approach and that healthcare requires some new ways of thinking and behaving, if we are to achieve safe high quality care.

Esther

Esther is a fictional, but ever present, 88-year-old Swedish woman, who has a number of chronic conditions, but nevertheless manages to live independently with a good quality of life. From 1998 onwards, clinicians and managers in Jonkoping in various settings have mapped Esther's journey through all the parts of the healthcare system, trying to see it through her eyes and structure it according to her needs. Seeing the process through the patient's eyes has been the foundation of a host of changes, including new admissions processes, more integrated communication, team based telephone conversations and a strong emphasis on patient involvement and self care.

Qulturum: centre for learning and culture

One of the most striking features of Jonkoping is the willingness, indeed hunger, to learn from others and to embed new and useful ideas and techniques within their system. Although Jonkoping now inspires others around the world, they continue to explore and maintain a continuous dialogue with external systems and individuals. For instance, a long relationship with the Institute for Healthcare Improvement has brought a range of improvement methodologies to Jonkoping, with an underlying emphasis on engagement of all staff. Paul Batalden has been a frequent visitor, collaborating on strategies for working on clinical microsystems.

Qulturum, led by Goran Henriks, is the learning and innovation hub of Jonkoping. Here staff come together for seminars, open discussion and conversation and here the new ideas are sifted, piloted and evaluated. Staff at Qulturum are usually clinical leaders and champions of quality improvement, though not necessarily senior people. They combine a sense of practicality with an interest in culture, theory and ideas. It is noteworthy that they use very few external consultants (as opposed to collaborators), always seeking to learn the new thinking themselves rather than buy it in.

Engagement and spread

The VA system engages staff in multiple improvement projects and creates time and resource to achieve particular goals. Jonkoping also does this, but their approach is more open and more fluid. Ross Baker quotes Karllson as saying:

We involve employees in lots of quality improvement projects and help them learn how to make changes and let them define how to create results using learning and innovation . . . results across the small parts of the system create results for the system and lots of winners. Big, high risk projects and changing structures in a traditional way . . . creates losers.
(BAKER *ET AL.*, 2008)

Rather than working within a framework of targets and goals, the Jonkoping approach has been to encourage staff to improve quality wherever they deem it important, guided by Esther and their own assessments of local needs. Rather than control the improvement process, they take a more organic approach, in which many small changes combine and build on each other to create wider gains. It is the complex adaptive system in action.

A quality strategy

While the improvements may initially stem from the staff themselves, they do need to be integrated into the broader strategy for the delivery of healthcare. This development came at a later stage, emerging from the more local activities. From 2001 onwards, Karllson and others initiated meetings of all senior leaders for five days over a year; he mirrored the open discussions he had fostered on the clinical level at the executive level. This has led to a model for system wide improvement, the Jonkoping Diamond, which explicitly links learning and innovation to both system improvement and to financial stability and discipline.

Styles and strategies for system improvement

Both the VA and Jonkoping have clearly approached the improvement of safety and quality with great integrity, strength of purpose and seriousness. Both have leaders, at all levels, committed to improvement, who have fostered a culture of aspiration and continuous improvement. Both systems have invested heavily in educating and training their staff in safety and quality improvement

Both the VA and Jonkoping have realized that if substantial progress is to be made staff must be given the time and resources to do it. This sounds blindingly obvious, and it is; in practice however, improving safety and quality is often of marginal concern at the higher levels of an organization. In the British National Health Service for instance, many posts cover such matters as patient safety, quality, risk and governance with varying job titles and responsibilities. Remarkably however, few of these people are concerned with improvement; they may be as individuals, of course, but their responsibilities seldom allow them to work on improvement. Their days are dominated by meeting standards, regulations and dealing with incidents and the occasional disaster. This is a slight caricature, but only slight. Improvement work is fitted in around other responsibilities and is extremely vulnerable to other priorities and events.

While there are similarities of approach between the VA and Jonkoping, we can also see that the strategies adopted by these two systems, whether consciously or not, have prioritized different features of the quality and safety journey. Both the VA and Jonkoping would identify performance measurement and organizational learning as critical to safety and quality improvement; however, measurement is more to the fore in the VA, and learning in Jonkoping. Leadership has been critical in both systems, but the styles of leadership have been different; in the VA there has been a strong element of monitoring and performance management, while in Jonkoping there has been more emphasis on staff empowerment and disseminated decision making. If we reviewed other systems studied by Ross Baker, Paul Bate and other researchers, we would see more variants on these and other themes. How should we interpret these different styles? Should we see them as necessary adaptations or do the approaches vary because we just don't yet fully understand how to make change on such a massive scale.

Bate, Mendel and Robert (2008) have provided us with a valuable perspective on the issue of variety in strategic approach, drawing on the 'universal but variable' thesis common in the social sciences, which essentially states that:

There are only a limited number of basic human problems to which all people at all times and in all places must find solutions, but the number of possible solutions to them is unlimited.

(BATE, MENDEL AND ROBERT, 2008)

Bate and colleagues suggest that the healthcare systems they studied face six core challenges – the basic human problems of the formulation above. These are:

- *Structural* – structuring, planning and co-ordinating quality efforts;
- *Political* – engaging the relevant parties, negotiating conflict and relationships;
- *Cultural* – the challenge of giving quality a shared collective meaning, value and significance within an organization;
- *Educational* – creating and nurturing the learning process;
- *Emotional* – inspiring and energizing people;
- *Physical and technological* – designing physical systems and technological infrastructures that support improvement and the delivery of safe, high-quality care.

These common challenges are met in different ways by organizations; what works in one setting might not work for another organization. However, although Bate and colleagues emphasize that the journeys are different, they are clear that the challenges are non-negotiable and an organization neglects them at their peril. No matter how wonderful your technology, you still need to inspire people. Conversely, the most charismatic leadership will not get you far, unless backed by education, training and technical understanding. This last scenario was common in the early days of patient safety, when 'changing the culture' was held by some to be the royal road to patient safety.

If the factors for successful improvement are reasonably well understood, then why have healthcare systems not made more progress? Ross Baker and colleagues pose this incisive question in the introduction to their book on high performing systems. In part it is that every healthcare system that takes this journey is finding its way, although obviously inspired and guided by those taking similar journeys. Knowing the factors is, as Ross Baker puts it, a static understanding and does not show you the strategies, how to deploy the resources, the nature of the leadership and so on (Baker *et al.*, 2008). However, to continue the journey metaphor, it also depends on where you are starting from and the resources available. One organization may be culturally ready, because they have reviewed and discussed safety and quality issues for years, but may not have developed formal organizational structures necessary for larger-scale transformation. Another may have the structures and the techniques, but a punitive and repressive culture which means that any attempts to engage staff are viewed with suspicion and even hostility. There are also a host of local circumstances which either support or impede these larger-scale activities. These range from the personalities of senior people in the organization, the huge range of other priorities that take resources from improvement, the fact that a merger has occupied the attention of senior staff for a year, a new building programme, and changes and the interest and knowledge that the wider staff have in safety and quality. There is, therefore, an awful lot to juggle and, just as there are many routes to success, there are innumerable ways of failing.

Investing for the long term

Many organizations do appear to have found a way of combining all the necessary aspects and making a sustained and long-term commitment to safety and quality improvement. There is, however, still some doubt as to how far this has translated into improvements for patients. This is partly because much of the data that might inform a response to this question has not been made public or reported; the VA for instance, clearly has large volumes of data but little of it is in the public domain. There is also, as we have seen, heated debate about the quality of data, the extent to which local improvement data reflects real improvement and whether it is necessary to ground all assessments in a formal clinical trial framework (Brown and Lilford, 2008). Measurement has also not been a strong point in even some of the finest programmes. John Ovretveit and Anthony Staines, clearly admirers of Jonkoping's achievements, commented that despite the embedded culture of quality improvement, the extensive and effective learning and the consistent improvement work in many settings:

Jonkoping County Council still has little improvement data that would be credible to many researchers or clinicians. We noted the lack of a strong culture of measurement, we observed fewer measurement systems and activities than expected and relatively little specialised support to teams for designing, collecting, analysing and presenting data.
(OVRETVEIT AND STAINES, 2007)

Do we assume that patients are seeing the benefits or do we pessimistically conclude, as some do, that the safety and quality rhetoric far outstrips the evidence of real change? This depends on how we see the whole quality improvement process; is it like the action of a drug on a disease or is it a more organic, evolutionary process? Ovretveit and Staines point out that in the case of Jonkoping in particular, with a strong emphasis on staff engagement and change at ground level, the quality improvement process is likely to take time to produce results, but when they are seen they should be widespread. Conversely, if you plough all your resources into a small number of critical targets, such as waiting times in the emergency department, then you will see results but probably only in very specific areas (Bevan and Hood, 2006).

Ovretveit and Staines suggest that, although leaders hope for rapid change, there is probably a necessary period of building a quality infrastructure. There may even be a threshold to achieve before real improvements are seen. In the first phase then, perhaps lasting some years, it is necessary to invest in a 'quality infrastructure', but not to expect any immediate return on investment. In the short term one hopes for engagement and enthusiasm and the sense of embarking on a journey; in this phase one is building awareness, leadership and freeing up resources to create the capacity for improvement. In the subsequent phase, one aims for some signs of improvement in specific areas; these may be incomplete, inconsistent and may be hard to distinguish in the face of other changes and developments. In the longer term, when measurement and capacity are mature, then patient experience and outcomes begin to improve in a sustainable manner; they suggest that this could take as long as ten years, even in as successful a system as Jonkoping.

The idea that a period of investment is necessary before returns are seen potentially makes sense of some of the conflicting evidence. Enthusiasts are not being naïve in seeing real change in an organization, even if more sceptical observers believe that patients are no better off. However, the enthusiasts need to understand that there is much further to go than they anticipated. The timescales we have discussed, however, are not absolute, but more reflect the current understanding of large-scale quality improvement. Only a very few systems have probably understood the nature and scale of capacity development that is actually needed; most have relied on enthusiasm, culture change and on people doing quality improvement in their non-existent spare time. If we trained people properly, gave them time and resources, and set up proper economic and clinical evaluations, then the period between initial investment and tangible patient outcomes could be a great deal shorter.

Making a Swiss watch from a Swiss cheese

If this book has succeeded in its aims you will, I hope, be convinced that patient safety is critically important for both patients and healthcare staff in every setting throughout the world. Hopefully too, something has been conveyed of the landscape of patient safety, the central concepts and an understanding of the nature, causes and prevention of error and harm. Perhaps you will also agree with the assertion in the preface that patient safety is a tough problem.

At the end of the first edition, I wrote that we had many good ideas and concepts, some solid evidence and many promising avenues to explore, but we were nevertheless still at the beginning of the safety journey. Although we understood the problem quite well, many interventions were haphazard in nature and their effects uncertain. Furthermore, we did not understand how to integrate the various safety interventions and components of safety into a coherent whole. As I hope the later chapters have shown, the last five years have brought considerable progress on many fronts and there is now reason for real optimism about what can be achieved. The earlier years of patient safety were mainly devoted to uncovering innumerable holes in the healthcare Swiss cheese. Now we can envisage the possibility of attaining the reliability and resilience associated with the classic Swiss watch.

Above all, for anyone who has read this book, working or associated with healthcare in whatever capacity, I would hope that you feel that patient safety is a subject worthy of your attention. Understanding and creating safety is a challenge equal to understanding the biological systems that medicine seeks to influence. While the challenge is immense, it is clear that we are making some progress in awareness, in understanding and on action to prevent harm and care for those affected. Treating patients one at a time brings obvious and immediate benefits, but working to improve the safety of healthcare as a whole may ultimately benefit many more.

References

Baker, G.R., Macintosh-Murray, A., Porcellato, C. *et al.* (2008) *High Performing Healthcare Systems. Delivering Quality by Design*, Longwoods, Toronto.

Barling, J., Loughlin, C. and Kelloway, E.K. (2002) Development and test of a model linking transformational leadership and occupational safety. *Journal of Applied Psychology*, **87**, 488–496.

Bass, B.M. and Avolio, B.J. (1991) *The Multifactor Leadership Questionnaire*, Consulting Psychologists Press, Palo Alto CA.

Bate, P., Mendel, P. and Robert, G. (2008) *Organising for Quality. The Improvement Journeys of Leading Hospitals in Europe and the United States*, Radcliffe Publishing, Oxford.

Berwick, D. (1999) Taking action to improve safety. How to improve the chances of success, in *Enhancing Patient Safety and Reducing Errors in Healthcare*, National Patient Safety Foundation, Chicago IL, pp. 1–11.

Bevan, G. and Hood, C. (2006) Have targets improved performance in the English NHS? *British Medical Journal*, **332**(7538), 419–422.

Brown, C. and Lilford, R. (2008) Evaluating service delivery interventions to enhance patient safety. *British Medical Journal*, **338**, 159–163.

Ferlie, E.B. and Shortell, S.M. (2001) Improving the quality of health care in the United Kingdom and the United States: a framework for change. *Milbank Quarterly*, **79**(2), 281–315.

Flin, R. and Yule, S. (2004) Leadership for safety: industrial experience. *Quality and Safety in Health Care*, **13**(Suppl_2), ii45–ii51.

Ovretveit, J. and Staines, A. (2007) Sustained improvement? Findings from an independent case study of the Jonkoping quality program. *Quality Management in Health Care*, **16**(1), 68–83.

Westrum, R. (1997) Social factors in safety-critical systems, in *Human Factors in Safety-Critical Systems* (eds R. Redmilland J. Rajan), Butterworth-Heinemann, Oxford, pp. 233–256.

Index

Page numbers in *italics* represent figures, those in **bold** represent tables.

Patient Safety, 2nd edition. By Charles Vincent. Published 2010 by Blackwell
Publishing Ltd.